Neuromorphic and Brain-Based Robots

Neuromorphic and brain-based robotics have enormous potential for furthering our understanding of the brain. By embodying models of the brain on robotic platforms, researchers can investigate the roots of biological intelligence and work towards the development of truly intelligent machines.

This book provides a broad introduction to this ground-breaking area for researchers from a wide range of fields, from engineering to neuroscience. Case studies explore how robots are being used in current research, including a whisker system that allows a robot to sense its environment and neurally inspired navigation systems that show impressive mapping results. Looking to the future, several chapters consider the development of cognitive, or even conscious, robots that display the adaptability and intelligence of biological organisms. Finally, the ethical implications of intelligent robots are explored, from morality and Asimov's three laws to the question of whether robots have rights.

JEFFREY L. KRICHMAR is an Associate Professor in the Department of Cognitive Sciences and Computer Science at the University of California, Irvine. His research interests include neurorobotics, embodied cognition, biologically plausible models of learning and memory, and the effect of neural architecture on neural function.

HIROAKI WAGATSUMA is an Associate Professor in the Department of Brain Science and Engineering at Kyushu Institute of Technology (KYUTECH) in Japan. His research interests include theoretical modeling of brain oscillations, the memory integration process of experienced episodes, and the implementation of oscillatory neural networks into neurorobotics.

Neuromorphic and Brain-Based Robots

Edited by

JEFFREY L. KRICHMAR
University of California, Irvine, USA

HIROAKI WAGATSUMA
Kyushu Institute of Technology, Japan

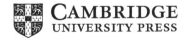

CAMBRIDGE
UNIVERSITY PRESS

University Printing House, Cambridge CB2 8BS, United Kingdom

One Liberty Plaza, 20th Floor, New York, NY 10006, USA

477 Williamstown Road, Port Melbourne, VIC 3207, Australia

314-321, 3rd Floor, Plot 3, Splendor Forum, Jasola District Centre, New Delhi - 110025, India

79 Anson Road, #06-04/06, Singapore 079906

Cambridge University Press is part of the University of Cambridge.

It furthers the University's mission by disseminating knowledge in the pursuit of education, learning and research at the highest international levels of excellence.

www.cambridge.org
Information on this title: www.cambridge.org/9781108826204

© Cambridge University Press 2011

First published 2011
First paperback edition 2020

A catalogue record for this publication is available from the British Library

Library of Congress Cataloging in Publication data
Krichmar, Jeffrey L.
  Neuromorphic and brain-based robots / Jeffrey L. Krichmar, Hiroaki Wagatsuma.
    p. ; cm.
  Includes bibliographical references and index.
  ISBN 978-0-521-76878-8 (hardback)
  1. Neural networks (Computer science)   2. Brain–Computer simulation.   I. Wagatsuma, Hiroaki.   II. Title.
  [DNLM: 1. Neural Networks (Computer)   2. Robotics.   3. Biomimetics.   4. Brain.
  5. Cognition.   6. Models, Neurological. WL 26.5]
  QA76.87.K75 2011
  006.3′2–dc23   2011018861

ISBN 978-0-521-76878-8 Hardback
ISBN 978-1-108-82620-4 Paperback

Additional resources for this publication at www.cambridge.org/9781108826204

Contents

Contributors

Keith Abney

Philosophy Department, California Polytechnic State University, San Luis Obispo, CA, USA

Minoru Asada

Adaptive Machine Systems, Osaka University, Osaka, Japan

Emilia I. Barakova

Faculty of Industrial Design, Eindhoven University of Technology, Eindhoven, The Netherlands

George A. Bekey

Department of Computer Science, University of Southern California, Los Angeles, CA, USA, and College of Engineering, California Polytechnic University, San Luis Obispo, CA, USA

Kenji Doya

Neural Computation Unit, Okinawa Institute of Science and Technology, Kunigami, Japan

David B. Edelman

The Neurosciences Institute, San Diego, CA, USA

Gerald M. Edelman

The Neurosciences Institute, San Diego, CA, USA

Erdem Erdemir

Center for Intelligent Systems, Vanderbilt University, Nashville, TN, USA

Loe Feijs

Faculty of Industrial Design, Eindhoven University of Technology, Eindhoven, The Netherlands

Andrew Felch

Cognitive Electronics, Hanover, NH, USA

Jason G. Fleischer
The Neurosciences Institute, San Diego, CA, USA

Richard Granger
Department of Psychological and Brain Sciences, Dartmouth College, Hanover, NH, USA

Koh Hosoda
Department of Multimedia Engineering, Osaka University, Osaka, Japan

Zhengping Ji
Department of Computer Science and Engineering, Michigan State University, East Lansing, MI, USA

Frédéric Kaplan
EPFL-CRAFT, Lausanne, Switzerland

Kazuhiko Kawamura
Department of Electrical Engineering & Computer Science, Vanderbilt University, Nashville, TN, USA

Jeffrey L. Krichmar
Department of Cognitive Sciences, University of California, Irvine, CA, USA

Patrick Lin
Philosophy Department, California Polytechnic State University, San Luis Obispo, CA, USA

Jeffrey L. McKinstry
The Neurosciences Institute, San Diego, CA, USA

Michael Milford
School of Engineering Systems, Queensland University of Technology, Brisbane, Australia

Ben Mitchinson
Department of Psychology, University of Sheffield, Sheffield, UK

Pierre-Yves Oudeyer
INRIA Futur, Talence, France

Martin J. Pearson
Bristol Robotics Laboratory, Bristol, UK

Anthony G. Pipe
Bristol Robotics Laboratory, Bristol, UK

Tony J. Prescott
Department of Psychology, University of Sheffield, Sheffield, UK

Danil Prokhorov
Toyota Technical Center, Ann Arbor, MI, USA

Ruth Schulz
School of Information Technology & Electrical Engineering, The University of Queensland, St Lucia, Australia

Masayoshi Shibata
Faculty of Letters, Kanazawa University, Kanazawa, Japan

Eiji Uchibe
Neural Computation Unit, Okinawa Institute of Science and Technology, Kunigami, Japan

Hiroaki Wagatsuma
Department of Brain Science and Engineering, Kyushu Institute of Technology, Kitakyushu, Japan

Juyang Weng
Department of Computer Science and Engineering, Michigan State University, East Lansing, MI, USA

Janet Wiles
School of Information Technology & Electrical Engineering, The University of Queensland, St Lucia, Australia

Mitch Wilkes
Department of Electrical Engineering & Computer Science, Vanderbilt University, Nashville, TN, USA

Gordon Wyeth
Queensland University of Technology, Brisbane, Australia

Preface

The genesis for this book came about from a series of conversations, over a period of several years, between Jeff Krichmar and Hiro Wagatsuma. Initially, these conversations began when Krichmar was at The Neurosciences Institute in San Diego and Wagatsuma was at the Riken Brain Science Institute near Tokyo. They included discussions at each other's institutes, several conversations and workshops at conferences, and an inspiring trip to a Robotics Exhibition at the National Museum of Nature and Science in Tokyo. In these conversations, we realized that we shared a passion for understanding the inner workings of the brain through computational neuroscience and embodied models. Moreover, we realized that: (1) there was a small, but growing, community of like-minded individuals around the world, and (2) there was a need to publicize this line of research to attract more scientists to this young field. Therefore, we contacted many of the top researchers around the world in Neuromorphic and Brain-Based Robotics. The requirements were that the researchers should be interested in some aspect of the brain sciences, and were using robotic devices as an experimental tool to further our understanding of the brain. We have been thrilled at the positive response. We know we have not included everyone in this field and apologize for any omissions. However, we feel that the contributed chapters in this book are representative of the most important areas in this line of research, and that they represent the state-of-the-art in the field at this time. We sincerely hope this book will inspire and attract a new generation of neuromorphic and brain-based roboticists.

JLK – To Tom Vogl, my mentor and advisor.
HW – To Natsue Sekiguchi, my lifelong supporter and advisor.

Part I

Introduction

1 History and potential of neuromorphic robotics

Jeffrey L. Krichmar and Hiroaki Wagatsuma

Neuromorphic and brain-based robots are not encapsulated in a single field with its own journal or conference. Rather, the field crosses many disciplines, and ground-breaking neuromorphic robot research is carried out in computer science, engineering, neuroscience, and many other departments. The field is known by many names: biologically inspired robots, brain-based devices, cognitive robots, neuromorphic engineering, neurobots, neurorobots, and many more. Arguably, the field may have begun with William Grey Walter's turtles, created in the 1950s, whose simple yet interesting behaviors were guided by an analog electronic nervous system. Another landmark was the fascinating thought experiments in the book by Valentino Braitenberg, *Vehicles: Experiments in Synthetic Psychology*. Braitenberg's *Vehicles* inspired a generation of hobbyists and scientists, present company included, to use synthetic methodology (Braitenberg's term) to study brain, body, and behavior together. We like to think of synthetic methodology as "understanding through building" and it is certainly an apt mission statement for neuromorphic and brain-based robots.

It has been almost 90 years since the popular word "robot" first appeared in Karel Capek's play *R.U.R.* With the dawn of the twenty-first century, our expectations are high for a new scientific paradigm and a major technological advancement in the field of robotics. In this time robots have become prevalent in our society. Robots can be found in commercial, manufacturing, military, and entertainment applications. We now have robotic vacuum cleaners, robotic soccer players, and autonomous vehicles on the ground, in the sky, and beneath the ocean. Because of major technical and empirical advances in the brain sciences over the last few decades, the time appears right for integrating the exciting fields of robotics and neuroscience. This promising area of research and the subject of this book, which we term neuromorphic and brain-based robotics, may generate the paradigm shift for truly intelligent machines.

Robots are increasing our productivity and quality of life in industry, defense, security, entertainment, and household chores. However, the behavior of these robots pales compared with that of animals and insects with nervous systems. Biological organisms survive in dynamic environments and display flexibility, adaptability, and survival capabilities that far exceed any artificial systems. Neuromorphic and brain-based robotics are exciting and emerging research fields that investigate the roots of biological

Neuromorphic and Brain-Based Robots, eds. Jeffrey L. Krichmar and Hiroaki Wagatsuma. Published by Cambridge University Press. © Cambridge University Press 2011.

intelligence by embodying models of the brain on robotic platforms. Moreover, because neuromorphic and brain-based robotics follows a working model (i.e. the biological brain and body), we believe this field will lead to autonomous machines that we can truly call intelligent.

Neuromorphic and brain-based robots are physical devices whose control system has been modeled after some aspect of brain processing. Because the nervous system is so closely coupled with the body and situated in the environment, brain-based robots can be a powerful tool for studying neural function. Brain-based robots can be tested and probed in ways that are not yet achievable in human and animal experiments. The field of neuromorphic and brain-based robots is built on the notion that the brain is embodied in the body and the body is embedded in the environment.

In the real biological nervous system, this embodiment mediates all the sensations and governs motion, and is also crucial for higher order cognition, and notions of mind and self. The question of how our mind is constructed from physical substrates such as the brain and body are still a mystery. A synthetic approach occupies an important position in investigating how complex systems, such as the brain, give rise to intelligent behavior through interactions with the world. The concept is highlighted by "embodiment" in the fields of robotics, artificial intelligence, and cognitive science. It argues that the mind is largely influenced by the state of the body and its interaction with the world.

The neuromorphic and brain-based robotic approaches can provide valuable heuristics for understanding how the brain works both empirically and intuitively. Neurologists analytically investigate whether the brain is healthy or impaired due to neurological disorders. Neuroscientists probe different areas of the brain to determine which brain regions are necessary for a specific function. By using a synthetic methodology, neurobiologically inspired robots can constructively exhibit how the brain works through its interaction with the body, the environment, and other agents in real world situations. We believe that neuromorphic and brain-based robotics will provide the groundwork for the development of intelligent machines, contribute to our understanding of the brain and mind, as well as how the nervous system gives rise to complex behavior.

Neuromorphic and brain-based robotics is an exciting field of research that has a growing community of researchers with a wide range of multidisciplinary talents and backgrounds. We wrote this book as an introduction to the recent advances in neuromorphic and brain-based robotics. The contributing authors speculate how robots can be used to better understand brain science and what properties of the nervous system are necessary to produce truly intelligent robots.

We divided the chapters of this book into logical sections starting with physical robotic platforms, progressing to case studies using brain-based robots, to several articles on philosophical considerations with future brain-based robots, and finally important ethical issues as robots become so intelligent that we have to think about the mental state of the robots.

In Part II on neuromorphic robots, we directly consider how the body of a robot affects thinking and cognition. Hosoda from Osaka University describes an anthropomorphic hand, which he designed to be much more natural in its movement and sensing than a conventional robotic hand. Different types of objects can be recognized through the hand's movement and posture. This study is a direct demonstration of how the body shapes the way we think. Mitchinson and colleagues from Sheffield University have been studying the whisker system, which is the rat's primary means of sensing its environment. They used high-speed video of real rat whisker movements to guide the development of a complete robotic whisker system. The robot uses its artificial whisker system to switch between several behaviors. The mechanical and electrical design of the Osaka and Sheffield groups is extremely impressive. Many lessons remain to be learned through the construction of ingenious biomimetic devices. However, it is also important to make neuromorphic and brain-based robots available to a wider audience. Most computational neuroscientists are not mechanical engineers and do not have ready access to electronics and machine shops. Felch and Granger, who are computational neuroscientists with expertise in robot design, have developed the Brainbot to meet this need. The Brainbot has a visual system, reaching system, language system, and software packages to make neurobotics readily accessible to researchers who are not necessarily "gear heads."

In Part III on architectures and approaches, several authors present case studies on the embodied approach to neuroscientific study. Rats have exquisite navigational abilities that allow them to form cognitive maps of their environment. Wyeth and colleagues from the University of Queensland in Australia have used recent findings on place cells in the hippocampus and grid cells in the entorhinal cortex to develop a neurally inspired navigation system they call RatSLAM. They show impressive mapping results with RatSLAM on the streets of Brisbane, as well as navigation and communication of places between two robots with RatSLAM. Uchibe and Doya at the Okinawa Institute of Science and Technology have developed the CyberRodent project in which they use multiple robots to explore learning algorithms, neuromodulation, and robot interactions. In their chapter, they use the CyberRodent paradigm along with evolutionary algorithms to develop brain circuits that use both extrinsic and intrinsic rewards to develop autonomous behaviors. Wilkes and colleagues from Vanderbilt University review their work with the humanoid robot ISAC (Intelligent Soft Arm Control) as a means of developing a cognitive architecture. They present working memory and mental rehearsal experiments using this paradigm. Weng at Michigan State University has pioneered the field of autonomous mental development for cognitive robots. In their chapter, Ji, Weng, and Prokhorov present a model of the visual "what" and "where" pathways that could be used in neuromorphic systems for recognizing general objects from complex backgrounds, allowing a location- or type-command from a motor end to dynamically modify a network's internal neuromorphic operations. Barakova and Feijs, from Eindhoven University of Technology in the Netherlands, use various robotic paradigms to study autism spectrum disorder (ASD). Because children with ASD have difficulties with social interaction, Barakova and Feijs have used their robots as a form of therapy for these children with encouraging results.

In Part IV, we turn to more philosophical considerations. As brain-based and neuromorphic robots become more sophisticated, the possibility of truly intelligent machines is becoming a reality. The chapters in this section present frameworks for developing cognitive, or even conscious, robots. To reach this level of complexity, it will be impossible to program all the behaviors and intelligence into a robot. Some scientists are now looking at child development for inspiration in creating intelligent robots. Kaplan of EPFL in Switzerland and Oudeyer of INRIA-Futur in France present the concept of generic and stable kernels, and the notion of changing body envelopes to allow robots to develop on their own. A kernel can be thought of as a learning algorithm, and the envelope is the sensorimotor space that the body explores. The kernel and envelope idea may not only allow robots to develop body plans and fluid movements, it may also serve as a means to study our own development. Asada of Osaka University presents a framework for cognitive developmental robots. In particular, this chapter focuses on issues regarding the mirror neuron system for social cognitive development, and the development of a sense of self and others. Important to both developmental approaches is interaction with a rich real-world environment, as well as interaction with other agents. As an alternative to the developmental approach, Wagatsuma of the Kyushu Institute of Technology turns to dynamical systems to build neuromorphic robots. It is well known that brain oscillations and neural pattern generation are prevalent in the vertebrate brain. Moreover, it is thought that these dynamic patterns give rise to cognitive functions such as motor coordination, episodic memory, and consciousness. Wagatsuma presents a synthetic approach to studying the brain and uses embodied systems that emulate the brain's oscillatory dynamics. In the last chapter of this section, Fleischer and colleagues take on the ultimate goal of autonomous robotics: that is, machine consciousness. This group, which is led by Nobel laureate Gerald Edelman, has been studying consciousness for a number of years. Their chapter reviews prior work towards this goal, and presents a case for how to construct a conscious artifact, and how to test if the artifact is indeed conscious.

We feel strongly that the brain-based and neuromorphic approach will transform the field of autonomous robots to the point where we will have robots in our society that have the adaptability and intelligence that we attribute to biological systems. To paraphrase "Spiderman": with great power comes great responsibility.

The last section of the book deals with some very important ethical considerations. Bekey from the University of Southern California and his colleagues Lin and Abney from California Polytechnic State University discuss the ethical implications of intelligent robots and highlight the immediacy and urgency of the issue. They start by recapitulating Asimov's three laws of robotics and apply it to current military, healthcare, and other social robots. However, these laws fall short for present-day robotics, and the authors propose a hybrid approach toward achieving robot morality. In the final chapter, Shibata of Kanazawa University examines the ethical issue from a different point of view. He evaluates the argument that even though some people with autism lack a theory of mind or empathy towards others, we still need to grant these people the same rights as any member of the human race. Shibata then argues that we need to extend similar rights to intelligent robots if they have a theory of mind, even though they are not members of the human race.

The fact that *Neuromorphic and Brain-based Robotics* covers such a wide range of topics shows how unexplored this young field is at the present time. It is our sincere wish that scientists from other fields and a new generation of researchers find the chapters in this book thought provoking and inspiring. We have made our best effort to provide meaningful examples of prominent neuromorphic robots, present the philosophy behind this approach, and speculate on the construction of future robots with higher cognitive systems. These intelligent, brainy robots of the future will one day, very soon, be interacting and cooperating with human society. We strongly believe this research approach will advance science and society in positive and prosperous ways that we can only now imagine.

We hope you enjoy this survey of an exciting and groundbreaking area of research.

Part II

Neuromorphic robots: biologically and neurally inspired designs

2 Robust haptic recognition by anthropomorphic robot hand

Koh Hosoda

2.1 Introduction

We can easily manipulate a variety of objects with our hands. When exploring an object, we gather rich sensory information through both haptics and vision. The haptic and visual information obtained through such exploration is, in turn, key for realizing dexterous manipulation. Reproducing such codevelopment of sensing and adaptive/dexterous manipulation by a robotic hand is one of the ultimate goals of robotics, and further, it would be essential for understanding human object recognition and manipulation.

Although many robotic hands have been developed, their performance is by far inferior to that of human hands. One reason for this performance difference may be due to differences in grasping strategies. Historically, research on robotic hands has mainly focused on pinching manipulation (e.g. Nagai and Yoshikawa, 1993) because the analysis was easy with point-contact conditions. Based on the analysis, roboticists applied control schemes using force/touch sensors at the fingertips (Kaneko *et al.*, 2007; Liu *et al.*, 2008). Since the contact points are restricted to the fingertips, it is easy for the robot to calculate how it grasps an object (e.g. a holding polygon) and how large it should exert force based on friction analysis. However, the resultant grasping is very brittle since a slip of just one of the contacting fingertips may lead to dropping the object.

An artificial hand structure with sensors only at the fingertips would severely restrict the hand's ability to feel objects. A human hand, in contrast, is covered with soft skin and several kinds of receptors that are distributed across the hand. These receptors are not only for manipulating an object (sense for acting), but also the hand structure or pose allows for active exploration of the object and the accumulation of information (act for sensing) (Pfeifer and Bongard, 2006). During such exploration, we do more than touch and grasp the object statically. We also act on the object through exploratory procedures such as lateral motion, pressure, unsupported holding, and enclosure (Lederman and Klatzky, 1987). Soft skin with many receptors enables stable grasping by multifaced contact and gathering rich information on the object.

Neuromorphic and Brain-Based Robots, eds. Jeffrey L. Krichmar and Hiroaki Wagatsuma. Published by Cambridge University Press. © Cambridge University Press 2011.

To achieve human-like stable manipulation and robust recognition, we have built an anthropomorphic robot hand, called a Bionic Hand, which is covered with soft silicon skin and equipped with distributed tactile receptors. The Bionic Hand can realize stable grasping with the object and gather rich information on the object. It has the ability to reproduce the exploratory procedures of human hands and, eventually, could be a very good tool for understanding human object manipulation and recognition through the use of hands. So far, we have demonstrated the sensing ability of soft skin with distributed receptors in lateral motion and pressure (Hosoda *et al.*, 2006). In this chapter, we discuss one of the exploratory procedures on objects, known as enclosure, which obviously needs hand morphology.

Since the hand has so many receptors, small changes in the position and orientation of a manipulated object lead to large changes of the haptic pattern, and as a result, object recognition tends to be unstable. This is certainly the case with human haptic recognition. The goal of this chapter is to realize robust human-like haptic recognition by an anthropomorphic robotic hand. For stabilizing recognition, we propose to utilize physical interaction between the hand and the object through repetitive grasping. Thanks to several physical features of the hand, the Bionic Hand can recognize different object classes by a repetitive grasping scheme, which is demonstrated by experiments.

2.2   Design of the Bionic Hand

The Bionic Hand is designed for realizing human-like adaptive and robust haptics. It has an endoskeletal structure covered with soft skin in which many tactile receptors are embedded. It is driven by pneumatic actuators for realizing joint compliance. A photograph of a developed hand is shown in Figure 2.1.

2.2.1   Why human-like structure?

To understand human intelligence, it is very important to study manipulation and categorization by hands since they are typical of human intelligent behavior. However, the manner in which we recognize objects through the manipulative ability and function of our hands is still not clear. To understand the manipulation and categorization skill used in daily life, we propose that we have to reproduce the human-like hand structure and move the Bionic Hand in a similar manner to that in daily life situations.

Specifically, we discuss how the hand can be used for generating sensory stimuli from the object by exploring. This aspect of active object recognition is not as well studied as is using sensors for grasp control (Pfeifer and Bongard, 2006). To study active object recognition, the robot hand should have a certain structure that enables active grasping without sophisticated control so that the hand can be used for generating sensory stimuli. We assume that our hands have such morphology to facillitate sensory stimulation, with compliant skin, distributed receptors, underactuated fingers, and carpal structure.

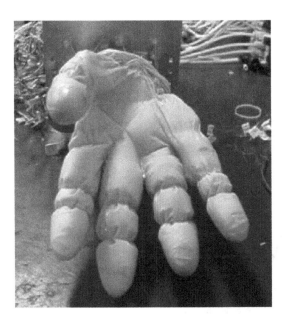

Figure 2.1   Photograph of the Bionic Hand. The hand has an anthropomorphic structure with sensitive skin and it is actuated by pneumatics.

2.2.2   Musculoskeletal structure

A prosthetic hand developed by Yokoi *et al.* (2004) is used as the skeletal structure of the hand (shown in Figure 2.2). The hand has 16 joints: the thumb has four joints, and the index, middle, ring, and little fingers have three joints each. The DIP (distal interphalangeal) and PIP (proximal interphalangeal) joints are driven by the same actuators via an underactuated tendon system. Underactuation, also found in the human hand, enables the fingers to adapt to the object shape (a similar structure is used in Fukaya *et al.*, 2000; Lee and Shimoyama, 2003; Biagiotti *et al.*, 2005; Saliba and Axiak, 2007; Dalley *et al.*, 2009). In total, 11 joints can be controlled independently. The fingers are fixed on the "carpals" plate. The plate bends in a curve so that the fingertips come closer together as the fingers bend (Takamuku *et al.*, 2007). This structure, which is inspired from human morphology (Kapandji, 1982), lets the manipulated object move into stable condition in the palm.

The hand is driven by 22 air cylinders that drive pairs of cables antagonistically so that the hand can realize joint compliance (Figure 2.3). Each cylinder is controlled by an ON/OFF valve. The valve is operated by a host computer via DI/O connection at 250 Hz. Pressured air from a compressor is fed into the actuators through valves. Sensing signals from the receptors are also sampled at 250 Hz.

2.2.3   Skin structure

Hosoda and colleagues developed anthropomorphic artificial skin consisting of multiple layers with two types of receptors (Hosoda *et al.*, 2006): one for sensing local strain and the other for sensing strain velocity. The same structure can be observed in human skin

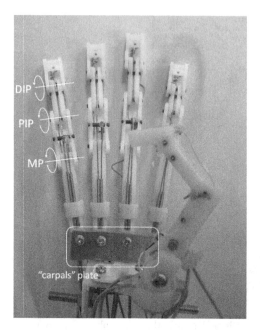

Figure 2.2   Skeletal structure of the Bionic Hand developed by Yokoi *et al.* (2004). Distal interphalangeal (DIP) and proximal interphalangeal (PIP) joints are underactuated; driven by the same set of actuators. The fingers are fixed on the carpals plate that has a particular curvature. The fingertips come closer together when the fingers bend. MP, metacarpophalangeal joint.

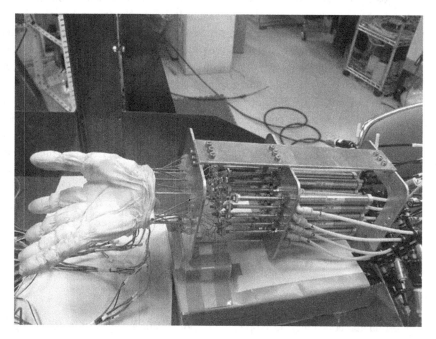

Figure 2.3   Pairs of cables in the Bionic Hand are driven antagonistically by 22 air cylinders. The pressure of each cylinder can be observed by pressure sensors.

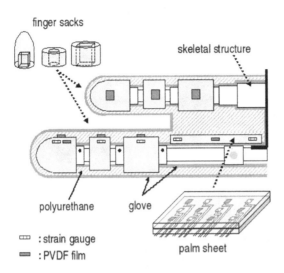

Figure 2.4   Skin structure. The figure shows a thumb (upper) and an index finger (lower), and the palm.
The skeletal structure is covered with a glove. Finger sacks and palm sheets made of relatively
stiff polyurethane material are mounted, which we call a cutis layer. Strain gauges and
polyvinylidene fluoride (PVDF) films are embedded in the sacks and sheets. Another glove is
put on the hand and soft polyurethane material is poured in between.

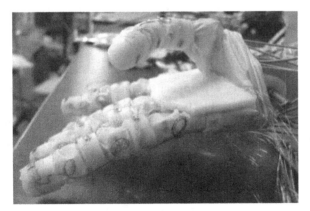

Figure 2.5   Structure of the inner flesh. The photograph shows the inner flesh of the Bionic Hand, called a
cutis layer. Strain gauges and PVDF films are embedded into this layer.

(Miller *et al.*, 1958). It shows high sensitivity for detecting textures (Hosoda *et al.*, 2006)
and slippage (Tada and Hosoda, 2007). Bionic Hand inherits the same structure not only
in the fingers but also in the palm (Figure 2.4). It has two layers: the inner one is relatively
hard (finger sacks in Figure 2.4; see Figure 2.5) and the outer layer is soft (hatched area in
Figure 2.4). We adopt strain gauges and PVDF films as receptors that sense local strain
and strain velocity, respectively. Every finger has three strain gauges and four PVDF
films. The palm has six strain gauges and six PVDF films.

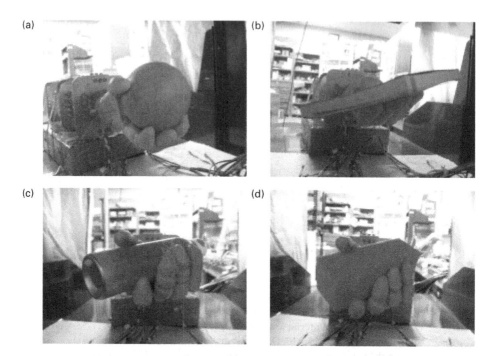

Figure 2.6   Adaptive grasping of various objects: Since the Bionic Hand has essential compliance in its actuation mechanism and skin, the hand can handle various kinds of objects: a ball, a book, a bottle, and a cube. In these experiments, the control parameters of the hand are fixed, and no feedback control is applied.

2.2.4   Adaptive grasping

First, we conducted a preliminary experiment to confirm the grasping ability of the hand for various objects. We gave objects with varying shape to the hand controlled with constant grasping actuation. It adaptively changes grasping posture through interaction even though the actuation does not change (several examples are shown in Figure 2.6). This demonstrates that rough control is enough to have proper grasps for various objects.

2.3   Stable recognition through repetitive grasping

The Bionic Hand has many receptors distributed in the skin like a human hand. Since each receptor gets only local information, such morphology induces another difficulty: small changes in position and orientation of the manipulated object cause large changes of sensation. We adopt a repetitive grasping strategy: the hand grasps the object and regrasps it several times. Since the hand has a curved carpal plate, and the joint and skin are compliant, the object is expected to move to a certain stable position and orientation after several iterations of grasping. As a result, the hand can get stable information on the object.

2.3.1 Repetitive grasping strategy

The repetitive grasping sequence is shown in Figure 2.7. Through (a) to (c), the hand grasps the object (in this case, a cube) over 9 seconds. Once it grasps the object, it partly releases the object (d) but does not release the object completely, and grasps it again (e) in 4.4 seconds. The hand repeats releasing and grasping through (d) to (e) several times. We applied a fixed valve sequence (an ON/OFF pattern) to realize the motion. Because of the morphology and compliance of the hand, the manipulated object moves to stable position/orientations without dropping during the process.

Transition of strain gauge output through the repetitive grasping is shown in Figure 2.8. At the beginning of the sequence, the strain gauge outputs are different between two different initial conditions. After a while, the outputs become similar as a result of the repetitive grasping. This intuitively demonstrates that the hand can recognize the object by a particular pattern of strain gauge outputs after several iterations of repetitive grasping. The manipulated object moves to a certain stable position/orientation without falling down through the process. In Figure 2.9, we show two pairs of initial and resultant final postures. Even though the initial postures are different (left), the object will move to almost the same posture after repetitive grasping (right).

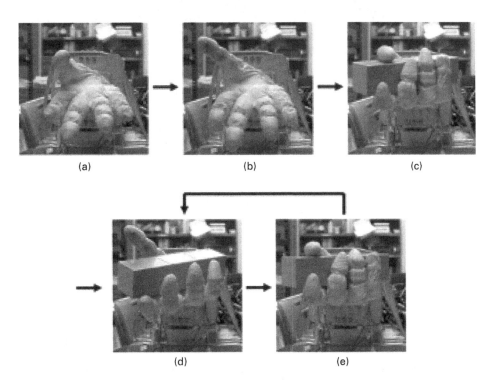

(a) (b) (c)

(d) (e)

Figure 2.7 A repetitive grasping sequence. Through (a) to (c), the hand grasps a cube over 9 seconds. Once it grasps the object, it begins to release the object (d) but does not release the object completely, and grasps it again (e) in 4.4 seconds.

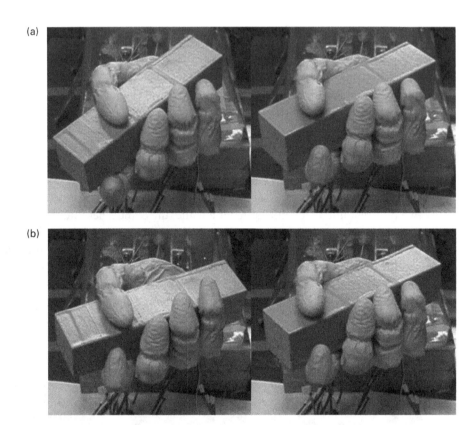

Figure 2.8 Adaptation through repetitive grasping by hand morphology. (a) The contact condition in the first grasp. (b) The contact condition in the tenth grasp.

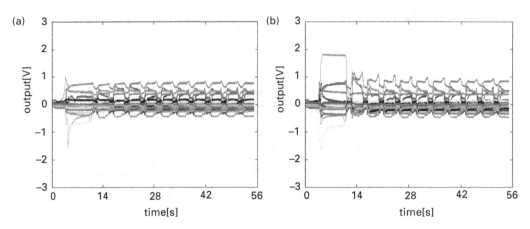

Figure 2.9 Strain gauge values during repetitive grasping. At the beginning of the sequence (a), the strain gauge outputs are different in the two different initial conditions. However, after a while (b), the strain gauge outputs become similar as a result of the repetitive grasping.

2.3.2   Classifying objects based on haptic sensory information

We investigated the ability to classify the shape of objects based on patterns of strain
gauges. At the beginning of the repetitive grasping sequence, the sensed pattern is not
stable since the initial postures differ across trials. After several iterations of grasping, the object settles into a stable posture thanks to the morphology and compliance
of the hand. The output pattern of the strain gauges is also expected to be stable.

The objects used for the grasping experiments are shown in Figure 2.10. We prepared four different objects to the hand: a cube, a cylinder, a bottle, and a ball. They are
hard and not deformable. One trial consisted of 10 iterations of grasping. We conducted
10 trials for each object, five of them started from roughly the same initial posture.
Therefore, we conducted 40 trials in total. First, we investigated within-class variance,
between-class variance (Figure 2.11), and variance ratio (Figure 2.12). Data from all 20
strain gauges were used for calculating variances. The within-class variance decreased

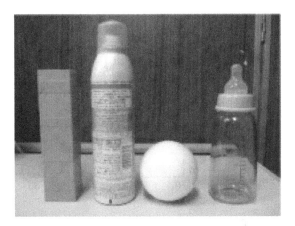

Figure 2.10   Photograph of the objects used in the experiment: a cube, a cylinder, a ball, and a bottle.

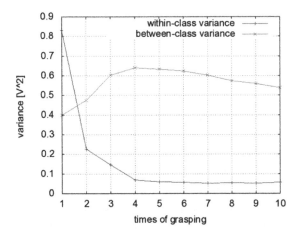

Figure 2.11   Within-class variance and between-class variance.

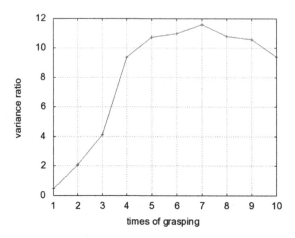

Figure 2.12   Variance ratio.

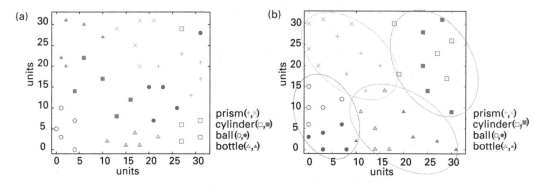

Figure 2.13   Result of SOM clustering. We adopt a 2D self-organizing map for visualization. (a) The solid and hollow symbols represent two different initial postures for grasping the same object. At the first grasp, the solid and hollow symbols form two separate clusters, which means that the hand grasped the bottle (see triangle symbols) roughly from two different initial postures. In this stage, the hand cannot distinguish the objects. (b) By the tenth grasp, there is one cluster for each object despite the different initial conditions.

while between-class variance did not change as much over iterations of grasping. As a result, the variance ratio increased, which meant that after several times of grasping, the hand can differentiate these objects.

For visualizing the result and understanding it intuitively, we applied a self-organizing-map (SOM) technique to decrease the 20-dimensional strain vector. The size of SOM was 32 × 32. The result is shown in Figure 2.13. Because we roughly started the trials from two initial postures, we can see that there are two clusters for each object at the first grasp. For example, solid and hollow triangle symbols in the figure form two separate and distant clusters at the first grasp, which means that the hand grasped the bottle roughly from two different initial postures. In this stage, the hand cannot distinguish the objects. By the tenth grasp, these two clusters converge into one cluster for each object. This means that after 10 times of repetitive grasping, the hand can distinguish the objects even from different initial postures.

These experimental results demonstrate how the hand can distinguish objects through repetitive grasping despite differences in the initial postures.

2.4   Discussion and future work

The analysis of variance and visualization by a self-organizing map both show that the sensed pattern of strain gauges obtained during grasping converges into discriminative clusters representative of each object. Since the actuation pattern for the repetitive grasping does not change through experiments, the differences in the clusters must be due to the morphology and compliance of the hand. Therefore, we can conclude that the idea of robust haptic recognition through repetitive grasping by virtue of morphology of the anthropomorphic hand is supported.

The objects used in the experiments are rigid but the robot hand can manipulate soft objects as well because of its compliance. In such a case, however, the interaction between the hand and the object becomes more complicated. We could use proprioceptive sensors such as joint angle sensors and apply proprioceptive feedback for controlling the hand to modulate the interaction. We plan to investigate such interaction as well, and show that the hand and proposed strategy can be applied for soft objects.

We did not use PVDF films directly for distinguishing the objects in this chapter. In another paper, we have shown that these receptors can be utilized to sense materials by two types of exploratory procedures: lateral motion and pressure (Hosoda *et al.*, 2006). We predict that the combination of these receptors and exploratory procedures would lead to more sophisticated sensing of the object. Moreover, tactile sensing in combination with other sensations, such as vision, would enable the robot to build a concept of objects. It could gather rich information on the object in different modalities and construct multimodal associations. Such association is supposed to be the key to building the concept of objects (Pfeifer and Bongard, 2006). Eventually, our work with the Bionic Hand may shed light on understanding how humans construct the concept of the objects in a constructivist approach.

References

Biagiotti, L., *et al.* (2005). Development of UB Hand 3: early results. In *Proceedings of the IEEE International Conference on Robotics and Automation, ICRA 2005*, pp. 4488–4493.

Dalley, S. A., *et al.* (2009). Design of a multifunctional anthropomorphic prosthetic hand with extrinsic actuation. *IEEE/ASME Transactions on Mechatronics*, 1–8.

Fukaya, N., Toyama, S., Asfour, T., and Dillmann, T. (2000). Design of the TUAU/Karlsruhe humanoid hand. In *Proceedings of the IEEE/RSJ International Conference. on Intelligent Robots and Systems*, pp. 1754–1759.

Hosoda, K., Tada, Y., and Asada, M. (2006). Anthropomorphic robotic soft fingertip with randomly distributed receptors. *Robotics and Autonomous Systems*, **54**(2), 104–109.

Kaneko, K., Harada, K., and Kanehiro, F. (2007). Development of multi-fingered hand for life-size humanoid robots. In *Proceedings of the IEEE International Conference on Robotics and Automation*, pp. 913–920.

Kapandji, A. I. (1982). *The Physiology of the Joints*. Vol. 1: *Upper Limb*. 5th edn. Edinburgh, UK: Churchill Livingstone.

Lederman, S. and Klatzky, R. (1987). Hand movements: a wind into haptic object recognition. *Cognitive Psychology*, **19**, 342–368.

Lee, Y. K. and Shimoyama, I. (2003). A skeletal framework artificial hand actuated by pneumatic artificial muscles. In Hara, F. and Pfeifer, R. (eds.), *Morphofunctional Machines: The New Species*. Berlin: Springer, pp. 131–143.

Liu, H., Meusel, P., Heuzinger, G., *et al.* (2008). The modular multisensory DLR-HIT-Hand. *IEEE/ASME Transactions on Mechatronics*, **13**(4), 461–469.

Miller, M. R., III, H. J. Ralston, and Kasahara, M. (1958). The pattern of cutaneous innervation of the human hand. *American Journal of Anatomy*, **102**, 183–197.

Nagai, K. and Yoshikawa, T. (1993). Dynamic manipulation/grasping control of multifingered robot hands. In *Proceedings of the IEEE International Conference on Robotics and Automation*, pp. 1027–1032.

Pfeifer, R. and Bongard, J. (2006). *How the Body Shapes the Way We Think*. Cambridge, MA: MIT Press.

Saliba, M. A. and Axiak, M. (2007). Design of a compact, dexterous robot hand with remotely located actuators and sensors. In *Proceedings of 15th Mediterranean Conference on Control and Automation*, pp. 1–6.

Tada, Y. and Hosoda, K. (2007). Acquisition of multi-modal expression of slip through pick-up experiences. *Advanced Robotics*, **21**(5), 601–617.

Takamuku, S., Gomez, G., Hosoda, K., Pfeifer, R. (2007). Haptic discrimination of material properties by a robotic hand. In *Proceedings of 6th IEEE International Conference. on Development and Learning*, pp. 1–4.

Yokoi, H., Hernandez, A., Katoh, R., *et al.* (2004). Mutual adaptation in a prosthetics application embodied artificial intelligence. In Iida, F., *et al.* (eds.), *Embodied Artificial Intelligence*. Berlin: Springer-Verlag, pp. 146–159.

3 Biomimetic robots as scientific models: a view from the whisker tip

Ben Mitchinson, Martin J. Pearson, Anthony G. Pipe, and Tony J. Prescott

3.1 Introduction

Why build robot models of animals and their nervous systems? One answer is that in building a robot model of a target organism, which mimics sufficiently some aspects of that animal's body, brain, and behavior, we can expect to learn a good deal about the original creature. Synthesis (engineering) is quite different from analysis (reverse-engineering), is often easier, and teaches fascinating lessons (Braitenberg, 1986). Another answer is that a robot model should allow us to conduct experiments that will help us better understand the biological system, and that would be impossible or at least much more difficult to perform in the original animal (Rosenblueth and Wiener, 1945). In this chapter our target organism is the rat and our specific focus is on the sophisticated tactile sensory system provided by that animal's facial whiskers (vibrissae). Neurobiology shows us that the brain nuclei and circuits that process vibrissal touch signals, and that control the positioning and movement of the whiskers, form a neural architecture that is a good model of how the mammalian brain, in general, coordinates sensing with action. Thus, by building a robot whisker system we can take a significant step towards building the first robot "mammal." Following a short review of relevant rat biology, this chapter will describe the design and development of two whiskered robot platforms – Whiskerbot and SCRATCHbot – that we have constructed in order to better understand the rat whisker system, and to test hypotheses about whisker control and vibrissal sensing in a physical brain-based device. We provide a description of each platform, including mechanical, electronic, and software components, discussing, in relation to each component, the design constraints we sought to meet and the trade-offs made between biomimetic ideals and engineering practicalities. Some results obtained using each platform are described together with a brief outline of future development plans. Finally, we discuss the use of biomimetic robots as scientific models and consider, using the example of whiskered robots, what contribution robotics can make to the brain and behavioral sciences.

Neuromorphic and Brain-Based Robots, eds. Jeffrey L. Krichmar and Hiroaki Wagatsuma. Published by Cambridge University Press. © Cambridge University Press 2011.

3.2   The rat whisker system

Rats are endowed with prominent facial whiskers (Figure 3.1) which they use to explore the environment immediately surrounding their head. This tactile sense is generally considered to be primary in rats in the way vision is primary in primates – to the untrained eye the behavior of blind rats can appear indistinguishable from that of sighted animals.

One group of whiskers are the long "macrovibrissae" that are arranged into a regular grid of rows and columns set into the "mystacial pads" on each side of the snout. These are moved back and forth, when the animal is actively sensing its environment, in a behavior known as "whisking." A second group, shorter and less regularly organized, is distributed over the front and underside of the snout, and is referred to as the "microvibrissae." These whiskers do not have a musculature. This physical and functional dichotomy is reflected in the different uses to which the animal seems to put the two groups. The primary role of the macrovibrissae appears to be locating environmental features, whilst fine investigation is performed, in large part, by the microvibrissae, in concert with the other sensory apparatus around the front of the snout (the teeth, lips, tongue, and nose) (Welker, 1964; Brecht *et al.*, 1997).

The whisker system has become very popular as a model sensory system in neuroscience owing to its discrete organization from the sensory apparatus (the whisker shaft) all the way to the sensory cortex (Petersen, 2007), its ease of manipulation, and, not least, its presence in the laboratory rat. Our approach to this system begins with neuroethology, wherein we study neural systems holistically, including the observation of natural behavior as well as comparative and evolutionary data, and leading to computational models. We then expose these models to the complexities of real world operation, and the demands of functional robotics, revealing shortcomings that are not

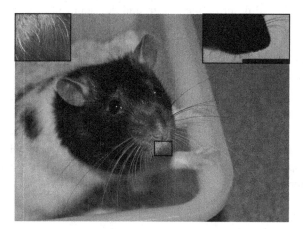

Figure 3.1   Macro and microvibrissae. Left inset shows a close-up of the microvibrissal region centered around the upper lip (see outlined region on main image). The right inset shows the microvibrissae being used to investigate a coin lying on the floor. Note the regular grid-like organization of the actuated macrovibrissae.

manifested in simulation. This engineering process feeds back, raising questions that are not raised (or addressed) by current biological data, and guiding us in the design of future biological experiments. Along the way, we hope to show that whiskers can be a useful robotic sensory system.

Below, we briefly review the neuroethology of the rat whisker system, including results from behavioral experiments conducted in our own laboratory. We then go on to describe two robotic platforms that we have developed, "Whiskerbot" and "SCRATCHbot." Whiskerbot was our first attempt to develop a biomimetic model of the rat whisker system and was, consequently, the more primitive mechanically. Investigations focused on embedded models of neural processing as well as our first efforts to build and control artificial whiskers. SCRATCHbot[1] is our latest platform and still a work-in-progress. Compared with Whiskerbot, the new robot is more refined mechanically and electrically and has more degrees of freedom. The sensor transduction and whisker actuation mechanisms have been redesigned based on insights drawn from our earlier attempt. SCRATCHbot's control system uses a mixture of neural-like and arithmetic computation with a focus on modeling motor control and sensory processing at a relatively abstract level. Its whisker system is also much closer to being a practical artificial sensory system, with possible applications in autonomous robotics.

Our work builds on, and was inspired by, a large number of previous research efforts in robotic tactile sensing systems, including, but not limited to, other whiskered robots that have been developed (Fend *et al.*, 2004; Kim and Möller, 2004; Seth *et al.*, 2004a; Russell and Wijaya, 2005; Solomon and Hartmann, 2006). We have recently provided an extensive review of artificial whisker systems (Prescott *et al.*, 2009); therefore, related projects are mentioned below only where they are of direct relevance to the design decisions that we made in developing our own robot platforms. Our wider goal, through this review, is to describe the development of a research program in neuromorphic robots, including the trade-offs made between accurate biomimicry and the need to engineer functioning systems at reasonable cost. We aim to show that, despite these constraints, the robotics provides insights to the biology; we will illustrate this using examples, and discuss the matter at the end of the chapter.

3.3 Neuroethology of the rat vibrissal system

3.3.1 Morphology, sensory transduction, and whisker actuation

Rat macrovibrissae are made of keratin, are tapered from base to tip, are curved (Figure 3.1), and are typically between 20 mm and 50 mm long (length varying regularly with location on the face) (Brecht *et al.*, 1997). Their frequency response and other mechanical characteristics have been quantified both *in vivo* and *ex vivo* (Hartmann *et al.*, 2003; Neimark *et al.*, 2003), and mechanical response seems to play a key role in signal transduction (Lottem and Azouz, 2009).

---

[1] The name of the robot is derived from the acronym Spatial Cognition and Representation through Active TouCH.

Each macrovibrissa is mounted in a modified hair follicle, a roughly ellipsoidal capsule around 1 mm in diameter and 3 mm long (Rice *et al.*, 1986), which is responsible for transducing mechanical signals into neural signals. A rich variety of mechanical signals are transduced – around 150–200 sensory nerves serve each follicle, and seven or more anatomically distinct classes of "mechanoreceptor" (the mediators of biological tactile transduction) are found distributed throughout the follicle (Ebara *et al.*, 2002). Amongst this range of signals, transverse whisker deflections have been the most studied and are known to generate strong signals in a large proportion of sensory cells (Lichtenstein *et al.*, 1990; Shoykhet *et al.*, 2000) (deflection cells). Cells that transduce something related to whisker angular position (Szwed *et al.*, 2003) (angle cells) and longitudinal deflections (Stüttgen *et al.*, 2008) have also been observed.

The principal, and first-described, component of whisker kinematics is the periodic, forward-backward (anterior-posterior, AP) motion of all macrovibrissae together (Welker, 1964; Zucker and Welker, 1969), a behavior known as "whisking". A smaller, synchronized, up-down (dorsal-ventral, DV) component to this motion (Bermejo *et al.*, 2002) has been identified (that is, a typical "whisk" is reminiscent of a "rowing" action), as has a torsional rotation of the shaft during the whisk cycle (Knutsen *et al.*, 2008). Furthermore, the whisker columns move at somewhat different speeds, with the net effect that the angular separation, or spread, between the whiskers varies significantly within each whisk cycle (Grant *et al.*, 2009). Finally, the whiskers do not always move in concert on the two sides of the face (Sachdev *et al.*, 2003; Mitchinson *et al.*, 2007), and the mystacial pad moves substantially during whisking (Hill *et al.*, 2008). Nonetheless, AP motion of all whiskers together describes a large proportion of overall whisker motion (Grant *et al.*, 2009).

The "intrinsic" muscles are found under the skin of the pad, wrap around each follicle, and are anchored to the skin and/or to neighboring follicles (Dörfl, 1982). These drive "protraction" (forward angular motion) of whiskers individually, by rotating the follicle around a lower pivot point beneath the skin (Dörfl, 1982; Wineski, 1985). Whisker "retraction" (rearward angular motion) is partly passive, due to the elastic properties of the skin, and partly active, driven by the "extrinsic" muscles to the rear of the pad (Carvell *et al.*, 1991). These muscles pull the pad backward, causing all the follicles to rotate around an upper pivot point (Berg and Kleinfeld, 2003). A more recent study reports a contribution to protraction from another set of extrinsic muscles forward of the pad (Hill *et al.*, 2008).

3.3.2   Whisker motion and active sensing behavior

Rats generally whisk when they are exploring an environment or attempting most forms of tactile discrimination. Studies of neural responses to "passive" whisker deflection (deflecting the whiskers of an anaesthetized rat) are therefore beginning to give way to studies of more natural "active" deflection where moving whiskers encounter stationary obstacles. These studies show that whisker motion plays a key role in signal formation. There is no evidence of proprioception in the whisker musculature but angle cells may provide equivalent information (Szwed *et al.*, 2003). Either these cells, or the temporal

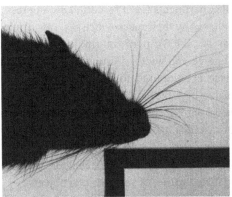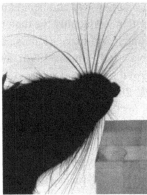

Figure 3.2 Whisking asymmetry induced by contact with a surface. Frames from two example high-speed video sequences recorded in our laboratory, showing exploring rats with whiskers at the maximum protraction phase of the whisk cycle, but with the whiskers ipsilateral to an object of interest held back towards the cheek, whilst the contralateral whisker field pushes forward towards the surface. Electromyograph recordings from the whisking muscles confirm that the contralateral whiskers are driven significantly harder than the ipsilateral ones (Mitchinson *et al.*, 2007). We interpret behavior such as this as evidence for a "Minimal Impingement, Maximal Contact" (MIMC) active sensing control strategy.

relationship between whisker motion and whisker deflection, are thought to provide the information necessary to transform deflections of moving whiskers into an appropriate head-centered reference frame (Ahissar and Arieli, 2001; Szwed *et al.*, 2003).

Whisking motor patterns vary substantially with behavioral circumstance, but discernible "bouts" of more-or-less periodic whisking at 6–10 Hz interspersed by periods of inactivity are typical. Whisk frequency tends to be relatively constant within a bout (Hill *et al.*, 2008) but other kinematic parameters can vary substantially, driven, apparently, by both internal and external variables. The strongest observed external influence is whisker–environment contact, which rarely fails to modulate whisking (Mitchinson *et al.*, 2007; Grant *et al.*, 2009). For instance, a unilateral unexpected whisker–environment contact generally leads to suppression of protraction ipsilaterally (i.e. on the side the contact was made) and to increased protraction amplitude contralaterally (Figure 3.2). We hypothesize that this is the outcome of a control policy we term "Minimal Impingement, Maximal Contact" (MIMC), which tends to maximize the count of whisker–environment contacts, while keeping the depth of those contacts within a managed range to maintain signal quality. A further observation (Grant *et al.*, 2009) that spread between whisker columns is reduced during environmental contact is consistent with this policy, with rearward, noncontacting whiskers brought forward to meet an ipsilateral obstruction. Another, internal, modulatory influence is head rotation, whereby the animal appears to preempt upcoming head rotations by moving its whiskers backward (forward) on the side to which (away from which) the head will turn (Towal and Hartmann, 2006). In addition to these asymmetries, a temporary loss of bilateral synchrony in whisker movements is often observed following a unilateral contact (Mitchinson *et al.*, 2007), while repeated contacts with the environment can lead to longer periods of desynchronization (unpublished results from our laboratory).

Psychophysical and behavioral experiments (see Prescott *et al.*, in press, for review) show that, using only the data gathered by their macrovibrissae, rats can locate objects accurately in space (Knutsen *et al.*, 2006), perform fine textural discriminations (Carvell and Simons, 1990), and judge gap widths (Krupa *et al.*, 2001), and that both macrovibrissae and microvibrissae are required for effective prey capture (Anjum *et al.*, 2006). However, a reasonable hypothesis is that macrovibrissae are primarily used for locating objects, and then microvibrissae are brought to bear for close investigation (Brecht *et al.*, 1997). For instance, the microvibrissae seem to be used preferentially in a shape-discrimination task (Brecht *et al.*, 1997; Fox *et al.*, 2009) and in our own laboratory, where we do not constrain the animal's behavior, we consistently see the microvibrissae used for close investigation of surfaces and objects.

As a consequence of these findings, and from inspecting many in-house video recordings of rats exploring environments and objects, we consider the "orient" behavior, in which a rat positions its head such that the front of its snout is brought to bear on its apparent focus of attention (Figure 3.1, inset top right), to be a key component of active sensing. Indeed, orienting should perhaps be considered as the primary active sensing strategy employed by the animal, with repetitive whisker motion (whisking) adding a second component that provides wider coverage of space, contact–detach cycles without head motion, and more precise control over the nature of contacts. Observing that the body must also be moved if the rat is to orient its snout to locations a little distance away, we could consider that locomotion of a rat in a novel environment may be well described as a stream of orients of the snout to one location after another. That is, the rat shifts its focus of attention and the head, whiskers, and body follow. Thus, we might consider orienting to constitute the foundation of exploratory behavior in general, and therefore to be a prerequisite for effective active sensing in any whiskered entity, animal or robot. Note that, in a familiar environment, episodes of locomotion with a specific destination in mind, as opposed to a series of orients to immediately sensed features, are also seen. In such conditions, where locomotion is not motivated by sensing, we might expect different whisking behavior, attuned more to supporting locomotion (e.g. to ensure a sound footing and avoid collisions) rather than to maximizing the gain of new sensory information. Experiments to establish whether rat whisking behavior is noticeably different in these circumstances are currently in progress in our laboratory.

Orients are generally observed to occur on the timescale of one or two whisking periods (Prescott *et al.*, 2009). Contact usually occurs during whisker protraction, and repositioning of the snout may complete quickly enough such that the battery of contacts due to the subsequent protraction sample the neighborhood of the attended object. Supplementary Video 3.1 shows an example orient that completes in about one whisking period (all supplementary videos are available at www.cambridge.org/9780521768788). In this clip, the orient has begun by 40 ms following contact, and completes around 160 ms after contact (with the peak of the subsequent protraction occurring about 120 ms after contact). Some orients may take two (perhaps, more) whisks to complete – for instance Supplementary Video 3.2 shows an orient completed in the space of two whisks.

After orienting, the animal will often keep its snout near to an attended object for a few whisks in order to investigate it more closely using the sensory equipment around the snout. This activity can be complex, and is thus less easy to describe, but we often see an investigative behavior we refer to as "dabbing", whereby the microvibrissae are lightly touched or brushed against the object in synchrony with macrovibrissal protractions (Hartmann, 2001; Prescott *et al.*, 2005). The result is that tactile information is obtained at high spatial density towards the center of the dab, through the microvibrissal array, while, within the same narrow time window, surrounding surfaces are sampled in a sparser fashion by the macrovibrissae. Supplementary Video 3.1 shows the animal, immediately following the orient, performing five "dabs" at the attended feature (the corner of a block) before appearing to move on, whisking and dabbing across the wider extent of the object. The whole operation, from contact through orient and dabbing to moving on, is completed within three quarters of a second.

3.3.3 Neurobiology of the rat vibrissal system

Anatomical loops at multiple levels are present in the rat whisker system (Kleinfeld *et al.*, 1999) (Figure 3.3). Within this complex circuit, the most studied pathway is that carrying whisker signals upstream from the follicle, through the trigeminal complex, and ventro-posteromedial and posteromedial thalamic nuclei (known as "VPM" and "POm," respectively), to the primary ("barrel") somatosensory cortex (S1; Waite and Tracey, 1995). This, and related, cortical pathways are likely to be involved in extracting behaviorally relevant features from vibrissal signals, and have been shown to be required for some whisker-driven tasks (Krupa *et al.*, 2001). However, it is important not to overemphasize the role of this feedforward pathway to the cortex. As is clear from the diagram, the more general character of the system is that it consists of a set of nested closed loops which likely have different, though overlapping, functional roles. Each of these loops connects sensation to actuation at relatively short latencies, particularly at the lower levels of the neuraxis.

For instance, the pathway via the trigeminal complex to the facial nucleus, which contains the motoneurons that drive the intrinsic and extrinsic whisking musculature, provides a fast and direct, brainstem-only pathway through which contact information could affect the ongoing movement of the whiskers (Nguyen and Kleinfeld, 2005; Mitchinson *et al.*, 2007). A midbrain loop through the superior colliculus (SC) (Drager and Hubel, 1976) is likely to underlie whisker-initiated orienting and avoidance responses (Sahibzada *et al.*, 1986). The latency for whisker deflection signals to reach the SC may be as short as 5 ms (Cohen *et al.*, 2008), thus providing the capacity for very rapid orients as might be required, for instance, when the source of the stimulus is a moving prey animal. From the S1 cortex signals pass to the motor cortex (MCx) which has a substantial area devoted to the whisker system (Haiss and Schwarz, 2005). Although it is known that the MCx sends a large projection to the brain areas involved in whisking pattern generation (Kleinfeld *et al.*, 1999), its precise role in modulating or initiating whisking is poorly understood. Areas such as the trigeminal complex, SC, and S1 also project to two brain subsystems that perform more general purpose roles

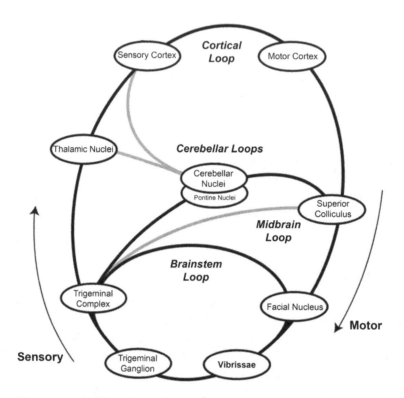

Figure 3.3   Neuroanatomical loops in the whisker system of the rat (modified from Kleinfeld *et al.*, 2006). Loops through nonwhisker musculature (neck, shoulders, etc.) are not shown. Whisker sensory signals pass up from the vibrissae via the trigeminal nerves to the trigeminal sensory complex. From here, they pass along multiple loop paths, including: directly to the facial nucleus and back to the muscles driving the vibrissae; through superior colliculus; through cerebellar nuclei; through sensory and motor cortex via the thalamic nuclei.

within the brain architecture, the cerebellum, and basal ganglia (BG). The cerebellum is thought to function as an adaptive filter (Dean *et al.*, 2010) that could, for instance, use current state to predict future sensory signals. In contrast, the role of the BG seems to be to provide action selection (Redgrave *et al.*, 1999): that is, to decide which of the many possible behaviors available to the animal are engaged at any one time.

In the accounts of our whiskered robots that follow we will describe implementations that constitute embodied tests of functional hypotheses concerning several of the neural circuits and brain subsystems mentioned here.

3.4   Whiskerbot

Our first foray into whiskered robotics was Whiskerbot (2003–2007) (Pearson *et al.*, 2007b), which ran simultaneously with an effort to model neural components of the rat whisker sensory system. Computational models were developed of transduction in the whisker follicle (Mitchinson *et al.*, 2004, 2008), processing in the trigeminal nucleus (Pearson *et al.*, 2007a), transformation of whisker signals into a head-centered reference frame, orienting to whisker contacts (Mitchinson *et al.*, 2006), and whisking pattern generation and its modulation by contact signals (Mitchinson *et al.*, 2007). A number of these models used arrays of artificial "leaky-integrate-and-fire" (LIF) neurons and were designed to run on embedded onboard digital hardware in real-time (Pearson *et al.*, 2006b, 2007a). The robot, including deployment of these models, is discussed in this section.

3.4.1 Robot

Whiskers and transducers

Since our control models are based on the neural systems of the rat, we expect them to work with signals of the type used by the rat. Where those systems are not fully understood, we cannot assume that they will work with signals with different characteristics. Our approach, therefore, is to engineer our whiskers to match those of the animal as closely as possible. Biological whiskers display an enviable combination of stiffness and damping, and even light contacts on the tip can elicit orienting, indicating that they effectively propagate mechanical deformation. Our hope was to design artificial whiskers for our robot with similar physical characteristics to their natural counterparts so that our robotic sensors would share these beneficial properties. Inevitably, however, since we were designing an engineered system composed of nonbiological materials, the desire to accurately mimic the properties of natural whiskers and of the tissues that support them was balanced against engineering practicalities, necessitating some compromises, described below.

In the past, potentiometers and springs have been used to measure torque at the whisker base (Russell, 1992; Ueno and Kaneko, 1994). More recently, real rat whiskers were bonded to the diaphragms of electret microphones to measure high frequency deflections as the whiskers were moved across textured surfaces (Yokoi *et al.*, 2005). In Whiskerbot, we chose resistive strain gauges bonded directly to the base of the artificial whiskers and configured to measure strain in two axes, which we denote x (AP) and y (DV) (Pearson *et al.*, 2007b). The advantages of this approach were two-dimensional measurement, high sensitivity, and large bandwidth (limited only by sampling speed). The disadvantage of strain gauges is that high strains can reduce bond integrity, leading to calibration drift. Similar gauges have also been used recently configured, as in Whiskerbot, to measure two-dimensional strain at the whisker base (Quist and Hartmann, 2008).

Given this gauge technology, manufacturing constraints (in particular, attaching the gauges securely) forced us to build our whiskers physically scaled up by a factor of four. Moreover, a complex robot of similar size to a rat would generate significant engineering challenges that we are not currently equipped to face. To mitigate the effect of this change on whisker dynamics, we adopted a temporal scaling-down by a factor of two (that is, our neural models ran at half wall-clock speed when deployed on the robot). This temporal scaling means that we match the animal's behavior by whisking at a more leisurely pace of around 3–4 Hz.

We tested a variety of materials for the whisker shaft. A major finding was that, to generate a strain at the base of the whisker that was well clear of the noise floor, we were forced to build from materials much stiffer than those of real whiskers. This compromise did not prevent useful modeling – indeed, experiments described later in this chapter demonstrate effective contact detection and texture discrimination using these whiskers. What remains to be discovered is whether additional, or higher quality, sensory information might be recovered from whiskers that are a closer physical match to biology. An active line of research in our own and other laboratories is mechanical modeling of whiskers, in an attempt to gain insight into this question (Birdwell *et al.*, 2007; Fox *et al.*, 2008).

Whisking

As we have seen, actuating the whiskers (whisking) seems to be key to sensing in the animal. Several groups have shown that moving artificial whiskers across surfaces can provide useful information about surface features such as texture or shape (Russell, 1992; Ueno and Kaneko, 1994; Wilson and Chen, 1995; Gopal and Hartmann, 2007). Some mobile platforms have used nonactuated whiskers for obstacle avoidance and perception (Jung and Zelinsky, 1996; Seth *et al.*, 2004b), and some have used actuated whisker arrays where all the whiskers, on both sides, are moved together (Fend *et al.*, 2004; Kim and Möller, 2007). Physical whisking mechanics as complex as that found in the biology (Hill *et al.*, 2008) would be very challenging to implement. However, we noted above that AP angular motion is sufficient to reproduce a substantial part of the whisker motion observed in the animal (Grant *et al.*, 2009). Our current robot platforms therefore reproduce just this degree of freedom for whisker motion. Although, unlike previous whisking robots, we do allow for independent AP movement of individual whiskers (Whiskerbot) or whisker columns (SCRATCHbot). Shaft encoders provide sensory data encoding the angle of each whisker carrier (denoted by θ), in analogy to biological angle cells.

The Whiskerbot platform was designed to have nine whiskers on each side. Shape-memory alloy wire was used to independently actuate each whisker to minimize weight and power consumption. Passing current through this material generates heat, causing a linear muscle-like contraction, which generated whisker protraction. Springs played the role of tissue elasticity, providing passive retraction (Dörfl, 1982). This system was able to whisk at up to 5 Hz, when fans were used to cool the actuating wires; however, operating in this region limited the lifetime of the wires significantly. Most experiments, therefore, were performed in the 1–2 Hz range.

Platform

The basic platform layout is a two-wheel differential drive unit, with the head fixed in relation to the body, and a "snout" area at the front of the head (no microvibrissae were included, but the area at the front of the head between the macrovibrissal fields was designated as the snout to act as the target area for orienting). The whiskers were mounted in rows on either side of the head. In common with most robotic platforms, the actuators were driven by local feedback controllers, in response to set-point signals

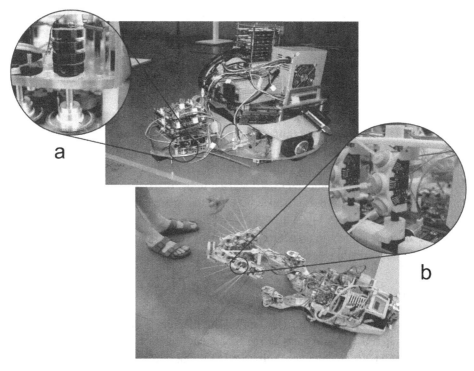

Figure 3.4 Photographs of whisking actuation technology used for (a) Whiskerbot, shape memory wire (protraction) and springs (passive retraction), and (b) SCRATCHbot, motor and gearbox driving each column.

(position or velocity) (Figure 3.4). This represents a significant departure from biological actuation, which is open-loop at short timescales. We contend, however, that this is an advantageous approach during early development, since it decouples actuation mechanics from motor control. Not only does this avoid the need to develop mechanics that are functionally similar to those of the biology, as well as nontrivial plant-tailored open-loop controllers, it also frees us to update our model of the mechanical plant (in the light of new results) without having to change the mechanics themselves. Thus, we can simulate any biological plant in software, and charge the servos with following its outputs. The disadvantage of this approach is that interactions between the plant mechanics and the mechanics of the environment are only indirectly modeled. Since these interactions could be a contributor to whisker transduction, we may seek to move away from artificial closed-loop control as our physical models of whiskers and whisking mature.

Computing

The ever-present constraint of any mobile robotics platform is power, which limits the amount of processing that can be deployed. This constraint is hardened by the fact that closed-loop controllers need to receive update signals on a regular period to avoid erratic behavior. Thus, software components must operate in strict real-time, constraining model complexity (size, resolution, scope, etc.). To mitigate this on Whiskerbot, we offloaded some of the large (but simple) neural models onto re-programmable hardware devices (Field Programmable Gate Arrays, FPGAs). Using parallel computing and function-specific hardware, in this way, we were able to run detailed spiking neural network models yet maintain strict adherence to the real-time constraint (Pearson *et al.*, 2006a, 2007a). Coordination of this processing architecture, incorporating both hardware and software components, was left to BRAHMS, a framework for integrated heterogeneous computing that we have developed in-house (Mitchinson *et al.*, 2010). The main control resource of the platform was a reconfigurable computing platform called a "Bennuey" PC-104+ motherboard (Nallatech, 2007). This consists of a PC-104 single-board computer (SBC) and a number of expansion slots for FPGA modules. One FPGA was used as a bridge between hardware communications systems and the PCI bus of the PC. Other FPGAs were configured for hardware acceleration of spiking neural models in a "neural coprocessor" and a "follicle coprocessor" (Pearson *et al.*, 2005, 2006b) (see Section 3.4.2).

3.4.2   Control architecture

An overview of the robot control architecture is illustrated in Figure 3.5, which we map loosely onto parts of the biological architecture of Figure 3.3; the figure shows the SCRATCHbot configuration. At the bottom left is the interface to the robot platform; this consists of the neural and follicle coprocessors (Whiskerbot) as well as the sensors (x, y, θ) and actuators (whiskers, wheels, neck). The remainder of the architecture can be described as an inner loop (small circular arrow) mediating whisking pattern modulation, and a middle loop (large circular arrow) mediating behavior. Higher loops (curved arrow to left) modeling cortical and hippocampal systems, for such competences as object discrimination and spatial mapping, are the subject of current work in our laboratory (Fox *et al.*, 2009) (see also Section 3.6 Discussion); the current architecture exhibits only immediate responses, and has no long-term memory. The Whiskerbot configuration is similar, but uses the spiking output of the follicle coprocessor to drive the coordinate transform (and does not perform reafferent noise removal) and implements the Whisker Pattern Generator as a spiking neuron model in the neural coprocessor, with modulation from the follicle coprocessor output.

Whisker pattern generation

The Whisker Pattern Generator (WPG) is a model of the central pattern generator present (Gao *et al.*, 2001) (though not yet located; Cramer *et al.*, 2007) in the rat brain and whose activity underlies the rhythmic whisker motions observed in the behaving animal. Although bilaterally asynchronous whisker movements are sometimes observed in animals, particularly following, or during, interactions with surfaces, movements of the two whisker fields generally appear to be tightly coupled such that perturbations are usually corrected within a small number of whisk cycles (often one). Likewise, within each whisker field some asynchronous movements have been observed, but this

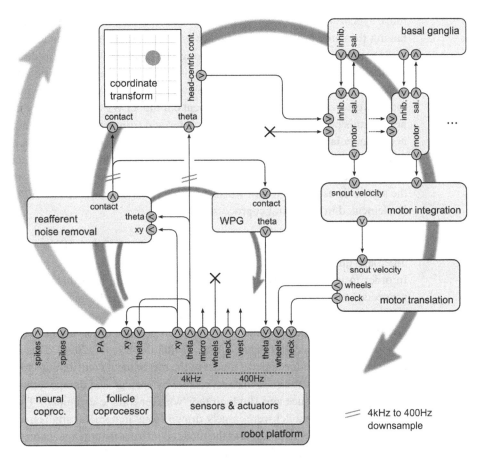

Figure 3.5 Overview diagram of control architecture of SCRATCHbot/Whiskerbot; SCRATCHbot configuration shown (see text for details). Straight arrowed lines represent numeric data streams at 400 Hz or 4 kHz; **xy** and **theta** are raw sensor data. Reafferent noise is removed from **xy** to generate **contact**, the clean per-whisker contact strength signal, which modulates the Whisker Pattern Generator (WPG). Contact is transformed into head-centric space using the instantaneous values of **theta**, and is passed to the actions. Competition between actions for the motors is mediated by the basal ganglia. Finally, the selected action sends snout velocity to the motor translation layer, which generates platform-specific control signals for the actuators.

has yet to be quantified or explained. Rather than address the issue of multiple coupled WPGs at the outset of our study, for Whiskerbot we chose to use a single WPG to generate the base whisking signal, and derive movement patterns for each whisker from this signal.

Typical whisking, as described above, can be broadly described as modulated periodic oscillations. Therefore, our model is based around modulation of periodic oscillators. The simplest possible model is a single oscillator generating the angular position of each individual whisker through a gain. In this model, the whiskers are constrained to move synchronously (all whiskers in phase), symmetrically (whisking on the two sides having the same profile), and periodically (each whisking cycle is identical). Each of these constraints is relaxed in a long-enough series of rat whisking, as described above; in the robot, we can relax these constraints to test the impact of different modulation strategies. Although not enough is known about the rat WPG to constrain a detailed model we nevertheless chose to implement our model WPG in a neurally inspired manner. For this purpose a base oscillator was formed from two, alternately active, spiking neuron populations, one population acting as the integrator and the other as the reset signal. An additional pair of populations, one on each side, relayed the oscillator activity to the actuator control board (and could be modulated; see below), where each of the signals is used to drive all whiskers on that side of the face. The WPG model was implemented in the neural coprocessor.

Sensory transduction through a model of the whisker follicle and trigeminal ganglion

In order to use the Whiskerbot platform to investigate embedded neural processing we needed to recode the x, y whisker deflections recorded using the strain gauges into spike trains in simulated sensory nerves. For this purpose we used a model of transduction that we developed in order to accurately reproduce observations made under both passive and active deflection conditions (Mitchinson *et al.*, 2004). This model was in two parts. First, we developed a model of the mechanical contributions to transduction consisting of six anatomical masses, related by springs and dampers that represented the response of tissues and fluids in the "whisker-follicle assembly." The parameters of this part of the model were largely drawn from anatomical studies, making direct connection with the anatomy, and the model confirms that the mechanics are substantially involved in signal formation. The second part of the model was a conventional noisy LIF cell model that was used to simulate the sensory cells within the trigeminal ganglion (these cells do not merely transmit the response of the mechanoreceptors, but play a key role in signal formation). The parameters of this second model, along with remaining parameters of the mechanical part, were chosen to balance plausibility (e.g. smoothness) with reproduction of the results of biological experiments (Lichtenstein *et al.*, 1990; Shoykhet *et al.*, 2000; Szwed *et al.*, 2003). Two distinct classes of deflection cell were modeled, "slowly adapting" (SA) and "rapidly adapting" (RA), reflecting a dichotomy widely described in the literature. These classes are defined by their responses to prolonged deflections: SA cells fire throughout these deflections, whilst RA cells fire only during their onset and offset. Both classes of cell are directionally sensitive, so information on the direction of whisker deflection is encoded. This model was computed on the Whiskerbot "follicle coprocessor", in FPGA (see Figure 3.5).

Our control architecture also included a population of model whisker angle cells (Mitchinson *et al.*, 2006) similar to those described in the animal by Szwed *et al.* (2003). For this purpose, angular position, as measured by each shaft encoder, was used to drive a bank of cells associated with each whisker. Each cell responded strongly only when the measured angle was near to its preferred angle, with some overlap between cells. Thus, the identity and response of the active cells implies the whisker angle, consistent with biological data.

Coincidence detection

Whisker deflection signals, in the animal and in the robot control architecture, are generated whenever the whiskers are obstructed during protraction. The contact signals from each whisker are provided in a "whisker-centered" frame-of-reference. In order to integrate information from multiple whiskers (and with information from other sensory modalities) signals therefore need to be transformed into a single reference frame (this is the "coordinate transform" of Figure 3.5). In the rat, it has been hypothesized that this is performed by neural mechanisms that detect coincidences between firing in deflection cells and angle cells (Szwed et al., 2003). In the Whiskerbot control architecture a sheet of LIF cells representing the head frame was driven by deflection cells and angle cells together, with innervation patterns calculated based on the known geometry. Thus, coincident firing generated activity in the correct location on the sheet (Mitchinson et al., 2006), and indicated contact at the encoded location. Since the architecture does not yet include a model to determine the distance along the whisker at which contact occurred (although extensions to allow this are possible, e.g. Birdwell et al., 2007; Evans et al., 2008), it is instead assumed that contact occurred close to the tip of the whisker. In practice, this assumption has proved adequate for the robotic experiments performed using the Whiskerbot platform, allowing us to defer the problem of computing radial distance to contact for later.

Action selection

A fundamental problem faced by all but the simplest organisms is deciding which action, of those possible, to take at one moment. Failure to efficiently select a unique action to perform can lead to confused use of the actuators (or muscles), and flawed behavior (Prescott et al., 2006, 2007). Appropriate action selection should take into account not just exteroceptive sensory signals, such as those derived from whisker–environment contacts, but also proprioceptive signals (odometry, for example) and internal indicators of homeostatic and motivational state. One proposal is that these different signals are integrated in a collection of brain nuclei called the basal ganglia (BG) whose intrinsic circuitry appears to be optimized to perform efficient and robust selection between competing behavioral alternatives (Redgrave et al., 1999). This theoretical proposal has been developed into a number of computational neuroscience models that have been evaluated both in simulation and on a robot platform (Gurney et al., 2004; Prescott et al., 2006). We use a version of this BG model to perform action selection within our robot control architecture. Briefly, each action that the robot can express "bids" for use of the motors by indicating its current "salience" – salience is higher when the action is strongly indicated by the current sensory input. The model BG chooses a winner, and allows that action to have use of the platform, avoiding mix-ups. Actions that Whiskerbot exhibited include: dead reckon (use odometry to reach a preprogrammed location, analogous to path integration in rodents; Etienne et al., 1996);

various forms of explore (random walk, whisking from side to side to detect obstacles); and orient (orient snout towards focus of attention). Since we are interested in viewing the majority of motor output (at least during exploratory behavior) as directly consequent to a desired positioning and orientation of the snout, all of these actions are designed to generate a desired snout velocity vector. Motor integration across actions, then, means simply summing the (snout) velocity vector from all active actions, relying on the BG to suppress motor output from nonselected actions. Note that we were not concerned with learning, here – the BG model has fixed weights and mediates between bids by actions, the salience of each of which is a preprogrammed function of current sensory inputs.

3.4.3   Whiskerbot experiments

The Whiskerbot platform was used to validate the embedded computational neuroscience models (i.e. to demonstrate that they could adequately perform their intended role), to evaluate active control strategies for vibrissal sensing, and to develop and test classification methods for texture discrimination using whisker signals.

An example of the type of experiment performed was our investigation of the likely consequences of a minimal impingement (MI) control strategy on the whisker deflection signals processed in the brain. As noted previously, our own behavioral observations in animals had indicated that whiskers rapidly cease to protract following contact with an object during exploration. We hypothesized that this result implied a control strategy that sought to minimize the extent to which whiskers were allowed to bend against surfaces. To implement MI in our robot control architecture the total activity across all whisker deflection cells on one side of the face was fed back to suppress activity in the ipsilateral WPG relay. This has the desired effect that protraction ceased rapidly after contact, as seen in the animal (Mitchinson *et al.*, 2007). Figure 3.6 shows how MI affects WPG output, the signals consequently generated in the strain gauges, and the response of the simulated deflection cells, during whisking against a stationary obstacle (examples of whisker movement and deflection with MI off and on are shown in Supplementary Videos 3.3 and 3.4, respectively). With MI enabled, the signals are cleaner and more closely match those observed in the animal (Mitchinson *et al.*, 2006; Pearson *et al.*, 2007b). This result is in line with our predictions for the effect of this control strategy on signal quality in the animal (Mitchinson *et al.*, 2007), and suggests that the whisker signals being relayed to the sensory cortex (and elsewhere) in awake, exploring animals will be quite different from those generated in the same animals in the absence of feedback control (as for instance, in whisker deflection experiments performed under anesthesia).

We also tested Whiskerbot's ability to orient to obstacles following contact. In these experiments the robot was allowed to proceed across a smooth floor and interact with one or more point obstacles (narrow cylinders). Initially, the robot control architecture selects the default explore behavior and the robot proceeds in a random walk, whisking as it goes. On detecting one of the obstacles, the robot switches to orient, and turns its snout to the obstacle before pausing – that is, it expresses an "orient." With no ability

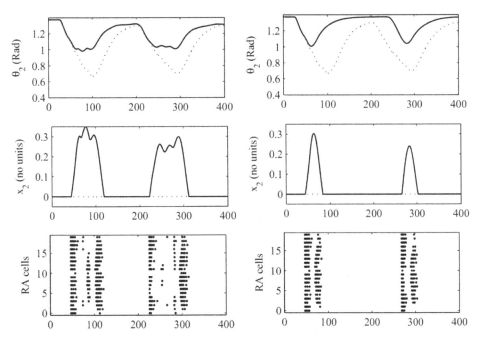

Figure 3.6   Signals recorded during two whisks where the rostral whiskers contact a stationary obstacle; left/right column of panels is without/with MI control. Top panels show rostral whisker column angles (solid line); dotted line is the same in both panels, and shows the output of the pattern generator (i.e. the requested column angle) for the unmodulated case. In the unmodulated case (top left), the whisker presses hard against the obstacle, and the column is physically prevented from moving further forward. In the modulated case (top right), the whisker briefly touches the obstacle, and the column is retracted by the MI policy. Other panels show strain gauge output (middle) and simulated rapidly adapting (RA) deflection cells (bottom, with each dot representing a spike). All panels reproduced from figures in Mitchinson *et al.* (2006).

to "dab" on this platform, orient concludes with the robot backing off and heading in another direction. An example, using a version of the platform equipped with only two whiskers, is shown in Supplementary Video 3.5.

On occasion an orient was performed when no obstacle had been contacted. Under high-speed video observation, we see complex whisker dynamics excited by the motion of the whisker carrier – that is, the whiskers "whip" around when they are moved. This generates a relatively high power noise signal in the *x* data stream, leading to spurious spiking in contact cells. These "ghost orients" were traced to this noise source (Pearson *et al.*, 2007b) and are considered further in Section 3.5 describing SCRATCHbot.

In addition to providing an embodied test-bed for neural models, an important goal for Whiskerbot was to investigate tactile feature extraction from artificial whisker signals. To that end, we have shown that simple Gaussian classifiers, together with either hand-picked or biomimetic features derived from whisker contact signals, can be used as the basis for effective robotic texture classification (Fox *et al.*, 2009). These results serve to further demonstrate the potential of vibrissal tactile sensing for applications in autonomous robotics such as navigation and spatial-mapping in darkness.

3.5   SCRATCHbot

SCRATCHbot constituted a fundamental redesign of many of the physical and mechanical aspects of our whiskered robot, and a more high-level approach to the development of the embedded brain-based control system. The following subsections summarize and explain the main changes and extensions.

3.5.1   Changes to the robot design

Signal transduction

One limitation of Whiskerbot was that the strain gauges used to measure whisker deflection were apt to come loose, such that repairing a snapped whisker, or reattaching strain gauges, was a laborious process. Therefore, an important practical improvement for SCRATCHbot was to move to a more robust (though less sensitive) method of transduction (Figure 3.7). In the new whisker assembly the whisker shaft is supported in a rigid hollow sleeve by a thick layer of relatively soft polyurethane around the base; thus, it returns elastically to its rest position when it is released. A small, axially magnetized, disk magnet is bonded to the very base of the whisker, and a miniature tri-axis Hall-effect sensor (HS) is positioned underneath. The HS generates two voltages linearly related to the displacement of the magnet in the two axes. This design took its inspiration from the work of Kim and Möller (2007). Each whisker assembly is calibrated after construction by programming the rest position and deflection limits in each axis into the HS. This effectively sets the sensitivity of the whisker to deflections, since the voltages generated by the HS are linearly scaled to the programmed deflection range. Figure 3.7 shows some typical voltage trace outputs from a calibrated whisker during a range of controlled displacements in one axis (deflection outside the programmed range results in saturation). Importantly, these sensory modules remain undamaged under large deflections. Where such deflections cause a whisker to break, a new whisker is simply inserted into the old module, and the HS recalibrated to return to normal operation.

A secondary consequence of this change was the freedom to explore alternative, less stiff, materials for the whisker shaft. Nonetheless, it has still proved difficult to match the simultaneous high sensitivity and high damping displayed by rat whiskers. Partly, this is an issue of materials: biological whiskers are highly composited, and achieve good energy absorption simultaneously with good signal transmission; reproducing such a material will require substantial further development. Partly, it is an issue of scale: the smaller the whisker, the less prone to prolonged oscillation; a substantially smaller (factor four) whisker/whisking assembly is currently under development in our laboratory – this will be a close match to the size of a rat's larger whiskers, and we expect to achieve a better sensitivity/damping trade-off as a result.

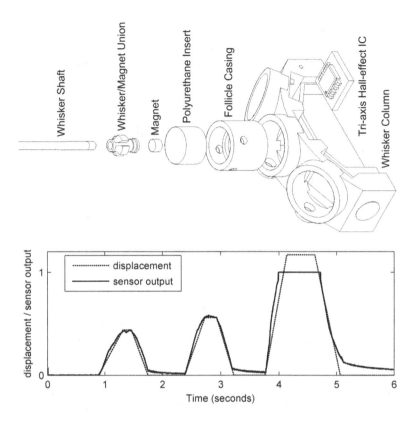

Figure 3.7 Exploded view of the Hall-effect-based macrovibrissae sensor assembly and an example output voltage plot taken from the sensor during three ramp–hold–release displacement profiles of varying magnitude. The voltage and displacement data have been normalized to the maximum output voltage (5V), calibrated for a 40-mm deflection of the whisker applied at a point 60% along the length from the base. Note that the magnitude of the third displacement profile exceeds the calibrated range resulting in the output voltage saturating.

Microvibrissae

An important enhancement over Whiskerbot is the addition of an array of microvibrissae, mounted at the center of the snout between the two actuated macrovibrissal arrays. The central array consists of nine short (80 mm) plastic whiskers, mounted at their base into a common polyurethane sheet, and again instrumented with magnets and Hall-effect sensors to measure deflections in two dimensions. These microvibrissae are able to initiate orienting in the same manner as the macrovibrissae if an obstacle is encountered snout-first. In addition, they are able to sample the object at a relatively high spatial resolution once the robot has oriented. The classifier systems originally developed for discriminating texture using Whiskerbot macrovibrissae are currently being adapted and extended for use with both the macrovibrissal and microvibrissal arrays (Evans *et al.*, 2009), and to distinguish other object properties such as orientation, distance, and velocity relative to the snout.

Whisker array geometry and actuation

A further issue that emerged with Whiskerbot was that the shape memory alloy actuators chosen for whisker actuation, although lightweight and low power, were fiddly to work with and tended to deteriorate rapidly with use. Therefore, we moved to more conventional whisker actuation by DC motor for SCRATCHbot. To reduce the number of motors required, three whisker carriers were mounted on either side of a light-weight plastic "head," with each carrier carrying three whiskers in a column. The geometry of the head was such that all the whiskers would point directly ahead of the robot when fully protracted. Each column can rotate (AP) through 120°, which is similar to the maximum angular range available to the rat. A second actuated axis of rotation (DV) was implemented on the SCRATCHbot platform, though this was limited to a single actuator for each side (three columns) and constrained to ± 15° of rotation about the vertical.

Head and body design and actuation

We argued earlier that active sensing in rats is as much a matter of positioning the head and body as of positioning the whiskers. The Whiskerbot platform, with its head fixed relative to its body and nonholonomic constraints on the body, was very restricted in this respect (Prescott *et al.*, 2009). With a view to opening up our investigations of the role of head and body positioning in sensing, SCRATCHbot was endowed with several additional degrees of freedom (DOF) – see Figure 3.8. The head is fixed to the top stage of a 3-DOF "neck" assembly (Elumotion; www.elumotion.com) with its base fixed to the body. This neck allows the head to be moved through axes referred to as elevation, pitch, and yaw, as well as providing a certain amount of "reach." In addition, the platform's three wheels can be turned through 180°, approximating a holonomic platform.

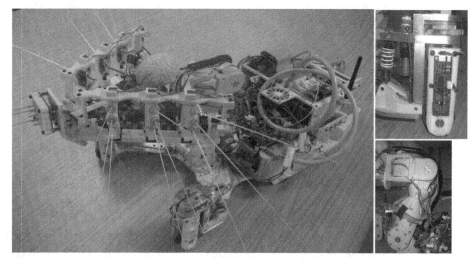

Figure 3.8 Photograph of the SCRATCHbot platform with detailed view of the front right motor drive unit (top right panel) and the three degree of freedom neck assembly (lower right panel).

Computing

Finally, although demonstrating embedded onboard processing for neural models was a key goal in the development of Whiskerbot, this was less of a core objective in the design of SCRATCHbot. Onboard FPGA coprocessors have been retained to allow for the possibility of computationally intensive onboard processing; however, we have also added a wireless signal link allowing the inclusion into the control architecture of asynchronous heavy-duty off-board processing. Three levels of computation are thus available on the new platform: short-latency, relatively inflexible (onboard FPGA); medium-latency, limited computational power, synchronous (in the PC-104); high-latency, high computational power, asynchronous (off-board PC). This gives a range of computing options that are well suited to implement aspects of the lower, middle, and upper loops of the neural architecture.

3.5.2   Changes and additions to the control architecture

On SCRATCHbot, we have so far chosen not to model the encoding of x, y (whisker deflection signals), and θ (whisking angle) in simulated spiking neurons. Rather, these signals are propagated as continuously valued numeric variables to other parts of the control architecture. Consequently, the brain-based models investigated in SCRATCHbot should be thought of as more abstract approximations to the computations performed by the rat vibrissal system than some of the spike-based models previously investigated in Whiskerbot. Modeling at this higher level, we believe, can allow us to make more rapid progress in identifying the computations that are performed by whisker-related circuitry in the rat brain. We remain very interested, however, in understanding how these more algorithmic models might be implemented in neural tissue. Indeed, for problems such as whisking pattern generation, we are currently conducting investigations at multiple levels of abstraction. We are using more detailed neurally based models to explore, in simulation, the role of particular cell populations (such as the whisking motoneurons in the facial nucleus) whilst, at the same time, employing more abstract algorithmic WPG models to generate whisker movement patterns on the robot platform that are more directly comparable to rat whisking behavior.

Naturally, we have an extensive list of additions that we hope to make to the SCRATCHbot control architecture. The following subsections summarize some changes that have already been implemented, and also provide a brief outline of where we expect this work to go in the near future.

Using MIMC to control whisker spread

Predictable variation in whisker spread (the angular separation between the whiskers) was noted previously as a characteristic of animals that are exploring surfaces (Grant *et al.*, 2009). To investigate the possible causes of this variability we extended the modulation options of SCRATCHbot's WPG by implementing a separate relay for each column (rather than having just one for each side of the head, as in Whiskerbot). Whisker–environment contact excites all of these relays, whilst suppressing only those relays driving the whiskers that contacted the environment. The result is that, in addition to the per-side MIMC elicited in Whiskerbot, more rearward whiskers move more rapidly than they would otherwise, and are thus brought forward to meet a contacted obstacle. The net result is a reduction in intercolumn spread following contact, as seen in the animal. Another way of putting this is that, by implementing MIMC at the per-column level, "control" of whisker spread appears as an automatic consequence of this general active sensing strategy – the whiskers are brought forward to meet the environment wherever possible, whilst being restrained from bending too far against it.

Head and body movement

A key task for the motor system is to generate control signals for the wheels and neck that achieve the desired snout movement; this takes place in the motor translation layer (MTL) of our control architecture. Conventional robotic approaches to controlling multi-DOF systems (e.g. potential-field or sampling-based) can be expensive to solve, may suffer from local minima, may not be robust, and are not generally bioplausible. We use, instead, an algorithm we call "Snake," which takes a bio-inspired approach, causing free (uncontrolled) nodes of the mechanics to follow adjacent, controlled, nodes according only to mechanical constraints (that is, there is no explicit motion planning). Thus, actuators are "recruited" to contribute to the movement in a distal-first pattern, as has been seen in the animal during fictive orienting (Sahibzada *et al.*, 1986), and more massy central nodes tend to be moved less than lightweight peripheral nodes. This algorithm results in motion that appears quite natural to the human observer. Furthermore, nodes are moved no more than necessary to achieve the target velocity of controlled nodes, and the computations for each node are local to that node and cheap, all of which are bio-plausible characteristics. The algorithm can be inferior to explicit motion planning under some conditions; for instance, the trajectory of the overall plant may pass through illegal configurations, or uncontrolled nodes may intersect obstacles. We hypothesize that, in biology, failures of this class are easier to deal with (reactively) than is computationally heavy proactive global motion planning. In SCRATCHbot, usually only the snout node is controlled (snout location being the hypothesized goal), and the joints and base of the neck follow as if the robot was being led by a ring through its nose.

Predicting and canceling sensory signals due to self-movement

Other than the increased complexity of the motor translation layer (due to the increased degrees of freedom in the head and neck), and the abstraction away from the spiking neuron level, SCRATCHbot initially employed similar algorithms for generating orienting responses to those used in Whiskerbot. The robot therefore displayed "ghost orients" just as Whiskerbot did, for the same reason that movements of the robot body, head, or whiskers can induce large transients in the transduced whisker signals.

To mitigate this problem, we took inspiration from a hypothesis of motor-reafferent noise removal in cerebellum (Anderson *et al.*, 2009; Dean *et al.*, 2010), and used a bank of linear adaptive filters, one for each whisker, to attempt to predict this noise signal based on the whisker angle signal measured from the shaft encoder attached to each column. After learning the parameters of the filters independently for each whisker from example data, this noise removal proved to be very effective. The nature of the motor-reafferent noise generated at the transducers depends both on the whisker material and length, so it would appear that both the animal and the robot would benefit from mechanisms, such as efficient damping, that can act to minimize this noise at source.

Work in progress

We are currently working on a range of extensions to the robot control architecture. These include systems for tactile spatial mapping (modeled on the rat hippocampus), for feature detection (modeled on S1 cortex), and for improved decision making by BG. In the longer term we also plan to explore the role of the whisker motor cortex (MCx) in initiating and modulating whisking bouts, and of further cortical areas involved in somatosensory processing such as the S2 cortex. The cerebellum is known to be involved in a number of distinct loops with the vibrissal system that may each implement a similar computation (adaptive filtering) but in a context that fulfills a quite different role with respect to the behavior of the animal. For instance, one hypothesis that we wish to explore is that the cerebellum may be involved in predictive tracking of a moving target that would allow a whiskered predator to track rapidly moving prey using only their vibrissae. Another is that cerebellum may be involved in the tuning of open-loop motor control operations, such as the orient action implemented on the robot.

3.5.3   Scratchbot experiments

Observing general SCRATCHbot behavior (locate and orient), we typically use 30–60 second runs in a featureless flat arena, with one or more obstacles, or an experimenter's hand. On start-up, a behavior called "unpark" bids strongly to the BG, and is given control of the robot, whilst other actions (and whisking) are suppressed. The neck axes are driven such that the head is moved from its "park" position to an unstable point we call the "unpark" position. On arrival, unpark stops bidding, the default explore behavior is given control, and whisking begins. At the preset end time, software control ceases, and the low-level controllers automatically return the neck to the park position.

Figure 3.9 and Supplementary Video 3.6 illustrate what happens when contact is made by one or more of the macrovibrissae. The deflection of the whisker due to the whisker coming into contact with the experimenter's hand (Figure 3.9 and Frame 1) causes the salience of orient to increase. If the salience of orient is held for long enough (a few tens of milliseconds), the BG switches, selecting the new action by inhibiting the output of explore and disinhibiting the output of orient. The orient action pattern consists of two phases: first, the snout is oriented to the point of contact; second, this pose is maintained for a period of time suitable for fine-scale exploratory behavior with the microvibrissae (currently being implemented). Note that the salience of the second phase of orient is lower than that of the first; thus, the robot can be more easily interrupted while exploring the object than while completing the orient itself. When orient completes, it stops bidding for the plant, explore is again selected, and the robot straightens up as it resumes its exploration. The removal of motor reafferent noise is very effective, and SCRATCHbot does not express ghost orients.

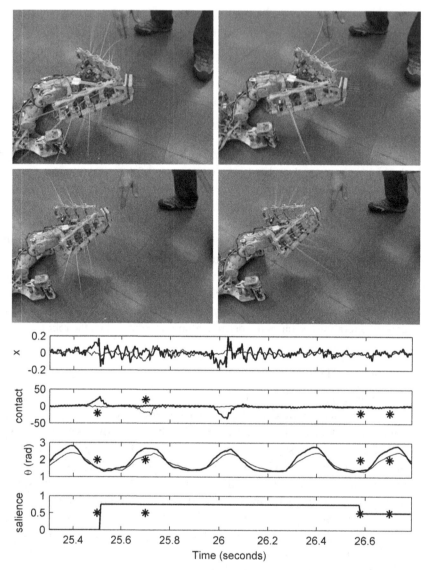

Figure 3.9   Graphs show data from SCRATCHbot during an orient to a whisker contact. Upper three plots show data from fifth whisker (middle whisker row/column, thick line) and seventh whisker (top whisker row, rear column, thin line) on the left. (Upper) Raw x-component of whisker sensory signal. (Second) Reafferent noise removed, greatly improving the signal-to-noise ratio. (Third) Angular position (θ) of middle/rear columns (π radians indicates straight ahead). (Lower) Saliency of orient. Frame timing is indicated in plots by star symbol. Contact on whisker 5 during retraction (Frame 1, top left) is followed by increase in orient salience and action selection. Additional contacts on whisker 7 (Frame 2) and 5 during the orient are ignored. Snout arrives at the point of initial whisker contact (Frame 3, lower left), completing the orient; saliency is reduced. The second phase of orient (Frame 4) is a placeholder, during which the microvibrissae will be used for fine inspection of the contacted feature, in future work.

Currently, as described (and shown in Supplementary Video 3.5 for WhiskerBot, Supplementary Video 3.6 for SCRATCHbot), locomotion during robot exploration results from switching between explore and orient. As described in Section 3.3.2, we hypothesize that rat locomotion in similar circumstances might be viewed as a series of orients, with the focus of attention being constantly shifted, often ahead of the animal. In future, we will test this hypothesized approach to locomotion using SCRATCHbot, removing explore and generalizing orient, such that the robot can "attend to" (thus, orient to) a more general target, which may not be something immediately detected as interesting, but rather a location about which it intends to gather sensory information.

We have also tested the effect of the addition of control of whisker spread on the nature of signals collected by the whiskers. In Whiskerbot, we showed that MI implemented on each side of the face effectively cleaned up contacts between a single whisker and the environment. In SCRATCHbot, we were able to demonstrate that per-column MIMC was effective in (a) cleaning up contacts on multiple whiskers and (b) generating more whisker–environment contacts than would otherwise have occurred. An example of this new version of MIMC is illustrated in Figure 3.10 and Supplementary Video 3.7. For this experiment we fixed the robot head in a position facing a stationary "wall," similar to that typically recorded using the experimental set-up described by

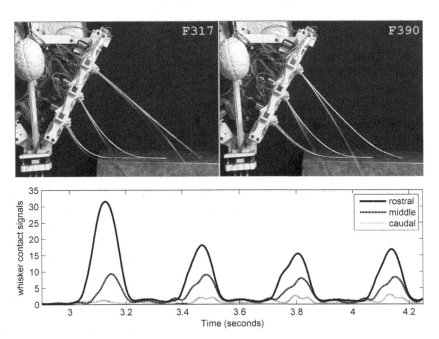

Figure 3.10 Investigating the impact of per-column MIMC on whisking patterns and data collection (see text). Upper panel shows two frames taken from a high-speed video of a trial of whisking against a wall. The frames are taken from the moment of peak whisker protraction in the first whisk (left) and in the second (right); in the second whisk, modulation has taken effect, and the contacts of each column with the wall are normalized. Lower panel shows the contact signals retrieved from the center whisker in each of the three columns, during the first four whisks of the same trial – signals are normalized in second, and later, whisks.

Grant *et al.* (2009). In each trial, the first whisk against the wall is unmodulated (left upper panel), and shows that the more rostral column whiskers are heavily deflected, whilst the most caudal column whiskers do not touch the wall at all. On the second whisk, the MIMC modulation has taken effect (right upper panel), the rostral whiskers are less protracted and thus are deflected less heavily, and the caudal whiskers are brought forward and generate contacts with the wall (i.e. whisker "spread" is reduced). The effect of this modulation on the contact signals collected can be seen in the lower panel of the figure – across the three columns, there is a tendency towards normalization of contact depth.

3.6   Discussion

3.6.1   Why build robot models of animals and their nervous systems?

When neuroscientists think of model systems they usually think, not of robots, but of using one animal as a model of another (e.g. the rat as a model of a human); of an animal in an altered condition (e.g. under anesthesia, or awake but immobilized) as a model of the awake, behaving one; or of an isolated part, such as a brain slice or a muscle, as a model of that component within the intact, functioning system. However, consider the task that our research group is attempting, which is to understand the whisker system of the rat. Some of the biological models that are available to us, the properties that they share with our target system, and their amenability to experimental investigation of their internal processes are summarized in Table 3.1.

The right-hand column of Table 3.1 qualitatively illustrates the difficulty of studying the internal processes of the mammalian nervous system in each of the available models. This is hardest to do in the awake, freely moving animal (the behaving rat as a model of itself) and becomes progressively easier as we move to the restrained preparation, then anesthetized, then to an isolated brain slice. Despite recent advances in embedded, wireless chronic recording systems, which are making more naturalistic experiments possible, access to the neural processes of unrestrained behaving animals will always be very limited. The problem, however, as illustrated in the other columns of the table, is that as we move from the target animal to the more amenable biological models, we progressively lose many of the interesting properties that we wish to understand – how the free-moving animal controls its head and body so as to optimize sensing; how sensorimotor loops are closed through the environment; and how the component parts operate within an integrated and intact system. The more restricted animal preparations can still be useful, of course, but insight concerning these properties will need to be inferred where it cannot be obtained directly. As a consequence we may then ask how the compromises made to create a particular model (e.g. treatment with anesthesia) have impacted on the results and on the inferences drawn.

Now, examine the bottom line of Table 3.1. All of the interesting properties just listed are, or could be, exhibited in a robot model of the behaving animal in a system that is highly amenable to investigation of its internal processes, indeed, far more so

Table 3.1 Comparison of material models of the awake, free moving rat

| System | Properties | | | | Amenable to experimental investigation of internal processes |
	Similar substrates	Intact and integrated	Closed loop	Capable of active control	
Awake, free-moving rat (target organism)	*****	*****	*****	*****	*
Animal models: Awake, restrained rat	*****	*****	*****	***	**
Anesthetized rat	*****	*****	***	*	***
Rat brain slice	*****	*	**	*	****
Whiskered robot	*	*****	*****	*****	*****

Asterisks signify an arbitary rating scale from 1 to 5 stars, with 5 stars the highest.

than any of the available animal models. The snag, and of course it's a big one, is that the robot's physical and computational substrates – its body and its brain – may not approximate the target animal in an adequate way. Thus the results obtained from experiments with the robot may not be valid when translated back to the animal. But note that this is not too different from the situation with the animal models: in both cases, animal and robot, we have had to compromise and allow some aspects of the model to differ significantly from our target. What we have with robotics, at least, is the possibility that we can continue to refine the model, so that if we are worried that some aspect is substantially wrong we can fix it and re-run the experiment to see if the result changes. As the biomimicry improves, we can expect richer and more convincing insights into the properties of the biological system we are trying to understand.

But how good does the biomimicry need to be to make the model useful? According to the pioneer of cybernetics Norbert Wiener "the best material model of a cat is another, or preferably the same, cat" (Rosenblueth and Wiener, 1945, p. 320). But this is "best" in the sense of most accurate, not most useful. That is, if you want to be really fussy about the fidelity of the model compared with the target, then you will end up coming back to the original system (the same cat, or, in our case, the awake, free-moving rat) as the only model that is good enough. In practice, and this is exactly the point that Wiener was making, all systems that are useful as models will only approximate their target. Indeed, Rosenblueth and Wiener (1945) suggested that, for a useful model, sufficient and necessary conditions are not that it should be accurate in every detail (some degree of abstraction is decidedly a good thing), but that it should translate the problem into a domain we understand better, and it should allow us to conduct experiments with relative ease. We contend that – for exploring the relationships between brain, body, and behavior – robotics, which translates problems in biology into problems in computing and engineering, meets these requirements well.

3.6.2   Insights from whiskered robots into the biology of the rat vibrissal system

We would like to conclude by reviewing some of the contributions that we believe robotics can make to neuroethology, illustrating each with an example from our research on whiskered robots.

Discovering important questions

We have discovered, as the consequence of our collaboration, that the engineer's mindset is really very different from that of the experimentalist, and that both can gain from the interchange of ideas and experience. When an engineer is asked to design a robot that mimics some aspect of animal behavior, his or her first questions are likely to include "What is your specification for this robot?" and "What would you like it to do?". The biologist is then likely to reply that they can specify some aspects of the design, and of the desired behavior, but not all, since much of the biology is still unknown at this stage. Further, of those things they can specify, much of what they can tell you is approximate or qualitative and some of it is disputed. At this point the engineer may wonder if the problem is adequately posed! If both sides are still keen to pursue the collaboration the experimentalist might then ask what is it that the engineer needs to know in order to create a sufficient specification, and the ensuing list of questions can then be integrated into the ongoing program of empirical work. Often the questions that the engineer will ask are very different from those that have hitherto been addressed by any experiment. This is because the task of synthesis differs radically from that of analysis (Braitenberg, 1986). Synthesis often imposes an order on design decisions which makes the answers to some questions more important, or at least more urgent, than others. For instance, when we began to design our first whisking robot one of the first questions from the engineers was "What happens to the whiskers once they touch a surface – do they keep moving and bend against the object, or do they stop?". A simple enough question, but when we looked at the experimental literature that existed at that time there was no clear answer. Thus began a program of experimental work that showed that, during exploratory whisking, protraction ceases rapidly following contact, leading to our hypothesis of the "minimal impingement" whisker control strategy (Mitchinson *et al.*, 2007).

Testing the sufficiency of theories

Many good reasons for building models, in simulation or in robots, have been nicely summarized by Epstein (2008). One of the most important of these is that a model allows us determine whether our theories are adequate to account for the behavior we are trying to explain. If the robot can replicate the behavior of the animal then there is no longer any question of whether the theory is sufficient (although we can still ask whether it does the task as well as the animal or in the same way). As it turns out, some of the tasks that look easy are harder to replicate than you would expect, and some apparently hard tasks turn out to be relatively easy. For instance, orienting to a whisker contact sounds easy, but when we implemented it we found that the robot was easily distracted by ghost contacts generated by its own movement. Resolving this problem using an adaptive filter was nontrivial and suggested a new theory about the role of vibrissal loops through the cerebellum. A theory of vibrissal orienting without noise cancellation was an insufficient theory, but this was not apparent until we built the robot model and tried it out.

Suggesting new hypotheses

The task of devising an effective solution to whisker-guided orienting has also suggested a new hypothesis concerning the representations of vibrissal stimuli in the midbrain superior colliculus (SC). In mammals, the SC is known to be a seat of spatially organized sensory information, and to drive rapid orienting and aversion responses (Dean et al., 1989). It is also well evidenced that SC is an important locus for cross-sensory integration of spatial information (Sparks, 1986). Recent histological and electrophysiological measurements indicate that, in the rat, there are strong neural projections from the brainstem trigeminal nuclei to the intermediate layers of SC (Kleinfeld et al., 1999), providing a substrate for whisker–visual integration. In visual animals, SC uses a retinocentric coordinate system; in the rat, retinocentric and head-centric are very closely related, since eye movement is minimal. If spatial information from the whiskers is also integrated in SC, the coordinate transform modeled in Whiskerbot (from whisker to head-centered reference frame) must take place either in SC itself, or on the way to it (i.e. in the trigeminal nuclei). Whisker representations in SC in the anesthetized animal are very broad (Drager and Hubel, 1976), particularly in the AP direction, with individual whiskers having representations almost as large as the whisker rows to which they belong. From our modeling work we contend that these broad, AP-biased, fields are to be expected. Specifically, if accurate integration is to be performed between visual and vibrissal stimuli then, since whiskers move relative to the head as the result of whisking, their representations must also move around with respect to the head-centered map in SC, leading to broad overall fields. Recording from multiple cells in an animal while the whiskers move, it should be possible to show that the strongest response to individual whiskers moves around in SC in a manner consistent with this hypothesis. Whilst we can only be confident of this prediction in the awake animal, it might also be observed in a lightly anesthetized animal, with whisking invoked electrically.

Investigating the role of embodiment

It is increasingly recognized that behavior is the consequence of the interaction between the brain, the body, and the environment (Chiel and Beer, 1997; Chiel et al., 2009) and that robotics may be one of the most cost-effective ways of studying this interaction. Current simulations of real-world physics are not up to the task of adequately capturing all of the dynamical properties (e.g. collision elasticity, surface friction) of the interaction between two objects such as a whisker shaft and a moving or irregular surface (Fox et al., 2008); thus the world remains its own best model for this aspect of our work. As noted above, our recent efforts to build artificial vibrissae fall short of producing artifacts with all the desirable mechanical properties of the rat whisker-shaft/follicle.

Therefore, our current approach combines simulation, to better understand the biomechanics of natural whiskers, with robotic experiments to determine what properties of surfaces can be effectively discerned through artificial vibrissal sensing. Through this combined approach we hope to be able to better identify the contribution of the morphology to the task of tactile sensing for this system.

Investigating "What if?" scenarios

Robots do not have to mimic the biology, and one way to find out why the biology is as it is might be to build a system that works differently and compare. For instance, we can directly contrast the sensing properties of whiskers that do not taper or do not curve with those that do, in order to better understand why natural whiskers have evolved to do both. Likewise, we can investigate ways of controlling the movement of the whiskers that are either natural or unnatural and observe the consequences of these different movement strategies for the type, quality and quantity of tactile information obtained by the robot (animal).

Doing the experiments that cannot be done

One of the most important uses of a physical model is that it can allow experiments to be performed that could not be done on the animal, or at least would be very difficult to do *in vivo* given our current knowledge and available methods. For example, what impact does minimal impingement (MI) control of vibrissal movement (Mitchinson *et al.*, 2007) have on the sensory signals ascending from the whiskers to higher processing centers such as the S1 cortex? This question is important because much of the research conducted on the cortex is performed in anesthetized animals, or even in brain slices, using input signals that are intended to mimic the effects of natural contacts. Unfortunately we cannot perform a straightforward experiment in the animal where we turn off MI control and see the difference that this makes to signals (in the anesthetized preparation we can replace natural whisker motion with a form of fictive whisking (Szwed *et al.*, 2003); however, there are differences here from the awake, behaving animal that could make interpretation of the findings problematic). In contrast, in the robot model, the required experiment is trivial to perform (see Figure 3.6), and we can exactly compare the contacts resulting from movement, with and without MI, and the spike trains that these contacts generate in the simulated trigeminal nerve (which, in the animal, is just two synapses away from the signals arriving at the S1 cortex). These robot experiments can therefore help neuroscientists to select more plausible signal trains with which to stimulate animal models during *in vivo* or *in vitro* experiments.

Evaluating the usefulness of biological solutions to problems in robotics

Finally, one of the benefits for engineers of engaging in this kind of interdisciplinary collaboration is to determine whether the biological system has a solution to an existing practical problem that they might usefully copy. The rat is a successful and versatile mammal that uses its whiskers in a range of tasks from object detection and recognition, through guidance of locomotion across all kinds of terrain, to prey capture (Prescott *et al.*, in press). In mammals more generally, tactile hairs are widely deployed across the body (e.g. on the legs, paws, or back) for detecting unexpected contacts and for tactile discrimination of surface properties. A sensory capacity that has proved so effective for animals could lead to increased flexibility and performance when deployed on robots. Indeed an artificial whisker system could prove particularly useful for robots that must operate in environments where vision systems can provide only degraded or ambiguous input, such as in smoke- or dust-filled buildings or for covert operations in darkness. Towards this end, the next stage in the development of SCRATCHbot will be to devise tactile-based strategies for environment exploration and local and global navigation. For instance, we plan to incorporate a spatial memory based on current understanding of the rat hippocampal formation. By associating odometry and head-centered contact information with tactile sensory features, such as texture and object shape, a spatial map will be constructed as the robot explores. For the biologists, this will allow investigation into how tactile sensory information is presented to long-term memory systems. For the roboticists, this will provide valuable insight into how a touch-based platform could be effectively deployed for robot guidance in the absence of vision.

References

Ahissar, E. and Arieli, A. (2001). Figuring space by time. *Neuron*, **32**(2), 185–201.

Anderson, S. R., Porrill, J., Pearson, M. J., *et al.* (2009). Cerebellar-inspired forward model of whisking enhances contact detection by vibrissae of robot rat. *Society for Neuroscience Abstracts*, 77.2.

Anjum, F., Turni, H., Mulder, P. G., van der Burg, J., and Brecht, M. (2006). Tactile guidance of prey capture in Etruscan shrews. *Proceedings of the National Academy of Sciences of the USA*, **103**, 16 544–16 549.

Berg, R. W. and Kleinfeld, D. (2003). Rhythmic whisking by rat: retraction as well as protraction of the vibrissae is under active muscular control. *Journal of Neurophysiology*, **89**(1), 104–117.

Bermejo, R., Vyas, A., and Zeigler, H. P. (2002). Topography of rodent whisking. I. Two-dimensional monitoring of whisker movements. *Somatosensory and Motor Research*, **19**(4), 341–346.

Birdwell, J. A., Solomon, J. H., Thajchayapong, M., *et al.* (2007). Biomechanical models for radial distance determination by the rat vibrissal system. *Journal of Neurophysiology*, **98**, 2439–2455.

Braitenberg, V. (1986). *Vehicles: Experiments in Synthetic Psychology.* Cambridge, MA: MIT Press.

Brecht, M., Preilowski, B., and Merzenich, M. M. (1997). Functional architecture of the mystacial vibrissae. *Behavioural Brain Research*, **84**, 81–97.

Carvell, G. E. and Simons, D. J. (1990). Biometric analyses of vibrissal tactile discrimination in the rat. *Journal of Neuroscience*, **10**(8), 2638–2648.

Carvell, G. E., Simons, D. J., Lichtenstein, S. H., and Bryant, P. (1991). Electromyographic activity of mystacial pad musculature during whisking behavior in the rat. *Somatosensory and Motor Research*, **8**(2), 159–164.

Chiel, H. J. and Beer, R D. (1997). The brain has a body: adaptive behavior emerges from interactions of nervous system, body and environment. *Trends in Neurosciences*, **20**(12), 553–557.

Chiel, H. J., Ting, L. H., Ekeberg, O., and Hartmann, M. J. Z. (2009). The brain in its body: motor control and sensing in a biomechanical context. *Journal of Neuroscience*, **29**(41), 12 807–12 814.

Cohen, J. D., Hirata, A., and Castro-Alamancos, M. A. (2008). Vibrissa sensation in superior colliculus: wide-field sensitivity and state-dependent cortical feedback. *Journal of Neuroscience*, **28**(44), 11 205–11 220.

Cramer, N. P., Li, Y., and Keller, A. (2007). The whisking rhythm generator: a novel mammalian network for the generation of movement. *Journal of Neurophysiology*, **97**, 2148–2158.

Dean, P., Redgrave, P., and Westby, G. W. (1989). Event or emergency? Two response systems in the mammalian superior colliculus. *Trends in Neurosciences*, **12**(4), 137–147.

Dean, P., Porrill, J., Ekerot, C. F., and Jörntell, H. (2010). The cerebellar microcircuit as an adaptive filter: experimental and computational evidence. *Nature Reviews Neuroscience*, **11**(1), 30–43.

Dörfl, J. (1982). The musculature of the mystacial vibrissae of the white mouse. *Journal of Anatomy*, **135**(1), 147–154.

Drager, U. C. and Hubel, D. H. (1976). Topography of visual and somatosensory projections to mouse superior colliculus. *Journal of Neurophysiology*, **39**(1), 91–101.

Ebara, S., Kumamoto, K., Matsuura, T., Mazurkiewicz, J. E., and Rice, F. L. (2002). Similarities and differences in the innervation of mystacial vibrissal follicle–sinus complexes in the rat and cat: a confocal microscopic study. *Journal of Comparative Neurology*, **449**(2), 103–119.

Epstein, J. M. (2008). Why model? *Journal of Artificial Societies and Social Simulation*, **11**(4), 12.

Etienne, A. S., Maurer, R., and Séguinot, V. (1996). Path integration in mammals and its interaction with visual landmarks. *Journal of Experimental Biology*, **199**(1), 201–209.

Evans, M., Fox, C. W., Pearson, M., and Prescott, T. J. (2008). Radial distance to contact estimation from dynamic robot whisker information. In *Barrels XXI, Society for Neuroscience Satellite Meeting*, Poster.

Evans, M., Fox, C. W., Pearson, M. J., and Prescott, T. J. (2009). Spectral template based classification of robotic whisker sensor signals in a floor texture discrimination task. In *Proceedings of Towards Autonomous Robotic Systems (TAROS)*, pp. 19–24.

Fend, M., Bovet, S., and Hafner, V. (2004). The artificial mouse – a robot with whiskers and vision. In *ISR 2004, Proceedings of the 35th International Symposium on Robotics*.

Fox, C., Evans, M., Stone, J., and Prescott, T. (2008). Towards temporal inference for shape recognition from whiskers. In *Proceedings of Towards Autonomous Robotic Systems (TAROS)*.

Fox, C. W., Mitchinson, B., Pearson, M. J., Pipe, A. G., and Prescott, T. J. (2009). Contact type dependency of texture classification in a whiskered mobile robot. *Autonomous Robots*, **26**(4), 223–239.

Gao, P., Bermejo, R., and Zeigler, H. P. (2001). Whisker deafferentation and rodent whisking patterns: behavioral evidence for a central pattern generator. *Journal of Neuroscience*, **21**(14), 5374–5380.

Gopal, V. and Hartmann, M. J. Z. (2007). Using hardware models to quantify sensory data acquisition across the rat vibrissal array. *Bioinspiration and Biomimetics*, **2**, S135–145.

Grant, R. A., Mitchinson, B., Fox, C. W., and Prescott, T. J. (2009). Active touch sensing in the rat: anticipatory and regulatory control of whisker movements during surface exploration. *Journal of Neurophysiology*, **101**, 862–874.

Gurney, K. N., Humphries, M., Wood, R., Prescott, T. J., and Redgrave, P. (2004). Testing computational hypotheses of brain systems function: a case study with the basal ganglia. *Network*, **15**(4), 263–290.

Haiss, F. and Schwarz, C. (2005). Spatial segregation of different modes of movement control in the whisker representation of rat primary motor cortex. *Journal of Neuroscience*, **25**(6), 1579–1587.

Hartmann, M. J. (2001). Active sensing capabilities of the rat whisker system. *Autonomous Robots*, **11**, 249–254.

Hartmann, M. J., Johnson, N. J., Towal, R. B., and Assad, C. (2003). Mechanical characteristics of rat vibrissae: resonant frequencies and damping in isolated whiskers and in the awake behaving animal. *Journal of Neuroscience*, **23**(16), 6510–6519.

Hill, D. N., Bermejo, R., Zeigler, H. P., and Kleinfeld, D. (2008). Biomechanics of the vibrissa motor plant in rat: rhythmic whisking consists of triphasic neuromuscular activity. *Journal of Neuroscience*, **28**(13), 3438–3455.

Jung, D. and Zelinsky, A. (1996). Whisker-based mobile robot navigation. In *Proceedings of the IEEE/RSJ International Conference on Intelligent Robots and Systems (IROS)*, **2**, pp. 497–504.

Kim, D. and Möller, R. (2004). A biomimetic whisker for texture discrimination and distance estimation. In *Proceedings of the Eighth International Conference on Simulation of Adaptive Behavior: From Animals to Animats 8*. Cambridge, MA: MIT Press, pp. 140–149.

Kim, D. and Möller, R. (2007). Biomimetic whiskers for shape recognition. *Robotics and Autonomous Systems*, **55**(3), 229–243.

Kleinfeld, D., Berg, R. W., and O'Connor, S. M. (1999). Anatomical loops and their electrical dynamics in relation to whisking by rat. *Somatosensory and Motor Research*, **16**(2), 69–88.

Kleinfeld, D., Ahissar, E., and Diamond, M. E. (2006). Active sensation: insights from the rodent vibrissa sensorimotor system. *Current Opinion in Neurobiology*, **16**(4), 435–444.

Knutsen, P., Biess, A., and Ahissar, E. (2008). Vibrissal kinematics in 3D: tight coupling of azimuth, elevation, and torsion. *Neuron*, **59**(1), 35–42.

Knutsen, P. M., Pietr, M., and Ahissar, E. (2006). Haptic object localization in the vibrissal system: behavior and performance. *Journal of Neuroscience*, **26**(33), 8451–8464.

Krupa, D. J., Matell, M. S., Brisben, A. J., Oliveira, L. M., and Nicolelis, A. L. (2001). Behavioral properties of the trigeminal somatosensory system in rats performing whisker-dependent tactile discriminations. *Journal of Neuroscience*, **21**(15), 5752–5763.

Lichtenstein, S. H., Carvell, G. E., and Simons, D. J. (1990). Responses of rat trigeminal ganglion neurons to movements of vibrissae in different directions. *Somatosensory and Motor Research*, **7**(1), 47–65.

Lottem, E. and Azouz, R. (2009). Mechanisms of tactile information transmission through whisker vibrations. *Journal of Neuroscience*, **29**(37), 11 686–11 697.

Mitchinson, B., Gurney, K. N., Redgrave, P., *et al.* (2004). Empirically inspired simulated electro-mechanical model of the rat mystacial follicle-sinus complex. *Proceedings of the Royal Society of London B Biological Sciences*, **271**(1556), 2509–2516.

Mitchinson, B., Pearson, M., Melhuish, C., and Prescott, T. J. (2006). A model of sensorimotor co-ordination in the rat whisker system. In *Proceedings of the Ninth International Conference on Simulation of Adaptive Behaviour: From Animals to Animats 9*. Berlin: Springer-Verlag, pp. 77–88.

Mitchinson, B., Martin, C. J., Grant, R. A., and Prescott, T. J. (2007). Feedback control in active sensing: rat exploratory whisking is modulated by environmental contact. *Proceedings of the Royal Society of London B Biological Sciences*, **274**(1613), 1035–1041.

Mitchinson, B., Arabzadeh, E., Diamond, M. E., and Prescott, T. J. (2008). Spike-timing in primary sensory neurons: a model of somatosensory transduction in the rat. *Biological Cybernetics*, **98**(3), 185–194.

Mitchinson, B., Chan, T.-S., Chambers, J., *et al.* (2010). BRAHMS: novel middleware for integrated systems computation. *Advanced Engineering Informatics*, **24**(1), 49–61.

Nallatech (2007). *PCI-104 Series: COTS PCI-104 FPGA computing stacks product brief (NT190–0331 Version 1.0)*. Available online: www.nallatech.com/mediaLibrary/images/english/6406.pdf.

Neimark, M. A., Andermann, M. L., Hopfield, J. J., and Moore, C. I. (2003). Vibrissa resonance as a transduction mechanism for tactile encoding. *Journal of Neuroscience*, **23**(16), 6499–6509.

Nguyen, Q. T. and Kleinfeld, D. (2005). Positive feedback in a brainstem tactile sensorimotor loop. *Neuron*, **45**(3), 447–457.

Pearson, M., Nibouche, M., Pipe, A. G., *et al.* (2006a). A biologically inspired FPGA based implementation of a tactile sensory system for object recognition and texture discrimination. In *Proceedings of the International Conference on Field Programmable Logic and Applications (FPL)*, pp.1–4.

Pearson, M., Nibouche, M., Gilhespy, I., *et al.* (2006b). A hardware based implementation of a tactile sensory system for neuromorphic signal processing applications. In *Proceedings of the IEEE International Conference on Acoustics, Speech and Signal Processing (ICASSP)*, Vol. **4**, p. IV.

Pearson, M. J., Melhuish, C., Pipe, A. G., *et al.* (2005). Design and FPGA implementation of an embedded real-time biologically plausible spiking neural network processor. In *International Conference on Field Programmable Logic and Applications*, pp. 582–585.

Pearson, M. J., Pipe, A. G., Mitchinson, B., *et al.* (2007a). Implementing spiking neural networks for real-time signal-processing and control applications: a model-validated FPGA approach. *IEEE Transactions on Neural Networks*, **18**(5), 1472–1487.

Pearson, M. J., Pipe, A. G., Melhuish, C., Mitchinson, B., and Prescott, T. J. (2007b). Whiskerbot: a robotic active touch system modeled on the rat whisker sensory system. *Adaptive Behaviour*, **15**(3), 223–240.

Petersen, C. C. H. (2007). The functional organization of the barrel cortex. *Neuron*, **56**, 339–355.

Prescott, T. J., Mitchinson, B., Redgrave, P., Melhuish, C., and Dean, P. (2005). Three-dimensional reconstruction of whisking patterns in freely moving rats. In *2005 Annual Meeting of Society for Neuroscience*, Poster 625.3.

Prescott, T. J., Montes Gonzalez, F. M., Gurney, K., Humphries, M. D., and Redgrave, P. (2006). A robot model of the basal ganglia: behavior and intrinsic processing. *Neural Networks*, **19**(1), 31–61.

Prescott, T. J., Bryson, J. J., and Seth, A. K. (2007). Introduction: modelling natural action selection. *Philosophical Transactions of the Royal Society of London B Biological Sciences*, **362**(1485), 1521–1529.

Prescott, T. J., Pearson, M. J., Mitchinson, B., Sullivan, J. C. W., and Pipe, A. G. (2009). Whisking with robots: from rat vibrissae to biomimetic technology for active touch. *IEEE Robotics and Automation Magazine*, **16**(3), 42–50.

Prescott, T. J., Mitchinson, B., and Grant, R. A. (in press). Vibrissal function and behavior. *Scholarpedia*.

Quist, B. W. and Hartmann, M. J. (2008). A two-dimensional force sensor in the millinewton range for measuring vibrissal contacts. *Journal of Neuroscience Methods*, **172**(2), 158–167.

Redgrave, P., Prescott, T. J., and Gurney, K. (1999). The basal ganglia: a vertebrate solution to the selection problem? *Neuroscience*, **89**(4), 1009–1023.

Rice, F. L., Mance, A., and Munger, B. L. (1986). A comparative light microscopic analysis of the sensory innervation of the mystacial pad. I. Innervation of vibrissal follicle–sinus complexes. *Journal of Comparative Neurology*, **252**(2), 154–174.

Rosenblueth, A. and Wiener, N. (1945). The role of models in science. *Philosophy of Science*, **12**(4).

Russell, R. A. (1992). Using tactile whiskers to measure surface contours. In *Proceedings of the IEEE International Conference on Robotics and Automation*, Vol. **2**, pp. 1295–1299.

Russell, R. A. and Wijaya, J. A. (2005). Recognising and manipulating objects using data from a whisker sensor array. *Robotica*, **23**(5), 653–664.

Sachdev, R. N., Berg, R. W., Champney, G., Kleinfeld, D., and Ebner, F. F. (2003). Unilateral vibrissa contact: changes in amplitude but not timing of rhythmic whisking. *Somatosensory and Motor Research*, **20**(2), 163–169.

Sahibzada, N., Dean, P., and Redgrave, P. (1986). Movements resembling orientation or avoidance elicited by electrical stimulation of the superior colliculus in rats. *Journal of Neuroscience*, **6**(3), 723–733.

Seth, A. K., McKinstry, J. L., Edelman, G. M., and Krichmar, J. L. (2004a). Active sensing of visual and tactile stimuli by brain-based devices. *International Journal of Robotics and Automation*, **19**(4), 222–238.

Seth, A. K., McKinstry, J. L., Edelman, G. M., and Krichmar, J. L. (2004b). Texture discrimination by an autonomous mobile brain-based device with whiskers. In *Proceedings of the IEEE International Conference on Robotics and Automation (ICRA)*, pp. 4925–4930.

Shoykhet, M., Doherty, D., and Simons, D. J. (2000). Coding of deflection velocity and amplitude by whisker primary afferent neurons: implications for higher level processing. *Somatosensory and Motor Research*, **17**(2), 171–180.

Solomon, J. H., and Hartmann, M. J. (2006). Biomechanics: robotic whiskers used to sense features. *Nature*, **443**(7111), 525.

Sparks, D. L. (1986). Translation of sensory signals into commands for control of saccadic eye movements: role of primate superior colliculus. *Physiological Reviews*, **66**(1), 118–171.

Stüttgen, M. C., Kullmann, S., and Schwarz, C. (2008). Responses of rat trigeminal ganglion neurons to longitudinal whisker stimulation. *Journal of Neurophysiology*, **100**, 1879–1884.

Szwed, M., Bagdasarian, K., and Ahissar, E. (2003). Encoding of vibrissal active touch. *Neuron*, **40**(3), 621–630.

Towal, R. B. and Hartmann, M. J. (2006). Right-left asymmetries in the whisking behavior of rats anticipate head movements. *Journal of Neuroscience*, **26**(34), 8838–8846.

Ueno, N. and Kaneko, M. (1994). Dynamic active antenna: a principle of dynamic sensing. In *Proceedings of the IEEE International Conference on Robotics and Automation*, Vol. **2**, pp. 1784–1790.

Waite, P. M. E. and Tracey, D. J. (1995). Trigeminal sensory system. In Paxinos, G. (ed.), *The Rat Nervous System*. New York: Academic Press, pp. 705–724.

Welker, W. I. (1964). Analysis of sniffing of the albino rat. *Behaviour*, **22**, 223–244.

Wilson, J. F. and Chen, Z. (1995). A whisker probe system for shape perception of solids. *Journal of Dynamic Systems Measurement Control*, **117**(1), 104–108.

Wineski, L. E. (1985). Facial morphology and vibrissal movement in the golden hamster. *Journal of Morphology*, **183**, 199–217.

Yokoi, H., Lungarella, M., Fend, M., and Pfeifer, R. (2005). Artificial whiskers: structural characterization and implications for adaptive robots. *Journal of Robotics and Mechatronics*, **7**(5), 584–595.

Zucker, E. and Welker, W. I. (1969). Coding of somatic sensory input by vibrissae neurons in the rat's trigeminal ganglion. *Brain Research*, **12**(1), 138–156.

4 Sensor-rich robots driven by real-time brain circuit algorithms

Andrew Felch and Richard Granger

4.1 Introduction

The analysis of particular telencephalic systems has led to derivation of algorithmic statements of their operation, which have grown to include communicating systems from sensory to motor and back. Like the brain circuits from which they are derived, these algorithms (e.g. Granger, 2006) perform and learn from experience. Their perception and action capabilities are often initially tested in simulated environments, which are more controllable and repeatable than robot tests, but it is widely recognized that even the most carefully devised simulated environments typically fail to transfer well to real-world settings.

Robot testing raises the specter of engineering requirements and programming minutiae, as well as sheer cost, and lack of standardization of robot platforms. For brain-derived learning systems, the primary desideratum of a robot is not that it have advanced pinpoint motor control, nor extensive scripted or preprogrammed behaviors. Rather, if the goal is to study how the robot can acquire new knowledge via actions, sensing results of actions, and incremental learning over time, as children do, then relatively simple motor capabilities will suffice when combined with high-acuity sensors (sight, sound, touch) and powerful onboard processors.

The Brainbot platform is an open-source, sensor-rich robot, designed to enable testing of brain-derived perceptual, motor, and learning algorithms in real-world settings. The system is intended to provide an inexpensive yet highly trainable vehicle to broaden the availability of interactive robots for research. The platform is capable of only relatively simple motor tasks, but contains extensive sensors (visual, auditory, tactile), intended to correspond to crucial basic enabling characteristics for long-term real-world learning. Humans (and animals) missing sensors and limbs can nonetheless function exceedingly well in the world as long as they have intact brains; analogously, Brainbot has reasonable, limited motor function and all necessary sensors to enable it to function at a highly adaptive level: that is, prioritizing sensorimotor learning over unnecessarily complex dexterity.

Brainbots are being tested with brain-circuit algorithms for hierarchical unsupervised and reinforcement learning, to explore perceptual, action, and language learning

Neuromorphic and Brain-Based Robots, eds. Jeffrey L. Krichmar and Hiroaki Wagatsuma. Published by Cambridge University Press. © Cambridge University Press 2011.

capabilities in real-world settings. We describe details of the platform and of the driving algorithms, and give examples of the current and planned abilities of the Brainbot system.

4.1.1   Background

Over the last several decades the capabilities of robot hardware have improved substantially; it can be argued that hardware is no longer the key bottleneck to achieving the grand challenge of cognitive robots. Remotely operated robots can now demonstrate useful and economically valuable tasks, and significant expectations have been placed on their autonomous capabilities (HR, 2000; DOD, 2005; Thrun *et al.*, 2006). The algorithms and computational architecture necessary to provide such autonomy, however, have not been derived and it is widely agreed that this presents the greatest barrier to achieving the promise of these robots (USN, 2004). Despite advances in artificial intelligence (AI), robots cannot yet see, hear, navigate, or manipulate objects without rigid restrictions on the types of objects, phrases, or locations they are presented with.

There are, of course, no actual specifications describing the processes of recognition, learning, recall, imitation, etc.; rather, these abilities are all defined solely by reference to observation of corresponding abilities in humans (and other animals). For instance, speech recognition performed by automated telephone operators is a widely deployed industrial application, which nonetheless fails a large percentage of the time. This failure rate might well have been the best possible performance for this task; the only reason for believing that much better performance can be achieved is that humans achieve it. Nothing tells us what minimal mechanisms or components will suffice to attain human-level performance; it is not known, for instance, whether natural language learnability requires at least one complementary sensory input (sight, sound, touch), or other supporting capabilities. This observation generalizes whenever we attempt to extend simplified systems to more complex tasks. Algorithms that work on toy problems (e.g. software simulations of robots) often fail to scale to more difficult environments such as those encountered by autonomous robots in the real world. Thus, algorithms for broad robotic use may have to be designed and tested on platforms that are sufficiently similar to the final robot, yet robots with the sensing, motor, and onboard processing power for advanced development are typically quite expensive (see Table 4.1). The Brainbot platform (Figures 4.1, 4.2) was fashioned to provide research laboratories with the option of affording one or more such robots to support the development of brain algorithms and other AI and machine learning methods.

Extant robot platforms (Table 4.1) feature a wide variety of capabilities and costs. The Surveyor Corporation's SRV-1 provides significant functionality such as mobility, wireless connectivity, and a digital camera at low cost. The iCub and MDS have high levels of dexterity, impressive standard features (though relatively fixed sensor options) at high cost. The Pioneer robot comes with few standard features but is quite extendable by the user and some options are available from the manufacturer.

In this context, Brainbot is sensor rich, easily extensible, and carries the most substantial onboard computer available on any extant platform. Brainbot leverages her

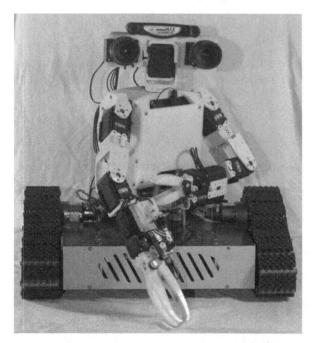

Figure 4.1 The design integrates off-the-shelf components with a minimum of customized pieces. The custom pieces include 27 printable plastic parts, 10 CNC machined Delrin pieces, 7 small printed circuit boards (PCBs), and 2 small machined aluminum pieces (see Figure 4.2).

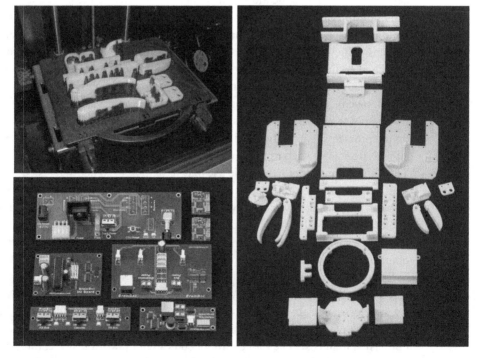

Figure 4.2 Gripper pieces approaching completion in the 3D printer (upper left), a complete layout of the printed plastic pieces (right) and custom printed circuit boards (PCBs, lower left) are shown. The power board, miniature IO boards (top), standard IO board, AX-12 bus board (middle), power switch board, and RX-64 bus board (bottom) can be seen.

Table 4.1. Comparison of existing robot platforms

Robot name	SRV-1	Pioneer P3-DX	Scout	Nao	Brainbot	MDS	iCub
Company	Survey or Corp.	Mobile Robots	Dr Robot	Aldebaran	Robozyme	MIT, Xitome Design, et al.	Consortium
Price	$495	$4200	$8750	$15,600	$28,000	~$200,000 (est.)	~$300,000 (est.)
Processor	Blackfin 500 mHz; 32 MB RAM; 802.11g	PC/104 (e.g. 1 GHz); USB	microcontroller; low-speed; 802.11g (912 kbps)	AMD Geode 500 mHz; 256 MB RAM; 802.11g	Core 2 Quad 2.83GHz; 4 GB RAM; 10 USB; 802.11g	PC/1041 GHz; USB	Celeron dual 2.13 GHz; 2 GB RAM; USB
Speech recognition	none	none	none	none	onboard	unknown if onboard	unknown if onboard
Speech synthesis	none	none	none	none	onboard AT&T Voices	unknown if onboard	unknown if onboard
Cameras	basic camera	optional	basic wireless camera	2 CMOS cameras	Prosilica GC-650c; up to 300 fps ROI	Stereo CCD	Point Grey DragonFly2
Expandable vision	not expandable	many options	second camera	not expandable	Prosilica GC, Tyzx Point Grey, etc.	not expandable	not expandable
Vision software	some onboard processing	some onboard vision processing; requires PC/104	not onboard	some onboard processing	RoboRealm software real-time onboard feature extraction; custom vision programmable	some onboard processing	some onboard processing
Manipulators	none	one 7-DOF arm	two 6-DOF arms	two 5-DOF arms; two 1-DOF grippers	two 4-DOF arms; two 1-DOF grippers; interchangeable grippers	two 7-DOF arms, 10 lb payload; two grippers, 4 digits each	two 7-DOF arms; two 9-DOF grippers
Manipulation sensors	none	none	touch pressure available	position; force	position; force; touch pressure	position; force; touch pressure	position; force; touch pressure
Sensors	sonar	many options; laser scanner, compass, tilt, etc.	microphone, IR, sonar	microphone; 5 axis IMU, sonar	any USB, GigE, or Atmel sensor; Sonar, Lidar, GPS, 9-axis IMU, compass, etc.	laser range-finder; balance sensors	microphone; IMU

The list is not exhaustive. Note that the Willow Garage PR2, carrying strong arms (4 lb/1.8 kg+), rich and extensible sensors similar to Brainbot, and multiple quad-core processors, was not available for purchase at time of publication. Pricing has been estimated to be more than $300 000 depending on sales' contribution to future R&D and pricing against similar robots.

computing and sensing capacity to integrate off-the-shelf voice, audition, and speech "middleware" with user-programmed intelligent real-time algorithms. The intent is to enable programmers to leverage the existence of existing support systems (visual feature extraction, speech recognition, speech production, motoric balance, etc.) to focus on advanced algorithms design and testing.

4.2   Platform

Brainbot has an open design with all source code and documentation available under an open source license including hardware designs and virtual Brainbot models for the widely used Webots simulation system. Intelligent algorithms that are written to control Brainbot's behavior have no open source requirements and can be closed source (private) or open sourced by their author, regardless of the commercial or research purposes for those algorithms, enabling the system to be used as a testbed for further research.

For actuation, 13 Robotis AX-12 servos provide 11 degrees of freedom (DOF) with 16 kg-cm holding torque, and a twelfth DOF providing tilt to the waist with double strength. The waist is also supported with springs, which were added to increase Brainbot's ability to lean over an object on the ground, pick it up, and lean back with the object in hand. Two Robotis RX-64 servos are embedded in the chest of Brainbot and provide each arm with a strong shoulder capable of 64 kg-cm holding torque. All of these servos include load, position, temperature, and voltage sensors. The servos are commanded, and their sensors polled, over the AX-12 bus and the RX-64 bus, which are each capable of 1 mbps transfer speeds. Interface to the servos is currently rate limited to commanding and polling all servos together at approximately 30 Hz due to the interfacing of Brainbot's computer to these buses through a USB adapter with approximately 1 ms latency. An alternative design utilizing one or more embedded processors to command and poll the servos directly over the AX-12 and RX-64 serial busses, and to present these servos to Brainbot's onboard computer as a whole, has been investigated and this design is believed to be capable of achieving 500 Hz to 1 kHz; this project may be pursued in the future. In sum, the 14 DOF are allocated as two grippers with 1-DOF, two wrists with 1-DOF, two elbows with 1-DOF, and two shoulders with 2-DOF each, in addition to one waist with 2-DOF, and one neck with 2-DOF each.

The standard Brainbot configuration uses a tracked base for locomotion (Figures 4.1, 4.3). Initial versions of Brainbot had bipedal locomotion; this, however, necessitated lower overall weight, which in turn limited the onboard processing power that could be carried. In addition, the legs were underpowered using the AX-12 servos, and an upgrade to RX-64 was not expected to raise maximum speed to human walking speed. In contrast, the Brainbot tracked base is able to travel at approximately human walking speed while still allowing objects on the floor to be reached and manipulated. Future research goals may necessitate a legged Brainbot, and the platform remains backward compatible with the legged design. It is worth noting that a leg design comprising the stronger EX-106 Robotis servos has been researched and is believed to

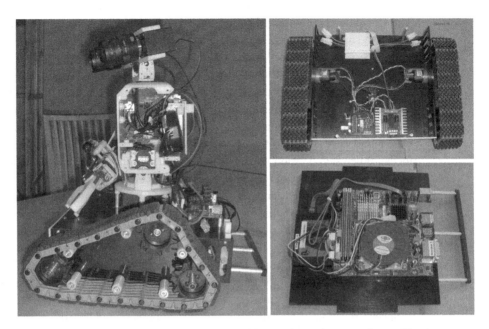

Figure 4.3 Internal chest and track views (left), and top and bottom base plates are shown. The chest houses three AX-12 servos, two RX-64 servos, an 18V voltage regulator, as well as the AX-12 and RX-64 USB bus adapters and the power switch board. The track motors are mounted to the track modules, and the rotation/distance encoders, IO board, and motor driver are mounted to the top plate, which is turned over for viewing (upper right). The PC motherboard and SSD drive are mounted to the bottom plate (bottom right).

be capable of carrying the standard quad-core Brainbot computer system and sensor complement while achieving speeds similar to human walking. These servos, which contain the same position and load sensing of all Robotis servos, allow perceptual bipedal algorithms to accurately estimate the force that is placed on a joint, and are complemented by these servos' capacity for high-frequency sensing and commanding, further improving the types of experiments that can be run when Brainbot is used as a bipedal balance and locomotion research platform.

Two Prosilica GC-series cameras can be used at the top of the neck, which can be synchronized to within a few microseconds for stereo vision algorithms. (A single camera can be used in cases where stereo vision is not of interest.) The cameras can operate with any C-mount or CS-mount lens. Alternatively, Point Grey, Tyzx or other cameras can be mounted in this position using GigE, USB, or Firewire (using a low-profile PCI Express Firewire card). The Prosilica GC650C gives Brainbot 659×493 resolution at 90 frames per second (fps) and provides uncompressed image data in RGB-24, Bayer-16, and some other user-selectable formats. Binning (resolution reduction) and regions of interest (ROI) can be specified, and when a 100×100 ROI is used, for example, the frame rate increases to 300 fps. This increased frame rate can greatly simplify real-time tracking algorithms by reducing the number of possible locations to search for an object, which increases quadratically with the inverse of the frame rate.

The Computar H2Z0414C-MP 4–8 mm f/1.4 varifocal lens has been selected for its ability to support wide angle (84.5° diagonal), zoom (2×, 44.1° diagonal), wide maximum aperture for reduced motion blur in low light (f/1.4), megapixel sensor resolutions, light weight (100 g), small size (50 mm × 40 mm), and a focal range suitable for visual inspection of items held by grippers. In particular, research that set out to find lenses for the GC650C that supported variable focus, low weight and a close minimum focal range was fortunate to find this Computar lens available, as the alternatives that were found were significantly less suitable (e.g. not sufficiently small, or lacking close focus). When stereo vision sensing is unnecessary, Brainbot has been designed to carry a camera blank and spare lens in the opposite robot eye position to maintain balance and to retain a matched lens pair for potential follow-on stereo vision research. The single camera design was inspired by the human ability to function exceedingly well with only one eye. An alternative purpose for a second camera is to function as a fovea, by applying zoom on the second camera lens either by adjusting the Computar lens to 8 mm, or with a higher zoom lens such as Fujinon's fixed-zoom lenses. This allows detailed visual features to be extracted that would otherwise (without zoom) require a 25 megapixel or greater camera.

Speech recognition is a difficult task for computers and several software vendors exist that claim various accuracy levels. In the case of English speech recognition, after considerable training it is quite possible for existing off-the-shelf software to achieve extremely good recognition accuracy on a limited vocabulary for most common accents. Given the human ability to understand speech at a range of distances it is perhaps unintuitive that computers perform much more poorly at speech recognition when a microphone is displaced at even a conversational distance of 1 meter, but the presence of noise substantially reduces the performance of most current speech processing systems. The typical solution is to place a headset on the speaker, thus providing a microphone at very close range. This solution also works with Brainbot; however, in real-world situations with multiple speakers and/or multiple robots it may be unsatisfactory. A larger, heavier, and typically more expensive alternative is to use an array microphone, which creates a virtual microphone beam aimed at the speaker using multiple built-in microphones and internal computation. Such a solution was judged to be too large and heavy to fit on board Brainbot. Thus, to achieve reasonable performance at conversational distances with off-the-shelf software, Brainbot integrates the Andrea Electronics SuperBeam SoundMax array microphone which achieves reasonable performance at very low cost by offloading the microphone array processing to the connected personal computer. This is an example of one of the multiple features that would be more expensive or not possible without the substantial processing power of the onboard Intel Core-2-Quad.

The Brainbot grippers were designed to manipulate many types of everyday objects. Initially a single gripper design was used for both grippers; however, a difficulty arose in that grippers optimized for pinching small items such as pencils were incapable of grasping relatively larger objects such as light bulbs or soda cans. This problem was exacerbated in initial designs by weak AX-12 based waist and shoulders, often resulting in overheating of shoulder servos and stalled reset of the waist servo. By

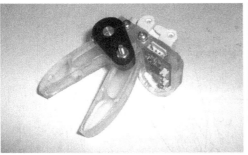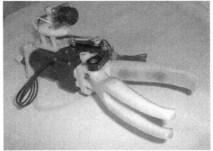

Figure 4.4 The pincher (left) and claw gripper (right) are shown with sonar and laser mounted (right).

strengthening the shoulders to be four times stronger and reinforcing the waist with springs and a servo pair with double strength, the grippers were enabled to lift and hold heavier objects, providing the impetus for a larger gripper that traded away abilities with small objects for large ones, coupled with a gripper able to manipulate smaller objects (Figure 4.4).

The grippers are fabricated by a 3D plastic printer and some aspects are not able to be fabricated without a dissolving system that removes support structure. For example, the pressure sensor wiring pathways internal to the gripper structure, as can be seen in the gripper fabricated in transparent plastic, are inaccessible to tools. Various types of pressure sensors can be placed on the surface of the gripper such as a combination of small circular sensors and a series of pressure-sensing strips that cover the entire interior surface. A layer of polyurethane is then placed over the sensors to provide stickiness. Each gripper is coupled with a miniature input–output (IO) circuit board that receives input from the pressure sensors. The miniature IO board also interfaces with other analog or digital sensors and outputs, such as the MaxBotix EZ0 sonar (interchangeable with EZ1–EZ4 to control volume characteristics), and a programmatically controlled laser pointer. The movement and force sensing of the gripper is provided by an AX-12, and the grippers are interchangeable by interfacing to the standard Robotis brackets for structural support and providing control and sensing through the mini IO board or by plugging directly into the AX-12 bus. It is also possible to mount a self-contained pressure sensor array to a gripper by routing the interface wire, typically USB, from the PC motherboard to the gripper.

Power and data are transferred between the electronic components of Brainbot over many pathways (Figure 4.5). Either wall power or battery power can be supplied to the power board, which provides power either directly or indirectly to all Brainbot systems. We have used a 17-amp 12-volt AC–DC converter for wall power, as well as NiMH 12V batteries with 200 watt-hours of capacity, which achieves 1–2 hours of run time. An important design goal was hot-swappability of power so that intelligent algorithms could be tested "in the wild" all day with a minimum of interference, and to facilitate transfer to/from the work bench. In this configuration, approximately three to four battery kits, allowing two to three to be simultaneously charging, has been sufficient to perform all-day testing without the use of wall power. The power board provides 12V

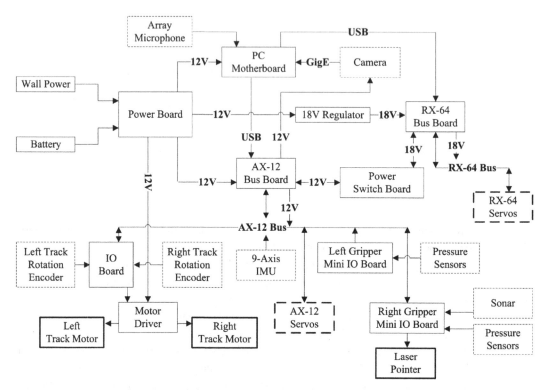

Figure 4.5   Brainbot electronics power and data flow. Bold boxes indicate outputs; dashed boxes indicate sensors.

supplies to the PC motherboard through a 150-watt DC–DC power supply. The power board also supplies 12V to the motor driver that powers the track motors. The RX-64 bus, which provides 18V power to all connected bus devices, receives power from the power board through an 18V step-up regulator. The AX-12 bus provides 12V power to all connected devices and receives 12V power from the power board. An additional 12V supply passes through the AX-12 bus board, which carries an interchangeable array of voltage regulators, such as two AnyVolt Micros from Dimension Engineering and one chassis-mounted AnyVolt-3 in order to power sensitive electronics such as cameras or a laser scanner. The RX-64 and AX-12 bus boards route their power supplies through a power switch board mounted to the back of the chest of Brainbot. In addition, the track motor driver power supply and the PC motherboard have power switches mounted on the power board.

The PC motherboard interfaces with the AX-12 and RX-64 bus boards via USB, through which all servos and bus-based sensors and devices (e.g. track motors, pressure sensors, sonar, laser pointer) can be communicated with. The microphone array and cameras interface directly with the PC motherboard, as is fitting for these higher-bandwidth sensors. The motherboard itself is mounted in the base of the chassis, which is slightly larger than a 19-inch half-rack space, with jacks presented in the back of the Brainbot chassis that include six USB, two gigabit Ethernet, audio, DVI, and eSATA ports. Internally, four additional USB ports and three SATA II ports are available, and the PCI-Express slot, typically providing the second gigabit Ethernet port, can be repurposed to allow connectivity to other interfaces such as Firewire. Behind the waist, the top of the chassis base serves as a mounting location for USB devices such as 802.11n.

4.2.1   Intelligent algorithm programming interface

BrainTalk provides a simple interface of ASCII over TCP/IP socket to allow any programming language on any operating system to access all of Brainbot's sensors, actuators, and output devices (Figure 4.6). The socket interface also allows algorithms to be executed onboard or externally on a desktop or supercomputer without requiring changes to the software. A difficulty arises in this type of interface, which is that the ASCII over TCP/IP interface is not the most efficient communication mechanism for the large amounts of sensor data collected by the camera or microphone, which can total hundreds of megabits per second in their uncompressed binary form. Two solutions have been implemented on Brainbot to simplify this issue. The first is that the microphone and speaker have speech-to-text voice recognition and text-to-speech voice production built into the BrainTalk interface. This allows programmers to retrieve text that has been spoken to Brainbot as ASCII text and avoids forcing programmers to integrate their own voice recognition to achieve interactivity. Similarly, ASCII text can be sent to Brainbot over the BrainTalk socket, which then uses the built-in text-to-speech software to speak this text over the onboard amplified speaker. The second solution integrates RoboRealm with the onboard camera(s). RoboRealm then provides vision options, such as feature extraction, with multiple interfacing options including TCP/IP, thus preserving the generic operating system and programming language capability of Brainbot. BrainTalk also interfaces with RoboRealm to simplify access to visual feature extraction data for the programmer if desired. Alternatively, the GigE

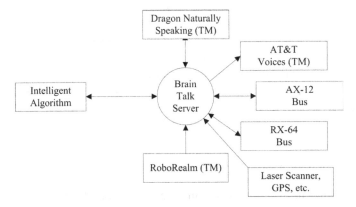

Figure 4.6   The BrainTalk server provides an interface to Brainbot hardware that is optimized for ease of programming.

camera protocol can be used to directly interface with the cameras, or Prosilica's free multiplatform SDK software can be used.

Because BrainTalk is ASCII over TCP/IP, a user can interact with the sensors, motors, etc. over a simple Telnet session. In this way it is possible for users to immediately get up and running with Brainbot, even before selecting a programming language. For example, a Telnet session might proceed in the way shown in Figure 4.7; server responses are indented, comments prefixed with "#".

4.2.2   Brainbot's interactive building blocks

Although Moore's Law has delivered computers with a million times more performance than they had 40 years ago, predictions of a future in which intelligent robots interact with humans in the real world have not yet come to pass. Implementing such creations is further complicated by the limited energy supply that can be carried on board robots. This has traditionally led mobile robots to be designed with low-power embedded computers that are not capable of executing the basic building blocks of intelligent interactive robots in real time (Table 4.2).

To support these building blocks, Brainbot's onboard computer utilizes an Intel Q9550S 65-watt (max) processor containing four Core 2 processor cores running at 2.83 Ghz, 4 GB of memory, and a solid-state hard drive (SSD) for storage. This system allows Brainbot to make at least one processor core available at all times for execution of intelligent algorithms. This arrangement also frees the intelligent algorithms from the low level details such as examining each camera pixel, microphone sample, or auditory frequency, and also frees programmers from having to interact with the low level API interfaces for microphones, speakers, and cameras.

4.3   Application example: a vision algorithm

Recently developed power-efficient algorithms and architectures for real-time visual processing (Felch and Granger, 2009) are being adapted to run with improved performance on hardware suitable for integration on board Brainbot. The vision-processing system extracts features from images and/or image sequences and processes these using a combination of bottom-up (features to abstractions) and top-down (abstractions to features) mechanisms to represent and recognize objects in the images (for background, see Rodriguez et al., 2004; Granger, 2006; Felch and Granger, 2009). Here we describe the algorithm as it is being developed for use and testing on the Brainbot platform.

4.3.1   Parallel computing for improved performance of mobile brain algorithms

Parallel processing has become increasingly common, and typical desktop computers now come standard with four processor cores. Although a sufficient number of transistors have been available to implement multiple cores in a processor for many

Speaker.say = "Hello, my name is Brainbot, and I am here to learn."

    Ok   #Brainbot says the above text

RightGripperSensor.laser = 1   #Activates laser

    Ok

{Camera.laserSpotX ; Camera.laserSpotY}

    { 632; 413}   #laser spot is believed to appear in upper right corner of camera view

RightWrist.val = 800   # Rotate servo at right wrist to position 800. Limits are 0-1023, 300 degrees of motion.

Dragon.buffer

    "I am talking to Brainbot and using telnet to retrieve the text she has heard"

Dragon.clearBuffer

{ io.quadA, io.quadB } #retrieve current odometry counts for the tracks, left and right respectively

    { 0; 0 }

{ io.leftSpeed=255; io.rightSpeed=255 }   #Tell motors to drive full speed forward

    Ok

{ io.quadA, io.quadB } #retrieve current odometry counts for the tracks, left and right respectively

    { 926321; 927123 }   #We have moved about 100-inches forward (approximately 9,265 ticks per inch)

{ io.leftSpeed=0; io.rightSpeed=0 }   #Tell motors to drive full speed backward

    Ok

{ io.leftSpeed=127; io.rightSpeed=127 }   #Tell motors to stop

    Ok

Compass.heading   #Which direction are we facing?

    137   #South East (0 = North, 90 = East, 180 = South, 270 = West)

{ Gps.longitude; Gps.latitude }   #Get GPS position.

    { 43.7040 N, 72.2823 W }   #We're at the corner of Wheelock St. and Park St., Hanover, New Hampshire

{ LeftWrist.val = 327; LeftElbow.val = 432; HeadPitch.val = 300 }   #Move servos to designated positions

    Ok

{ LeftWrist.val; LeftElbow; HeadPitch.val }

    {325; 436; 301}   #At desired position with a small error, typical of moving and sensing in the real world

Figure 4.7   This telnet session demonstrates the BrainTalk server's ability to access speech input/output, laser pointing and camera sighting, servo movement and sensing, track movement and sensing, and GPS and compass sensing.

Table 4.2. Examples of current state-of-the-art software building blocks for intelligent interactive robots

Ability	Example software	Requisite processing capacity for real time[a]	Requisite memory capacity
Speech recognition	Dragon naturally speaking	1 core	512 MB
Speech production	AT&T voices	1 core	256 MB
Visual feature extraction	RoboRealm	1 core	64 MB

[a] Assuming multigigahertz processor cores.

years, manufacturers of personal computer processors historically pursued better performance for single cores. In fact the transition to multicores was forced upon processor manufacturers when additional improvements to single core designs resulted in malfunctioning processors that consumed too much power and created too much heat to be effectively cooled.

By improving the power efficiency of processors, much more performance can be delivered under a given power envelope. Brains may well achieve their combination of high computational capacity and relatively low power requirements via the massive parallelism intrinsic to brain circuit design, incorporating billions of processing elements with distributed memory.

Moore's Gap refers to the difference between system hardware improvements versus system performance improvements. While Moore accurately predicted that hardware components of computer systems would grow exponentially, nonetheless this growth has not resulted in commensurate performance speed-up, measured as the ability of the hardware to carry out software tasks correspondingly faster. The gap arises from the difference between processor speed on one hand, versus the mapping of software instructions onto those processors on the other.

The phenomenon of Moore's Gap is consistent with, and indeed was in part predicted by Amdahl's Law, which can find the maximum expected improvement to a system as a function of an increased number of processors. If S is the fraction of a calculation that is inherently sequential (i.e. cannot be effectively parallelized), then $(1 - S)$ is the fraction that can be parallelized, and Amdahl's Law states that the maximum speed-up that can be achieved using N processors is:

$$\frac{1}{S + \frac{(1 - S)}{N}}$$

In the limit, as N gets large, the maximum speed-up tends toward $1/S$. In practice, price to performance ratios fall rapidly as N is increased: that is, once the quantity $(1 - S)/N$ becomes small relative to S. This implies differences in kind between tasks that can be effectively parallelized ($S \ll 1$) versus those that cannot ($S \approx 1$). Current architecture designs are tailored to $S \approx 1$ tasks such as large calculations, and perform notably poorly on $S \ll 1$ tasks.

Typical approaches to this problem are aimed at trying to modify tasks to be more parallelizable. For instance, recently Asanovic *et al.* (2006) have identified multiple classes of numerical methods that can be shown to scale well in parallel and yet are general methods with broad applicability to multiple domains. These methods are known to include many statistical learning, artificial neural net, and brain-like systems.

4.3.2 BrainBot as a brain-derived vision algorithm and hardware development platform

The vision system extracts features from images or image sequences, which is a preliminary step common to many vision systems. For example, two types of features that can be extracted are corner features and line segment features. The system is able to work with them interchangeably: that is, using relationships of corners to corners, corners to line segments, line segments to corners, and line segments to line segments. For explanatory purposes we will limit the discussion to corners; the system extends beyond this in a straightforward way.

The system uses a special data structure (Figure 4.8) to hold information about the types of corner configurations or "partial-constellations," which we will term atomic relations or atoms. An atom describes two or more subfeatures and their expected spatial relationship in the image plane. The data structures are used to identify substructures in an image that have been previously associated with objects that can be recognized. For example, an atom might relate the four corners of a windshield to each other so that windshields can be recognized and, once recognized, can cause the system to search for other features found on automobiles.

Each atom has a "center of gravity" (CoG), which is a point in the middle of the constellation to which all of the subfeatures relate. Each subfeature has an identity such as

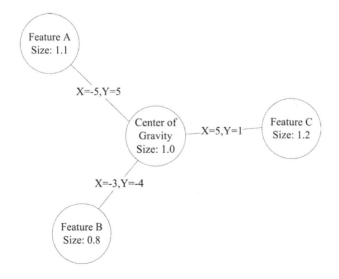

Figure 4.8

"feature A," "feature B," or "feature C," and an X,Y offset of the subfeature to the CoG given a certain size of the atom or subfeature. The process of deriving atom centers and sizes from subfeatures is called the hierarchical bottom-up process or HBU. The process of deriving subfeature x,y locations and sizes from an atom's CoG and size is called the hierarchical top-down process or HTD.

More rigorously, for a given feature detected in an image F_i with type T_{F_i} and size S_{F_i}, an atom data structure A_j with one sub-feature of type T_{F_i} having relational offset $\left(\bar{X}_{A_j, T_{F_i}}, \bar{Y}_{A_j, T_{F_i}} \right)$ and relational size $\bar{S}_{A_j, T_{F_i}}$ can derive its center of gravity location $\left(\tilde{X}_{F_i, A_j}, \tilde{Y}_{F_i, A_j} \right)$ using Equations 1 and equation 2 and center of gravity size $\tilde{S}_{F_i, A_j}$ using Equation 3.

$$\tilde{X}_{F_i, A_j} = X_{F_i} - \left(\bar{X}_{A_j, T_{F_i}} * \frac{S_{F_i}}{\bar{S}_{A_j, T_{F_i}}} \right), \tag{4.1}$$

$$\tilde{Y}_{F_i, A_j} = Y_{F_i} - \left(\bar{Y}_{A_j, T_{F_i}} * \frac{S_{F_i}}{\bar{S}_{A_j, T_{F_i}}} \right), \tag{4.2}$$

$$S_{F_i, A_j} = \frac{S_{F_i}}{\bar{S}_{A_j, T_{F_i}}}. \tag{4.3}$$

The HBU process derives the expected location and size for each relevant atom's CoG. Equations (4.1) to (4.3) are calculated for all incoming features and relevant atoms during the HBU process. The HTD process, by contrast, derives for each atom's CoG instance the expected locations and sizes of the other subfeatures within that atom. Equations (4.1) to (4.3) are solved for subfeature location/size derivation given a CoG location/size in Equations (4.4) to (4.6) respectively:

$$X_{F_i} = \tilde{X}_{F_i, A_j} + \left(\bar{X}_{A_j, T_{F_i}} * S_{F_i, A_j} \right), \tag{4.4}$$

$$Y_{F_i} = \tilde{Y}_{F_i, A_j} + \left(\bar{Y}_{A_j, T_{F_i}} * S_{F_i, A_j} \right), \tag{4.5}$$

$$S_{F_i} = S_{F_i, A_j} * \bar{S}_{A_j, T_{F_i}}. \tag{4.6}$$

Once expected locations for subfeatures have been calculated, the image can be compared with these expectations, and image features of the same type T_{F_i} can be measured for distance from the expected subfeature location. The minimum distance to the closest matching feature (same type) is summed with the other minimum distances to determine an overall match score for the atom A_j. Figures 4.9–4.14 give an example of calculating the overall expectation-deviation score (EDS).

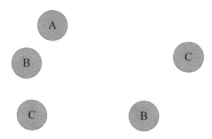

Figure 4.9

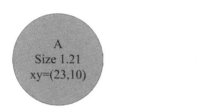

Figure 4.10

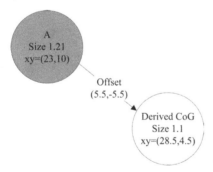

Figure 4.11

Corner features of types A, B, and C have been extracted from an image and are arranged as shown in Figure 4.9. Figure 4.10 shows the details of one of the feature instances, namely the A-type feature instance. Using the data structure of Figure 4.8 and Equations (4.1–4.3) the location and size of the CoG are derived as shown in Figure 4.11.

In Figure 4.12 the derived CoG location and size are used with Equations (4.4–4.6) to determine the location and size of the constituent type-B subfeature. In Figure 4.13 the expected location of subfeature B is compared with type-B features found in the image. Note that any image features not of similar size to the expected size (e.g. within 20%) will not be considered for the minimum-distance calculation. In this example, two type-B image features are of a size similar to the expected size and their distances to the expected location are calculated as 1.8 and 4.3. Thus, the minimum distance is 1.8 for the type-B constituent subfeature.

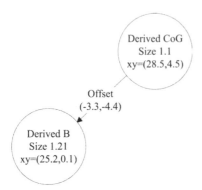

Figure 4.12

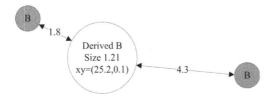

Figure 4.13

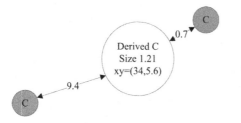

Figure 4.14

Figure 4.14 shows the minimum distance calculation for the type-C subfeature, calculated in a similar fashion to that of the type-B subfeature (Figures 4.12, 4.13). The minimum distance for the type-C subfeature is 0.7. Thus the overall expectation-deviation score, the sum of the minimum distances, is $0.7 + 1.8 = 2.5$.

The process of searching for all the implied atom instances in an input image is shown in Figure 4.15. When an input arrives (1201) the atom data structures that use the input feature's type in a subfeature are iterated through (1202) until finished (1203). It is also possible that the input feature is not a subfeature (1204) but is in fact the CoG of a specific atom (passed from a HTD process), in which case only the relevant atom data structure is retrieved. In the case that the input is a subfeature (not a CoG) the size (1206) and location (1207) are derived for the CoG using Equations (4.1–4.3), an example of which was shown in Figure 4.14. Next, the subfeatures of the atom are iterated through (1205). For each subfeature (1208) the expected size and location is

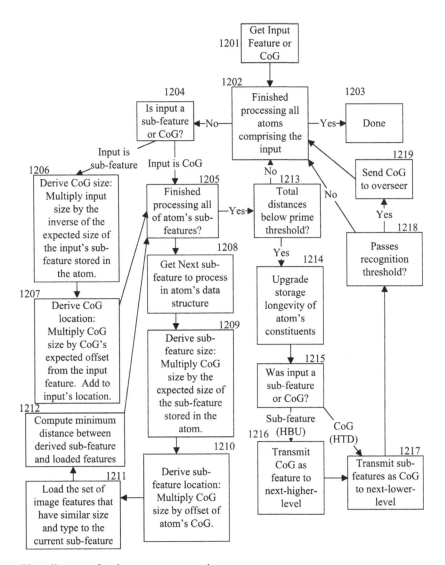

Figure 4.15 Flow diagram of node message processing.

derived using Equations (4.4–4.6), an example of which was shown in Figure 4.12. Next, the relevant image features (of the same type) that are within a certain maximum distance and which have a size within some percentage of the derived subfeature's size are processed (1211). The distance from the image feature's location to the current sub-feature's expected location is measured and the minimum distance (1212) is summed to the EDS running total for the current atom.

Once complete, the EDS is compared with a threshold (1213) and if the EDS is too high then processing the current atom has completed and the next atom (if not finished, 1203) is moved on to (1204). If the EDS is below the threshold, then the image features that achieved minimum distances are "refreshed" in memory so that when future image frames arrive the old features will still be accessible. Image features that are not refreshed by this process are removed from memory after input of the next or just a few new frames, and thus will no longer arrive in sets processed in step 1211. Note that if DRAM is used to hold the image features in memory then it may be possible to use DRAM's natural data leakage "forgetting" mechanism to implement this erasure.

If the EDS qualified for refresh, then additional signals are also sent depending on whether the input feature was a subfeature or CoG (1215). In either case the refreshed subfeatures are transmitted as CoGs to lower level processes (HTD). If the input was a subfeature (sent from an HBU process) then the CoG identified by the current atom and the size/locations derived in steps 1206 and 1207 is sent to higher-level processes (HBU) as a subfeature. Finally, if the EDS is below the "recognition threshold" (1218) then the CoG is transmitted to an overseer process (1219). The overseer process determines what object is being recognized by the input CoG and can act on this information such as navigating a robot to further investigate the object, to direct a grasping action, or to navigate around the object.

In summary, the system forms a hierarchy from the atoms found in an image. When initially detected features (corners) are found in a configuration expected by a particular atom, the atom acts as a "detected feature" to the next-higher level of processing. The next-higher level of processing performs exactly as if its input features are corners, but in fact they are atoms that identify constellations of corners. The atom data structures used in the next-higher level of processing describe relationships not between corners, but between atoms identified at the next-lower level of processing. This procedure allows identification of higher and higher feature levels, with each processing level called a layer. Once a hierarchy is formed in one of the higher levels, and the constituent atoms and corners have matched the input image well, a signal is sent to an overseer process indicating that a very high level feature has been identified. The overseer maintains a list that associates high-level atoms with object names, so that the overseer can determine what object has been identified based on the highest-level atom in the hierarchy.

A prototype of the above vision algorithm was tested on a class of difficult data (Figure 4.16) and performance was shown to closely match the current best system at the task (Carmichael, 2003; Felch et al., 2007); however, these tests took several days to compute. Research is being conducted in order to develop new computer hardware architectures that utilize the intrinsic parallelism of the algorithm to greatly improve performance while satisfying the low power requirements of mobile robots. Prior research into a related algorithm has shown performance-per-watt improvements on the order of $1000 \times$ (Furlong et al., 2007; Moorkanikara et al., 2009).

4.4   Task design and customization

4.4.1   Voodoo control

During development of intelligent algorithms, issues arise that must first be identified as an intelligence issue or a system issue. For example, the robot may repeatedly fail

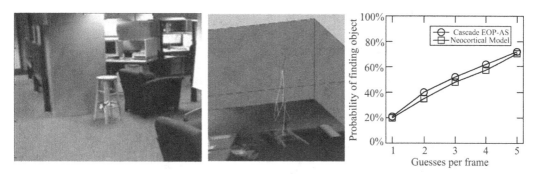

Figure 4.16   A representative wiry object (sitting stool) is recognized by the vision algorithm prototype (left). A 3D visualization of the hierarchy of abstract features is constructed through HBU and HTD processes (middle). Performance closely matches the best extant system at recognizing these objects.

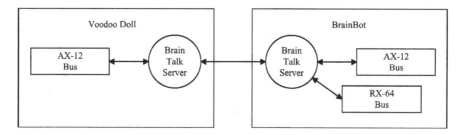

Figure 4.17   The hardware/software configuration of Voodoo control.

at a grasping task, and the issue may arise from a lack of dexterity or a lack of intelligence. An interesting aspect of the Brainbot platform is that the robot can be remotely controlled by a human using a controller, called the Voodoo bot, fashioned with the same shape and degrees of freedom as the Brainbot robot without the base component (Figures 4.17, 4.18). By first testing with Voodoo, it is possible to verify that a task is in fact possible for a given Brainbot configuration, and this is true in both the real and virtual world. Using a monitor also allows a first-person viewpoint that can help in identifying the degree of visual difficulty in a task.

Voodoo control has proven to be extremely useful in a number of ways, the most valuable of which in our experience has been its ability to weed out hardware and software bugs very early in development, before any advanced algorithms need to be written. Furthermore, a joystick has been integrated to allow driving of the tracks by wireless so that a large outdoor area can be tested for issues, such as for wireless interference. Voodoo was also very useful for testing and debugging the Brainbot virtual environment before the virtual model had been fully developed.

The Voodoo bot is constructed of AX-12 servos on all joints, and a laptop or netbook connects to the AX-12 bus using an AX-12 bus board (the bus board is powered by a local battery such as a 9.6V NiMH). Handles are attached at the head and gripper joints

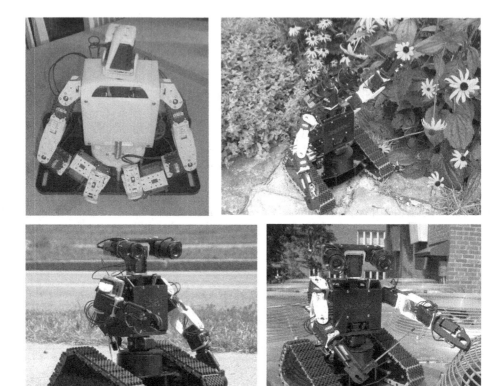

Figure 4.18   An experimental Brainbot design is tested through Voodoo control (Voodoo controller in upper left) for hardware capabilities at various tasks.

of the Voodoo bot to improve control, and the entire system is made wireless by using a shoulder strap to suspend the Voodoo bot in front of the user and placing the laptop in a backpack. A BrainTalk server runs on the laptop and frequently polls the position of the servos, which are then sent as position commands to the Brainbot robot designated in a configuration file which may be connected through a wireless network such as an ad-hoc 802.11n network connection.

4.4.2   Social cognition

Some problems can be better tackled by a group of robots rather than a single robot. Understanding the design principles that better enable robots to work together is an increasingly important research area. Multiagent systems have many properties that make the design of intelligent agents more difficult. These robots can have different sensor complements, morphologies, and locomotion, each more or less well suited for certain steps in the task at hand. The Brainbot platform has been studied for its suitability to multiagent tasks in which a team of robots collaborates to efficiently work together toward a common goal at the behest of a human or another robot. The result is that Brainbot appears quite amenable to multiagent tasks and may be especially suited for a difficult type of multiagent task in which a heterogeneous group of robots must work together in the changing and uncertain real world. The highly configurable nature of the Brainbot platform supports the creation of a diverse group of agents, each with different capabilities. For example, the extensibility of Brainbot allows each agent to be outfitted with different sensors such as a team that includes one member with a laser range scanner, one with stereo vision, and one with an infrared camera. The Brainbot platform provides all sensor data through TCP/IP sockets which, coupled with multiple USB wireless modules such as 802.11n, yields a high bandwidth mesh network that allows multiple robots to see the problem using a collection of sensors that no single robot is directly outfitted with.

Similarly, Brainbot's morphology can be easily changed through the reconfiguration of the arms, neck, or torso using the erector-set-like Robotis pieces that have been designed for this purpose, or by modifying the CAD files of the printer parts to enable 3D printing of new custom parts such as new grippers (Figure 4.19). The daisy-chain connection of new servos avoids excessive wiring issues (which plagued small robot servos prior to the AX-12), and the plastic Brainbot chassis is easily drilled/tapped to allow screw holes for attachment of additional appendages or instruments. Various Robotis servos can be added such as the AX-12 and RX-64 (shoulders) standard types, as well as the RX-28 and stronger EX-106 servos. Combined, this provides for configurations with joints ranging from 16 kg-cm to 106 kg-cm holding torque. Wheeled and legged locomotion arrangements have also been successfully tested in the laboratory in both virtual and real-world settings, allowing for truly diverse studies of social cognition using teams of Brainbots (Figure 4.20).

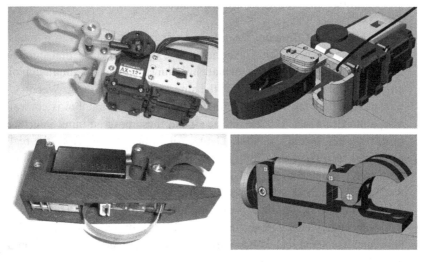

Figure 4.19 Virtual and real gripper designs.

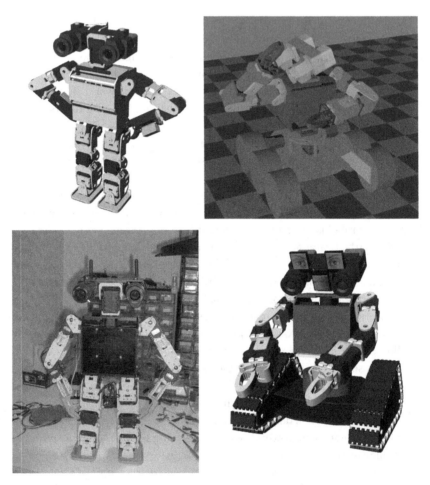

Figure 4.20   Various configurations of virtual and real Brainbot.

The low cost of Brainbot has allowed research laboratories to purchase teams for studies of social behavior. Furthermore, the open source virtual implementation of multiple Brainbots in a single virtual environment allows the simulation of social cognition experiments for the cost of the simulation program (e.g. Webots). Subsequent transition to the real world is facilitated because each Brainbot is controlled through a separate BrainTalk TCP/IP interface, and these programming interfaces are identical to the real-world Brainbot. The transition both to and from the real world may be further facilitated by using the Brainbot onboard computer as the simulation platform, since the onboard 2.83 GHz Quad-Core processor is fully capable of running the Webots simulator while also providing three cores for execution of driving algorithms. In this way, a brain algorithm can be transitioned between the virtual and real worlds by simply changing the designated BrainTalk server IP address. Discrepancies between virtual and real worlds will of course have interesting effects on robot behavior and algorithm performance.

4.5   Discussion

The real world is the ultimate arbiter of embodied perception and action; even carefully devised simulated experiments typically fail to transfer to real-world settings. Yet simulation is often preferable, due to the engineering requirements, programming minutiae, sheer cost, and lack of standardization of robot platforms. Current robot systems exhibit a wide range of dexterity, motor function, appearance, sensors, and computer power, but our interests were overwhelmingly aimed at the study of learning over time, accreting perceptual and motor abilities, in real-world settings. On many advanced computing tasks, including perceptual recognition, motor performance, and processing time-varying data, humans still substantially outperform even the best engineering systems. Living organisms acquire knowledge of the world, organize that knowledge in memories, and use those memories to perform in their learned environments, and transfer the knowledge to novel environments. This suggests that the underlying mechanisms of learning and knowledge organization still are key to identifying the biological mechanisms that so impressively achieve these real-world perceptual and motor tasks. Robot platforms for this research are thus most useful to the extent that they target these two overarching desiderata: extensive learning, occurring in real-world environments. This entails a sturdy (albeit simple) chassis, extensive sensors, and the most powerful possible onboard processors, while dispensing with most other features, especially any that add weight and/or increase power consumption or cost. This overall design decision is embodied in the Brainbot platform: a sensor-rich, lightweight robot with high onboard processing power, using open-source hardware designs and driving software. This powerful toolkit provides most low-level programming necessities, enabling testing of advanced algorithms ranging from learning and perception to reasoning and language, in real-world environments. Current testing includes mechanisms for visual and auditory recognition, real-time processing of time-varying input, performance in the presence of extensive noise, perceptual-motor learning in complex environments, construction of long-term hierarchical memories, exploratory learning in simulated and real settings, and accrual of knowledge over extended time periods.

4.5.1   Future work

The BrainTalk server is implemented in Squeak Smalltalk, a virtual environment that has been ported to many operating systems, such as ARM Linux. The availability of small, low-power systems that support Squeak allows the BrainTalk server to be installed on even very small systems. BrainTalk is currently being adapted to run on an AX-12 based robot with a bipedal dinosaur-like morphology as well as other designs, depicted in Figure 4.21. A miniature 6-inch submarine is also being examined for potential BrainTalk compatibility.

The BrainTalk server itself was designed for the purpose of providing a cross-platform interface for ease of initial programming; other robot operating systems, such

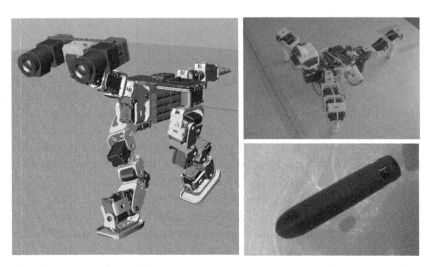

Figure 4.21   Brainbot platforms in development.

as ROS being developed by Willow Garage, or the URBI robot interface, include much more functionality. It is anticipated that the open Brainbot system can be readily ported to either of these (or other) platforms.

References

Asanovic, K., Bodik, R., Catanzaro, B., *et al.* (2006). *The Landscape of Parallel Computing Research*. Technical Report UCB/EECS-2006–183. Berkeley, CA: EECS Department, University of California.

Carmichael, O. (2003). *Discriminative Techniques for the Recognition of Complex-Shaped Objects*. Technical Report CMU-RI-TR-03–34. PhD thesis, The Robotics Institute, Carnegie Mellon University.

DOD (US Department of Defense) (2005). *Unmanned Aircraft System Roadmap 2005–2030*. Washington, DC: US Department of Defense.

Felch, A. and Granger, R. (2008). The hypergeometric connectivity hypothesis: divergent performance of brain circuits with different synaptic connectivity distributions. *Brain Research*, **1202**, 3–13.

Felch, A. and Granger, R. (2009). *Power-Efficient Computation of High-Level Computer Vision in Real Time*. U.S. Patent application.

Felch, A., Chandrashekar, A., Moorkanikara, J., *et al.* (2007). Accelerating brain circuit simulations of object recognition with a Sony Playstation 3. In *International Workshop on Innovative Architectures (IWIA 2007)*, pp. 33–42.

Furlong, J., Felch, A., Nageswaran, J., *et al.* (2007). Novel brain-derived algorithms scale linearly with number of processing elements. In *Proceedings of the International Conference on Parallel Computing (parco.org) 2007*, pp. 767–776.

Granger, R. (2006). Engines of the brain: the computational instruction set of human cognition. *AI Magazine*, **27**, 15–32.

HR (House of Representatives) (2000). H.R. 4205/Public Law no. 106–398 of October 30, 2000.

Moorkanikara, J., Felch, A., Chandrashekar, A., *et al.* (2009). Brain-derived vision algorithm on high-performance architectures. *International Journal of Parallel Programming*, **37**, 345–369.

Rodriguez, A., Whitson, J., and Granger, R. (2004) Derivation and analysis of basic computational operations of thalamocortical circuits. *Journal of Cognitive Neuroscience*, **16**, 856–877.

Thrun, S., Montemerlo, M., Dahlkamp, H., *et al.* (2006). Stanley: the robot that won the DARPA grand challenge: research articles. *Journal of Robotic Systems*, **23**(9), 661–692.

USN (U.S. Navy Unmanned Underwater Vehicle) (2004). *UUV Master Plan*, November 2004. Washington DC: US Department of the Navy.

Part III

Brain-based robots: architectures and approaches

5 The RatSLAM project: robot spatial navigation

Gordon Wyeth, Michael Milford, Ruth Schulz, and Janet Wiles

5.1 Introduction

Rats are superior to the most advanced robots when it comes to creating and exploiting spatial representations. A wild rat can have a foraging range of hundreds of meters, possibly kilometers, and yet the rodent can unerringly return to its home after each foraging mission, and return to profitable foraging locations at a later date (Davis, *et al.*, 1948). The rat runs through undergrowth and pipes with few distal landmarks, along paths where the visual, textural, and olfactory appearance constantly change (Hardy and Taylor, 1980; Recht, 1988). Despite these challenges the rat builds, maintains, and exploits internal representations of large areas of the real world throughout its two to three year lifetime. While algorithms exist that allow robots to build maps, the questions of how to maintain those maps and how to handle change in appearance over time remain open.

The robotic approach to map building has been dominated by algorithms that optimize the geometry of the map based on measurements of distances to features. In a robotic approach, measurements of distance to features are taken with range-measuring devices such as laser range finders or ultrasound sensors, and in some cases estimates of depth from visual information. The features are incorporated into the map based on previous readings of other features in view and estimates of self-motion. The algorithms explicitly model the uncertainty in measurements of range and the measurement of self-motion, and use probability theory to find optimal solutions for the geometric configuration of the map features (Dissanayake, *et al.*, 2001; Thrun and Leonard, 2008). Some of the results from the application of these algorithms have been impressive, ranging from three-dimensional maps of large urban structures (Thrun and Montemerlo, 2006) to natural environments (Montemerlo, *et al.*, 2003).

Rodents, by contrast, do not appear to represent their maps as geometrically organized arrays of features. The biological evidence gleaned from electrophysiological recordings from the rodent hippocampus and nearby brain structures indicate that the rodent encodes space by learning to associate sensory stimuli with places in space. The well-documented place cells of the rodent hippocampus (Tolman, 1948; O'Keefe

Neuromorphic and Brain-Based Robots, eds. Jeffrey L. Krichmar and Hiroaki Wagatsuma. Published by Cambridge University Press. © Cambridge University Press 2011.

and Dostrovsky, 1971; O'Keefe and Conway, 1978) are reliably active when the rodent is in a certain position in space. The activity of place cells can be triggered and maintained in the absence of external sensory cues, operating based on information from self-motion cues alone. Rearranging the cues in an environment will cause place cells to change where they fire with respect to rodent location, demonstrating the association between spatial representations and external sensory cues. The discovery of cells with further spatial abilities, such as head direction cells (Ranck, 1984) and grid cells (Hafting *et al.*, 2005), is slowly forming a more complete picture of the mechanisms used for spatial encoding in the rodent brain.

The core contrast between rats and robots lies in the rodent's ability to seamlessly integrate mapping, localization, and task execution throughout its lifetime, constantly building, maintaining, and using its spatial representations. The rat's mental representations of space remain consistent with its environment. This is despite the rat's lack of resolution and precision in measurements of the environment, compared with that of a robotic system. Current methods in robotic mapping, in contrast, build an initial map that is then not updated, and hence can rapidly become obsolete, despite the precise geometric information available from robotic range-measurement devices.

In our work, we have sought to build a system that captures the desirable properties of the rodent's method of navigation into a system that is suitable for practical robot navigation.

The core model, dubbed RatSLAM, has been demonstrated to have exactly the advantages described above: it can construct maps of large and complex areas from very weak geometric information, and it can build, maintain, and use maps simultaneously over extended periods of time (Milford *et al.*, 2004; Milford and Wyeth, 2008a, 2008b, 2010). The motivation behind development of the RatSLAM system contrasts with other work in hippocampal robot navigation models: where other research has sought biological authenticity (Burgess *et al.*, 1997; Arleo and Gerstner, 2000; Barakova and Lourens, 2005; Krichmar *et al.*, 2005; Cuperlier *et al.*, 2007; Barrera and Weitzenfeld, 2008; Giovannangeli and Gaussier, 2008), our approach has focused on the development of a practical robot system.

This chapter provides an overview of the functional neuroanatomy of the rodent hippocampus and surrounding brain regions that form the basis of the RatSLAM system. The RatSLAM model is described in detail highlighting the similarities to the biological data, and the concessions made for engineering pragmatism. We then overview three benchmark studies of the system:

1. *Mapping a complete suburb from a single webcam mounted on a car.* This study illustrates that the RatSLAM system can use very noisy and incomplete data to make a coherent map of a large, diverse, and complex environment.
2. *Navigating in an active office environment for two weeks.* This study shows that the spatial representations at the heart of RatSLAM remain stable in terms of functional use and computation requirements, despite changes in appearance and layout of the operating environment.

3. *Sharing a grounded lexicon to describe places.* This study shows that two robots, each with a uniquely grounded RatSLAM representation of space, can form a shared symbolic system for jointly navigating to previously visited places.

5.1.1 Neurophysiological background

Electrophysiological recordings from in and around the rodent hippocampus have demonstrated clear associations between electrical activity in certain cell groups and the location and orientation of the rodent in a test arena. By combining knowledge of cell function with that of the connectivity of cell groups derived from anatomical data, researchers have made considerable progress towards a neurophysiological model of spatial encoding in rodents. A review of the current understanding of the neural basis of spatial encoding can be found in McNaughton *et al.* (2006).

Cell types

The place cells are predominantly found in the CA1–CA3 regions of the hippocampus (Best *et al.*, 2001). Single cell recordings show that the firing rate of a single place cell is strongly correlated with the rodent's absolute place at the time of firing. Place cells tend to be direction invariant; it does not matter which way the rodent is facing, only where it is located. Figure 5.1a shows the firing rate of an idealized place cell with respect to place, and to absolute heading. The firing rate with respect to place (shown as intensity) forms a peak at a single location corresponding to the place within the testing environment that is associated with that place cell. The firing rate with respect to head direction (shown as the distance from the origin to the curve) is uniform for all directions, showing no association between head direction and cell firing. Recordings taken from other place cells within the same animal are selective to other places in the testing environment.

Head direction cells show a complementary property to place cells (Ranck, 1984; Taube *et al.*, 1990); they are place invariant and direction specific. Figure 5.1b shows an idealized head direction cell that is equally likely to fire at any position within the testing environment, but has a distinct peak in its firing activity at a particular orientation of the animal's head with respect to the global reference frame. As the name suggests, the head direction cell's firing is dependent on the direction of the animal's head, not the animal's body. Head direction cells are found in various brain regions around the hippocampus, particularly post-subiculum, retrosplenial cortex, and some regions of the thalamus.

Recently, a new type of spatial encoding cell called a grid cell has been discovered in the entorhinal cortex, an area closely related to the hippocampus proper (Hafting *et al.*, 2005). In the shallowest layers of the entorhinal cortex, grid cells show place-cell-like properties, but significantly show multiple firing fields tessellated with a hexagonal pattern across the environment. The shallowest layers show a tessellation in place, and no directional specificity, as shown in Figure 5.1c. In deeper layers, some cells have only head direction characteristics, while the deepest layers contain conjunctive grid cells that show the conjunction of grid and head direction characteristics as shown in Figure 5.1d.

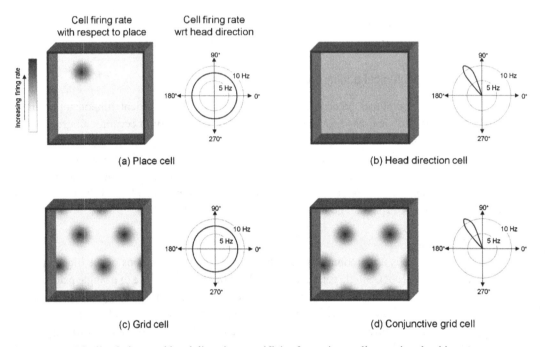

Figure 5.1   Idealized place and head direction specificity for various cell types involved in spatial encoding.

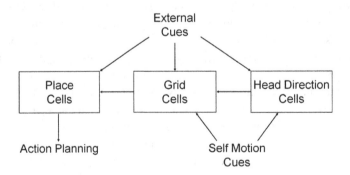

Figure 5.2   Connectivity of the brain regions containing various spatial encoding cell types.

Connectivity of regions

It is difficult to state categorically how the brain regions containing these cell types are connected, and how they connect to other parts of the brain. A recent review of spatial encoding behavior (Taube, 2007) constructed a map showing the principal connections between regions involved with the spatial encoding. On the basis of this more detailed diagram, one could broadly model the connectivity of the cell types involved in spatial encoding as shown in Figure 5.2.

Spatial encoding behavior

Spatially selective cells behave like a memory of the rodent's pose. Even when all sensory stimuli are removed from the rodent (including visual, auditory, and odor cues), the place cells and head direction cells continue to encode the position and orientation of the rodent (Quirk *et al.*, 1990). Furthermore, rodents use estimates of self-motion to update the pose estimate encoded by the firing of spatially selective cells. The internal representation of pose becomes less coherent over time in the absence of external cues (Knierim *et al.*, 1995), but can be reset when the rodent observes the layout of key features in the environment. No data exist on rodent performance with respect to loop closure and larger environments, as it is difficult to make these types of recordings due to constraints in terms of recording technique and the behavioral range of the caged laboratory rats.

The rat does not appear to build any geometrical representation of its surrounds; there is no map per se. Instead the rat relies on learned associations between external perception and the pose belief created from the integration of self-motion cues. Nor does the rodent appear to have any indication of a probability distribution in the activity in the cells. A roboticist versed in probabilistic SLAM might expect the activity in the head direction cells to represent a broader range of absolute heading in the absence of perceptual cues to correct bearing drift. Neural recordings, in contrast, show a consistent range of active head direction cells over all conditions. It is not clear whether the cell firings represent multiple or single estimates of pose – it is impossible to tell without recordings across all cells simultaneously – so it is hard to determine whether a rat tracks multiple hypotheses in the same way as probabilistic algorithms in robotics.

5.2   The RatSLAM model

RatSLAM emulates the rat's spatial encoding behavior using three key components: the *pose cells* which are analogous to the rodent's conjunctive grid cells, the *local view cells* which provide the interface to the robot's sensors in place of the rodent's perceptual system, and the *experience map* which functionally replaces the place cells found in CA1–CA3. The components of RatSLAM and the interactions of the components are illustrated in Figure 5.3, and described briefly in the following sections. Further details of the operation of RatSLAM can be found in Milford and Wyeth (2008a).

5.2.1   Pose cells

The pose cells are a three-dimensional Continuous Attractor Network (CAN) (Stringer *et al.*, 2002a; Stringer *et al.*, 2002b). The CAN, often used to model spatially selective cell networks, is a neural network that consists of an array of units with fixed weighted connections. The CAN predominantly operates by varying the activity of the neural units between zero and one, rather than by changing the value of the weighted connections. In rodents, spatially responsive cells such as place cells fire fastest when the rat is

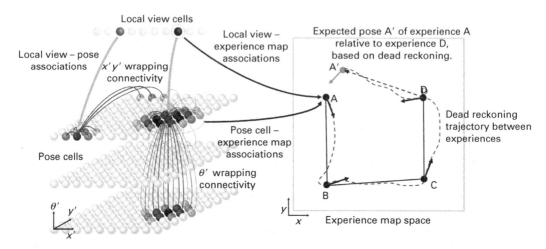

Figure 5.3   The RatSLAM system. Each local view cell is associated with a distinct visual scene in the environment, and becomes active when the robot sees that scene. A three-dimensional continuous attractor network forms the pose cells, where active pose cells encode the estimate of the robot's pose. Each pose cell is connected to proximal cells by excitatory (solid arrows) and inhibitory connections, with wrapping across all six faces of network. Intermediate layers in the (x', y') plane are not shown. The network connectivity leads to clusters of active cells known as activity packets. Active local view and pose cells drive the creation of experience nodes in the experience map, a semi-metric graphical representation of places in the environment and their interconnectivity.

at a certain location. In RatSLAM, the activation value of a neural unit increases when the robot approaches a location associated with that neural unit.

During operation, the pose cell network will generally have a single cluster of highly active units: the *activity packet*. The center of the activity packet provides an estimate of the robot's pose that is consistent with the pose cell network's rectangular prism structure, as shown in Figure 5.3. Each of the three dimensions of the prism corresponds to one of the three spatial dimensions x', y', and θ'. Primed coordinates are used to differentiate the space from that used with the experience map. The robot's pose in (x', y', θ') space maps to the active neural units in the rectangular prism structure. The dimensionality of the robot pose representation means the current RatSLAM implementation is suited to primarily flat environments.

The activity packet is self-maintained by local excitatory connections that increase the activity of units that are close in (x', y', θ') space to an active unit. Inhibitory connections suppress the activity of smaller clusters of activity elsewhere in the network. Connections wrap across all six faces of the pose cell network, as shown by the long thin arrows in Figure 5.3. The change in the cells' activity level ΔP is given by:

$$\Delta P = P * \varepsilon - \varphi, \tag{5.1}$$

where P is the activity matrix of the network, ε is the connection matrix, and $*$ is the convolution operator. As well as the inhibition in the connection matrix, the constant φ

creates further global inhibition. At each time step, activation levels in P are restricted to non-negative values and the total activation is normalized to one.

Path integration

Path integration involves shifting the activity packet in the pose cell network based on odometry information. At each time step, RatSLAM interprets the odometry informa- tion to displace a copy of the current activity state in the pose cell network. Like the excitatory and inhibitory weight matrices, the path integration process can cause a cluster of activity in the pose cells to shift off one face of the pose cell structure and wrap around to the other, as is shown in both packets in Figure 5.3, one of which is wrapping across the θ' boundary, the other across the y' boundary. Recording from a single cell under path integration will create firing fields with rectangular tessellations, similar to the triangular tessellations seen in grid cells (see Figure 5.1).

5.2.2 Local view cells

The local view cells represent a sparse classification vector based on what the robot is seeing. Each local view cell becomes active when the robot sees a distinct visual scene. Multiple local view cells can be simultaneously active to varying degrees in regions with perceptual aliasing, and there is no competition imposed between the cells.

RatSLAM increases the strength of connections between local view cells and pose cells that are active simultaneously. In other words RatSLAM learns an association between a visual scene and the robot pose. During a loop closure event, the familiar visual scene activates local view cells with learned connections to the pose cells rep- resenting the pose where the visual scene was first encountered. Due to the attractor dynamics of the pose cells, a single visual scene is not enough to force an immediate change of pose; several consecutive and consistent views are required to update the pose. The attractor dynamics temporally and spatially filter the information from the local view cells, providing rejection of spurious loop closure events.

The connections between local view cells and pose cells are stored in a connection matrix β, where the connection between local view cell V_i and pose cell $P_{x',y',\theta'}$ is given by:

$$\beta_{i,x',y',\theta'}^{t+1} = \max\left(\beta_{i,x',y',\theta'}^{t}, \lambda V_i P_{x',y',\theta'}\right), \qquad (5.2)$$

where λ is the learning rate. When a familiar visual scene activates a local view cell, the change in pose cell activity, ΔP, is given by:

$$\Delta P_{x',y',\theta'} = \frac{\delta}{n_{act}} \sum_i \beta_{i,x',y',\theta'} V_i, \qquad (5.3)$$

where the δ constant determines the influence of visual cues on the robot's pose esti- mate, normalized by the number of active local view cells n_{act}. Figure 5.3 represents the moment in time when a strongly active local view cell has injected sufficient activity into the pose cells to cause a shift in the location of the dominant activity packet. The previously dominant activity packet can also be seen, which is less strongly supported by a moderately activated local view cell.

5.2.3   Experience mapping for path planning

Over time, the (x', y', θ') arrangement of the pose cells corresponds decreasingly to the spatial arrangement of the physical environment. Often when a loop closure event occurs, the odometric error introduces a discontinuity into the pose cell's representation of space, creating two sets of cells that might represent the same area in space. Similarly, the wrapping connectivity leads to pose ambiguity, where a pose cell encodes multiple locations in the environment, forming the tessellated firing fields seen in grid cells in the rat. Planning with this representation is clearly not possible. Rather than try and correct these discontinuities and ambiguities within the pose cells, we combine the activity pattern of the pose cells with the activity of the local view cells to create a topologically consistent and semi-metric map in a separate coordinate space called the *experience map*.

The experience map contains representations of places combined with views, called experiences, e^i, based on the conjunction of a certain activity state P^i in the pose cells and an active local view cell V^i. Links between experiences, l^{ij}, describe the spatiotemporal relationships between places. Each experience is positioned at a location $\mathbf{p}^i$, a position that is constantly updated based on the spatial connectivity constraints imposed by the links. Consequently, the complete state of an experience can be defined as the 3-tuple:

$$e_i = \left\{ P^i, V^i, \mathbf{p}^i \right\}. \tag{5.4}$$

Figure 5.3 shows the region of pose cells and the single local view cell associated with the currently active experience A.

Transition links, l^{ij}, encode the change in position, $\Delta \mathbf{p}^{ij}$, computed directly from odometry, and the elapsed time, Δt^{ij}, since the last experience was active:

$$l^{ij} = \left\{ \Delta \mathbf{p}^{ij}, \Delta t^{ij} \right\}, \tag{5.5}$$

where l^{ij} is the link from the previously active experience e_i to the new experience e_j. The temporal information stored in the link provides the travel time between places in the environment which is used for path planning. Path planning is achieved by integrating the time values in the transition links starting at the robot's current location to form a temporal map. The fastest path to a goal experience can be computed by performing steepest gradient ascent from the goal experience to the current location.

5.2.4   Experience map maintenance

A score metric S is used to compare how closely the current pose and local view states match those associated with each experience, given by:

$$S^i = \mu_p |P^i - P| + \mu_v |V^i - V|, \tag{5.6}$$

where μ_p and μ_v weight the respective contributions of pose and local view codes to the matching score. If any experience matching scores are below the threshold, the lowest scoring is chosen as the 'active' experience, and represents the best estimate of the robot's location within the experience map.

If the activity state in the pose cells or local view cells is not sufficiently described by any of the existing experiences ($\min(\mathbf{S}) \geq S_{max}$), a new experience is created using the current pose and local view cell activity states. The odometry information defines the *initial* location in experience space of a newly created experience:

$$e_j = \left\{ P^j, V^j, \mathbf{p}^i + \Delta \mathbf{p}^{ij} \right\}. \tag{5.7}$$

When loop closure occurs, the relative position of the two linked experiences in the map will typically not match the odometric transition information between the two, as shown in the discrepancy between experience A and A' in Figure 5.3. The experience map relaxation method seeks to minimize the discrepancy between odometric transition information and absolute location in experience space, by applying a change in experience location $\Delta \mathbf{p}^i$:

$$\Delta \mathbf{p}^i = \alpha \left[\sum_{j=1}^{N_f} \left(\mathbf{p}^j - \mathbf{p}^i - \Delta \mathbf{p}^{ij} \right) + \sum_{k=1}^{N_t} \left(\mathbf{p}^k - \mathbf{p}^i - \Delta \mathbf{p}^{ki} \right) \right], \tag{5.8}$$

where α is a correction rate constant, N_f is the number of links from experience e_i to other experiences, and N_t is the number of links from other experiences to experience e_i. Equation (5.8) is applied iteratively at all times during robot operation; there is no explicit loop closure detection that triggers map correction. The effect of the repeated application of Equation (5.8) is to move the arrangement of experiences in experience map space incrementally closer to an arrangement that averages out the odometric measurement error around the network of loops.

5.3   Study 1: Mapping a large environment

The first study illustrates RatSLAM's capability in mapping very large and complex environments. We set out to map the entire suburb of St. Lucia in Brisbane, Australia (Milford and Wyeth, 2008a, 2008b), a challenging environment with many contrasting visual conditions: busy multilane roads, quiet back streets, wide open campus boulevards, road construction work, tight leafy lanes, monotonous suburban housing, highly varied shopping districts, steep hills, and flat river roads. The suburb is not only challenging in appearance, but also in structure. The road network includes over 80 intersections with some large roundabouts, forming a topological network with 51 inner loops of varying size and shape.

The images used to build the map of the road network were obtained from a built-in camera in a notebook computer on the roof of a car (see Figure 5.4a). The images were gathered at a rate of 10 frames per second from the camera, and saved to disk as a movie for offline processing. The car was driven at normal traffic speeds, and each street in St. Lucia was visited at least once, with most streets visited multiple times. The test took place on a typical fine spring Brisbane day starting in the late morning.

5.3.1   Interface to RatSLAM

RatSLAM requires an odometry measure to perform path integration in the pose cells, and an external perception system to selectively activate the local view cells. In this study, RatSLAM used only the captured images to generate the map; there were no GPS data, no inertial data, nor any connection to the vehicle systems. Each image was processed into a normalized one-dimensional vector formed by summing the intensity values in each pixel column (see Figure 5.4b), creating a scanline intensity profile (Pomerleau, 1997). The scanline intensity profile was used to estimate the rotation and forward speed between images for odometry. Rotation information was estimated by comparing successive scanline intensity profiles, and finding the pixel shift that maximizes the similarity between the profiles. Forward speed was estimated from the residual change in the successive profiles once rotation has been removed. The estimates of rotation and forward movement were used to control the movement of the activity packets in the pose cell network in the path integration process.

The scanline intensity profile was also used to compare the current image with previously seen images to perform RatSLAM's local view calibration process. By measuring the similarity between the current image's intensity profile and the intensity profiles stored with the current local view cells, the system determined whether the input image was already associated with a local view cell, or whether it should form the basis of a new local view. The consequent local view cell activity was then used to learn the association between pose cell activity and active local view cells (Equation 5.2), and to correct the pose cell activity for known local views (Equation 5.3).

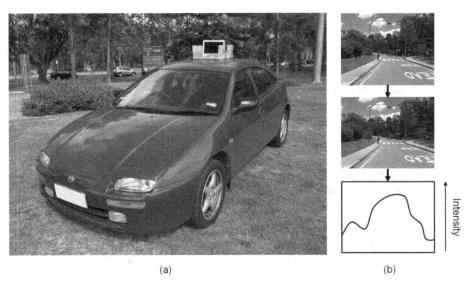

(a)   (b)

Figure 5.4   (a) The car with the laptop mounted on the roof and (b) the scanline intensity profile of a typical image.

5.3.2   Experience map

The experience map is the core global representation that forms the basis for navigation performance. The experience map was created using the RatSLAM algorithm by replaying the captured images offline. The algorithm ran in real time, with the time between images used to run the map correction step in Equation (5.8). Figure 5.5 shows the resultant experience map below an aerial photograph of the test environment with the route driven

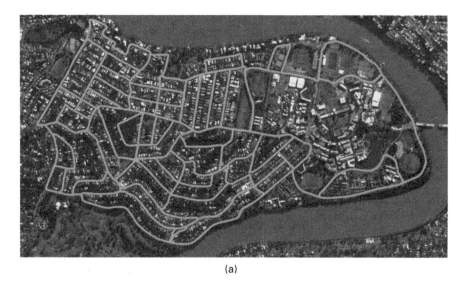

(a)

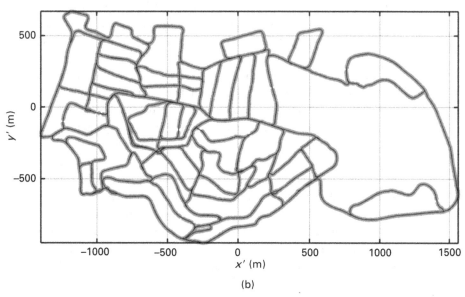

(b)

Figure 5.5   (a) Aerial photo of St. Lucia and (b) corresponding experience map (from Milford and Wyeth, 2008a). The map is topologically accurate but distorted in sections, such as in the central portion of the map where a high perceptual speed from moving through narrow pathways has enlarged the map representation.

in the experiment highlighted by a thick line. Each experience is plotted as a small circle at the (x, y) coordinates in the stored position **p** (see $(x, y) = (-1000$ m, -50 m) for an example of an experience in isolation). Linked experiences are joined with a line.

Clearly, the resultant map is consistent with the topology and structure of the real world that it represents, even capturing finer details such as curves, corners, and intersections. The consistency between the actual and inferred geometry is perhaps more remarkable given that the visual odometry system made no measurement of distance, but rather estimated the distance traveled from the degree of change in the scanline intensity profile. There are no incorrectly linked experiences, which would be clearly evident as lines stretched over the map.

The experience map contains 12 881 individual experiences, and 14 485 transitions between experiences. In creating the experience map, RatSLAM closed and organized multiple interlocking loops including one loop of over 5000 meters in length. When closing this long loop, the noisy visual odometry process had an accumulated odometric error of around 1200 m. Nevertheless the loop closed successfully, as RatSLAM relies on accumulated evidence of visual similarity, rather than global geometric consistency and optimality.

5.4   Study 2: Mapping over long periods

In this study, we show that the maps built by RatSLAM are readily maintainable in changing environments over an extended period. The challenge we set for RatSLAM was to build a map suitable to plan "deliveries" in two working office environments operating at all times in the 24 hour day/night cycle over a two week period. The robot was given an initial period to autonomously explore the first environment and generate a user readable map. The delivery locations were then marked on that map, and delivery requests randomly generated for over 1000 trials. While performing deliveries, the robot autonomously found and remembered the location of its charger, and autonomously recharged its batteries as required.

The system was deployed on a Pioneer 3-DX robot (shown in Figure 5.6) equipped with a panoramic imaging system, a ring of forward facing sensors, a Hokuyo laser range finder, and encoders on the wheels. All computation and logging was run onboard on a 2-GHz single core computer running Windows XP. The robot's typical operation speed was 0.3–0.5 ms^{-1}. The robot operated continuously for two to three hours between recharging cycles. Due to the need for supervision of the robot during operation (to ensure the integrity of the experiment), the total active time in a typical day was limited to one to four recharge cycles. In order to capture the effect of around-the-clock operation, experiments were conducted across all hours of the day and night.

5.4.1   Interface to RatSLAM

Odometry was calculated from the encoders on the robot's wheels. External perception for the local view system was driven entirely from the vision system, with the robot's

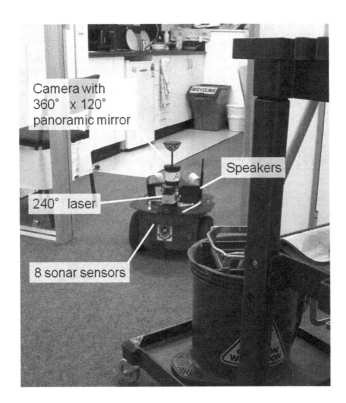

Figure 5.6   Robot in the indoor test environment.

laser range finder and sonar systems being used only to support obstacle avoidance and corridor centering behaviors for autonomous operation.

The vision system used panoramic images obtained from an IEEE-1394 camera, mounted at the central rotation axis of a Pioneer 3-DX robot and facing vertically upwards at a parabolic mirror. Automatic adjustment for global illumination changes was achieved in hardware through gain and exposure control, and patch normalization was used to reduce local variation. Since this is an indoor robot application, we assume that the ground surface is locally flat and that the robot is constrained to the ground plane. The recognition process starts with the current unwrapped, patch normalized 128×20 pixel panoramic image, with the long dimension aligned with the ground plane in the real world and the short dimension aligned with the vertical plane. Image similarities between the current image and template images are calculated using the cross correlation of corresponding image rows.

5.4.2   Experience map performance

The spatial coherence of the maps is evident from comparison with the floor plans shown in Figure 5.7. The maps are not globally accurate in a Cartesian sense as is evident from the change in scale, but global accuracy is not necessary for effective navigation. The

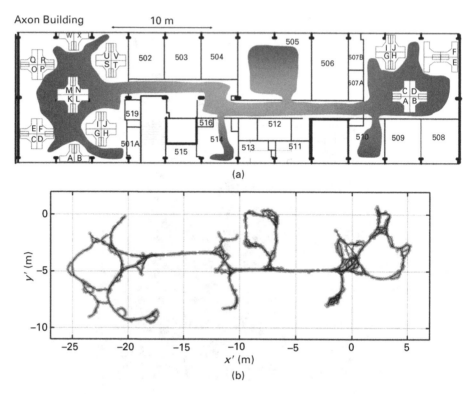

Figure 5.7　(a) Plan view of the testing environment. (b) The experience map state after five hours in the testing environment.

local spatial integrity of the map is important for selection of appropriate navigation behaviors, while global topological integrity is important for path planning.

5.4.3　Path planning performance

For the application of RatSLAM as an autonomous delivery robot, the most important indicator of performance is the success rate for planning and executing paths to the delivery locations. The robot roamed the office building for eight days, with 32 hours of active operation in both day and night cycles. During that time, the robot performed 1089 mock deliveries to six locations and autonomously navigated to and docked with its charger 21 times. The time to complete a delivery typically varied from one to three minutes, depending on the length of the path. Figure 5.8 shows the duration of each delivery task. The delivery duration is dependent on the distance from the robot starting location and the randomly chosen delivery location, so there is some degree of variation in the delivery time. The average trend data, plotted over the delivery time data, show that there is no increase in delivery times.

The robot failed to complete delivery trial number 579 (that is, to get close to the delivery location). This failure was due to an extended localization failure in room 505 (see Figure 5.7, between 504 and 506), resulting in the robot erroneously thinking it

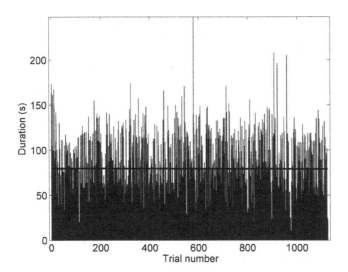

Figure 5.8   Navigate-to-goal durations for the navigation trials (deliveries and recharging) in the Axon building at the University of Queensland. Each thin vertical bar shows the delivery duration for that trial. A regression fit yielded $T = -0.00073n + 80$, with $P = 0.82$, and 95% upper and lower range bounds on the n coefficient of $[-0.0069, +0.0054]$, which includes zero.

was in the corridor outside the room when in reality it was in the corner of the room. Consequently, the robot became "stuck" in the corner, before eventually timing out the delivery attempt and reporting a delivery failure. Room 505 was one of the most challenging environments for the mapping system, because robot motion was relatively unconstrained in the large open space, leading to unique template sequences. The delivery accuracy and repeatability was worst for the delivery location in this room.

The RatSLAM algorithm does not have separate learning and recall cycles; it can update the map while being used to plan and enact navigation to goals. Because the use and update of the map operate in parallel, there is no need for user intervention to apply changes to the map, or to tell the robot to learn new features. In the experiment, the robot continuously updated and augmented its representations during operation over changes caused by day/night cycles, or by rearrangement of furniture and accessories in the office. The office environment was represented using approximately 1000 visual templates, and 1500 experiences. The complete RatSLAM algorithm, including visual processing and map updating, was continuously performed at around 10 Hz for the duration of the experiment. Further details of the results have been presented in our more detailed publication of this experiment (Milford and Wyeth, 2010).

5.5   Study 3: Grounding symbols in the map

The third study shows that maps built by RatSLAM can facilitate social interactions between the robots. The long-term results show that a mobile robot using RatSLAM is able to perform delivery to preset locations despite constant change in the environment.

The delivery locations were set by selecting experiences within the map of the robot, rather than selecting a more general location typically used by humans, such as "the kitchen" or "Ruth's desk." In this study, the challenge for the robots was to label locations in the world with symbols, which could be used as socially defined meeting places. The robots formed symbols that referred to locations in the world, or *toponyms*. Toponyms can be used to label locations, or to specify a distant location as a meeting place. To form symbols from their underlying representations, the robots played location language games in which they named their current location. The robot setup was identical to that used in the long-term studies, with additional language learning abilities.

The key issue when linking the symbolic (toponyms) with the subsymbolic (internal maps) is grounding (Harnad, 1990). Robots use grounding to link symbols with internal representations obtained from perceptions of the world. Each robot privately grounds its representations about the world – the map – through its unique perceptual sequence obtained from vision and odometry. When multiple robots use RatSLAM to map the same environment, each robot forms unique internal representations that can be used privately for navigation, but cannot be shared verbatim with the other robots. The challenge then was to socially ground common symbols that represent the world based on the robots' individual maps.

5.5.1   Language games for locations

In this study, the robots used social interactions to agree on symbols to refer to locations in the world. A methodology developing shared lexicons between agents is the playing of language games (Steels, 2001). The language games played in this study involve establishing shared attention, a speaker behavior, a hearer behavior, and acquisition of a new conceptualization. This experiment involved robots playing language games about locations. In a location language game, shared attention was achieved through co-location of the robots established by audible communication. With shared attention established through co-location, only the position of the robots was shared, with no restriction on the orientation of the robots. The robots had microphones and speakers with which they could emit and hear beeps, corresponding to signals for hand shaking and the words for the toponyms. Each toponym word comprised two syllables, where each syllable was a different beep. While exploring the world, the robots intermittently said "hello" and waited to hear an "I hear you" message from the other robot, indicating co-location. After shared attention was established, a game was played, with the robot who said "hello" assigned to the speaker role and the robot who said "I hear you" assigned to the hearer role.

The topic of a location language game was a location in the world, which could be the current location or a remembered location. The grammars of the location language games were predetermined: the robots knew the type of game and the type of concept referred to in each word in the utterance. Two location language games were played: the *where-are-we* game and the *go-to* game (see Figure 5.9). In a *where-are-we* game, the topic was the current location, which was shared by both robots through their shared attention of being within hearing distance. The resulting concepts were

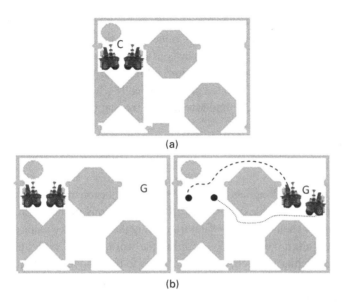

(a)

(b)

Figure 5.9   *Where-are-we* and *go-to* language games. (a) In a *where-are-we* game, the robots establish shared attention through co-location, the speaker determines the best word for the current location, C, and both robots update their lexicon tables. (b) In a *go-to* game, the robots establish shared attention through co-location, the speaker chooses a goal word, and both robots determine whether they can plan a path to the location specified by the goal word (left). If both robots can plan a path, they independently navigate to meet at the goal location (right).

toponyms, which could be used to identify an area in the world, and could be comprehended as an area or a point location. In word production and comprehension, only the position of each experience was considered. The toponyms formed in *where-are-we* games were direction invariant. In a *go-to* game, the robots started at the same location with the shared attention of hearing distance, and intended to end up near each other by meeting at a distant goal location. Toponyms were comprehended as point locations, corresponding to the experience most associated with the goal word. This experience was then set as the target location for the robot's navigation task.

Toponym concepts were distributed across the experiences of the robot, with experiences associated with words through a distributed lexicon table that extends the RatSLAM architecture. Every time a *where-are-we* game was played, both the speaker and the hearer increased the association between their current experience and the word used in the game. The internal representation of concepts was simply the set of associations between experiences and words. Word production and comprehension also relied on the currently active experience and the spatial relationships described in the experience map to determine the concept from these internal representations.

Once shared attention was established, the speaker determined which word was most appropriate for the current location. Concept elements in the distributed lexicon table were never considered in isolation, but in relation to each other. The speaker considered the associations between words and experiences located within the neighborhood (2 m) of the current experience in the experience plane. These associations were weighted by their distance from the current experience, with closer word–experience associations having greater weighting. The association values were then normalized by frequency of use to determine a confidence value. The confidence value indicated the confidence that the word referred to the current location, taking into account the associations of other words. New words were invented probabilistically when the speaker did not have a word for the current location, or had low confidence that the chosen word referred to the current location.

5.5.2   Evaluating the language

The resulting toponymic language can be evaluated by its coherence, which measures the similarity of the agents' lexicons over different locations in the world. Coherence can be calculated for each location by first translating the experience maps of the agents to obtain the best alignment, and determining the word used by both agents at each location. For a particular location, coherence refers to the proportion of the population that refers to the location by the same word. The overall coherence measure is an average of the coherence over all locations. The success of a series of *go-to* games can also be used to measure the coherence of the shared language.

The study involved three runs in which *where-are-we* games were played for 6 hours followed by 20 *go-to* games. The toponymic languages formed contained an average of 8.7 toponyms ($\sigma = 0.5$) with coherence at 30.4% ($\sigma = 15.4\%$) and *go-to* game success at 75.0% ($\sigma = 15.0\%$). The most coherent language had 9 toponyms with 43.9% coherence and 90% *go-to* game success (Figure 5.10). In this experiment, there was noise involved in using hearing distance to achieve shared attention. However, even with the noise, and with associations for words that spread over large areas in the world, the similarities between the languages can be seen, and the success of *go-to* games indicates that the languages were similar enough to be used for the task of meeting at other locations in the world.

5.6   Discussion

The neurophysiological evidence for the spatial encoding processes in a rat brain indicates some key contrasts in the way that rodents are thought to navigate compared with the way that robots are designed to navigate. RatSLAM is an attempt to take advantage of the points of difference highlighted by studies of the rat brain in order to build a better robotic navigation system. In this project, we found that building a mapping system based on an understanding of the highly competent spatial cognition system evidenced by the rat's remarkable navigation abilities has produced new insights into developing long-term and large-scale navigation competence in a robot. The outcome is a system that performs well at some of the most challenging problems in robotic navigation.

The spatial representations at the heart of the RatSLAM system bear many of the properties of the spatial representations encoded in and around the rodent hippocampus.

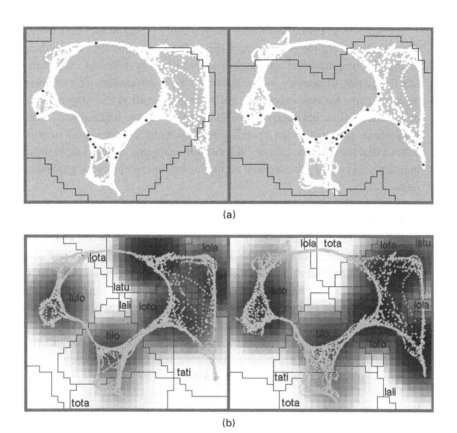

(a)

(b)

Figure 5.10 Word use for the two robots, one to the left, the other to the right. (a) The experience associations for the word "tilo." The entire experience map is shown in white, with the experiences associated with *tilo* in the distributed lexicon table shown in black. The area in which the word *tilo* has an association value greater than zero is outlined, using the 2-m neighborhood. (b) The usage of the word depends on the interactions with other toponyms. The experience map is shown in gray and the area in which each word is used is outlined and labeled. The background color indicates the confidence value of the word used in each location, with white indicating low confidence and black indicating high confidence. The usage of the word *tilo* is restricted to the triangular-shaped area in the center, corresponding to the area in which most of the experiences associated with the word are located.

The pose cell representation, inspired by the grid cells of the rat, forms a powerful spatiotemporal filter for the noisy data association information from the local view matching process, while providing a method for updating the pose belief based on information from odometry alone. The experience maps are inspired by the place cells in the hippocampus, decoding the ambiguous and redundant data in the pose cells and the local view cells into a representation that is useful for path planning and for the basis of symbolic interpretation. The experience map's flexibility in geometry helps to create a system that can cope with noisy input, deal with a changing environment, and accommodate increasing complexity.

The RatSLAM system continues to evolve as a practical tool for robotic navigation. We are combining the principles of flexibility developed thus far in the project with emerging computational approaches to probabilistic filtering. The aim is to quantify the quality of sensory information and the requirements for computation to build effective maps for task execution. Furthermore, we are continuing to explore methods of communication between robots, and between robots and humans, that can ground symbols in the distributed spatial representations encompassed in RatSLAM. We believe that the combination of a lightweight mapping, navigation, planning and communication systems are essential technologies for the emerging generation of mobile robots.

Similarly, the current RatSLAM system is being used as a reference model for new high-fidelity spiking models of regions in and around the rodent hippocampus. We are working closely with neuroscientists to bridge the gap between RatSLAM's abstract model of neural function, and the growing body of electrophysiological and anatomical data for the rodent brain. A complete model at this level requires each neuron to be modeled as an individual dynamical system, with attention to details such as the timing of spiking behavior, and the overlying brain oscillations such as the theta rhythm. Anatomical data for the numbers and connectivity of neurons and synapses must be accounted and appropriately incorporated in the model. By incorporating such a complete model into a robotic platform we hope to develop new understanding of spatial cognition in rodents and other mammals.

References

Arleo, A. and Gerstner, W. (2000). Spatial cognition and neuro-mimetic navigation: a model of hippocampal place cell activity. *Biological Cybernetics*, **83**(3), 287–299.

Barakova, E. and Lourens, T. (2005). Efficient episode encoding for spatial navigation. *International Journal of Systems Science*, **36**(14), 887–895.

Barrera, A. and Weitzenfeld, A. (2008). Biologically-inspired robot spatial cognition based on rat neurophysiological studies. *Autonomous Robots*, **25**(1–2), 147–169.

Best, P. J., White, A. M., and Minai, A. (2001). Spatial processing in the brain: the activity of hippocampal place cells. *Annual Review of Neuroscience*, **24**, 459–486.

Burgess, N., Donnett, J. G., Jeffery, K. J., and O'Keefe, J. (1997). Robotic and neuronal simulation of the hippocampus and rat navigation. *Philosophical Transactions of the Royal Society of London B Biological Sciences*, **352**(1360), 1535–1543.

Cuperlier, N., Quoy, M., and Gaussier, P. (2007). Neurobiologically inspired mobile robot navigation and planning. *Frontiers in Neurorobotics*, **1**(3), doi:10.3389/neuro.12/003.2007.

Davis, D. E., Emlen, J. T., *et al.* (1948). Studies on home range in the brown rat. *Journal of Mammalogy*, **29**(3), 207–225.

Dissanayake, G., Newman, P. M., Durrant-Whyte, H. F., *et al.* (2001). A solution to the simultaneous localization and map building (SLAM) problem. *IEEE Transactions on Robotics and Automation*, **17**(3), 229–241.

Giovannangeli, C. and Gaussier, P. (2008). Autonomous vision-based navigation: goal-orientated planning by transient states prediction, cognitive map building, and sensory-motor learning. In *IEEE International Conference on Intelligent Robots and Systems*, held in Nice, France, pp. 676–683.

Hafting, T., Fyhn, M., *et al.* (2005). Microstructure of a spatial map in the entorhinal cortex. *Nature*, **11**(436), 801–806.

Hardy, H. R. and Taylor, K. D. (1980). Radiotracking of *Rattus norvegicus* on farms. In Amianer, C. J., Jr. and MacDonald, D. W. (eds.), *A Handbook on Biotelemetry and Radio Tracking*. New York: Pergamon Press, pp. 657–665.

Harnad, S. (1990). The symbol grounding problem. *Physica D: Nonlinear Phenomena*, **42**, 335–346.

Knierim, J., Kudrimoti, H., *et al.* (1995). Place cells, head direction cells, and the learning of landmark stability. *Journal of Neuroscience*, **15**(3), 1648–1659.

Krichmar, J., L., Nitz, D.A., Gally, J. A., and Edelman, G. M. (2005). Characterizing functional hippocampal pathways in a brain-based device as it solves a spatial memory task. *Proceedings of the National Academy of Sciences of the USA*, **102**(6), 2111–2116.

McNaughton, B. L., Battaglia, F. P., *et al.* (2006). Path-integration and the neural basis of the cognitive map. *Nature Reviews Neuroscience*, **7**(8), 663–678.

Milford, M. and Wyeth, G. (2008a). Mapping a suburb with a single camera using a biologically inspired SLAM system. *IEEE Transactions on Robotics*, **24**(5), 1038–1053.

Milford, M. and Wyeth, G. (2008b). Single camera vision-only SLAM on a suburban road network. In *IEEE International Conference on Robotics and Automation*, held in Pasadena, CA.

Milford, M. and Wyeth, G., (2010). Persistent navigation and mapping using a biologically inspired SLAM system. *International Journal of Robotics Research*, **29**, 1131.

Milford, M. J., Wyeth G., and Prasser, D. (2004). RatSLAM: a hippocampal model for simultaneous localization and mapping. In *IEEE International Conference on Robotics and Automation*, New Orleans, LA.

Montemerlo, M., Thrun, S., Koller, D., and Wegbreit, B. (2003). FastSLAM 2.0: an improved particle filtering algorithm for simultaneous localization and mapping that provably converges. In *Proceedings of the 16th International Joint Conference on Artificial Intelligence*, held in Acapulco, Mexico.

O'Keefe, J. and Conway, D. H. (1978). Hippocampal place units in the freely moving rat: why they fire where they fire. *Experimental Brain Research*, **31**(4), 573–590.

O'Keefe, J. and Dostrovsky, J. (1971). The hippocampus as a spatial map: preliminary evidence from unit activity in the freely moving rat. *Brain Research*, **34**(1), 171–175.

Pomerleau, D. (1997). Visibility estimation from a moving vehicle using the RALPH vision system. In *IEEE Conference on Intelligent Transport Systems*, pp. 906–911.

Quirk, G. J., Muller, R. U., and Kubie, J. L. (1990). The firing of hippocampal place cells in the dark depends on the rat's recent experience. *Journal of Neuroscience*, **10**(6), 2008–2017.

Ranck, J. B. (1984). Head direction cells in the deep cell layer of dorsal presubiculum in freely moving rats. *Society Neuroscience Abstracts*, **10**, 599.

Recht, M. A. (1988). The biology of domestic rats: telemetry yields insights for pest control. In *Proceedings of the Thirteenth Vertebrate Pest Conference*, held in Lincoln, NE, pp. 98–100.

Steels, L. (2001). Language games for autonomous robots. *IEEE Intelligent Systems*, **16**(5), 16–22.

Stringer, S. M., Rolls, E. T., Trappenberg, T. P., and de Araujo, I. E. T. (2002a). Self-organizing continuous attractor networks and path integration: two-dimensional models of place cells. *Network: Computation in Neural Systems*, **13**(4), 429–446.

Stringer, S. M., Trappenberg, T. P., Rolls, E.T. and de Araujo, I.E.T. (2002b). Self-organizing continuous attractor networks and path integration: one-dimensional models of head direction cells. *Network: Computation in Neural Systems*, **13**(2), 217–242.

Taube, J. S. (2007). The head direction signal: origins and sensory-motor integration. *Annual Review of Neuroscience*, **30**, 181–207.

Taube, J. S., Muller, R. U., and Ranck, J. B., Jr. (1990). Head direction cells recorded from the postsubiculum in freely moving rats. I. Description and quantitative analysis. *Journal of Neuroscience*, **10**(2), 420–435.

Thrun, S. and Leonard, J. (2008). Simultaneous localization and mapping. In Siciliano, B. and Khatib, O. (eds.) *Springer Handbook of Robotics*, Vol. 1. Berlin: Springer.

Thrun, S. and Montemerlo, M. (2006). The GraphSLAM algorithm with applications to large-scale mapping of urban structures. *International Journal of Robotics Research*, **25**(5–6), 403–429.

Tolman, E. C. (1948). Cognitive maps in rats and men. *Psychological Review*, **55**(4), 189–209.

6 Evolution of rewards and learning mechanisms in Cyber Rodents

Eiji Uchibe and Kenji Doya

Finding the design principle of reward functions is a big challenge in both artificial intelligence and neuroscience. Successful acquisition of a task usually requires rewards to be given not only for goals but also for intermediate states to promote effective exploration. We propose a method to design "intrinsic" rewards for autonomous robots by combining constrained policy gradient reinforcement learning and embodied evolution. To validate the method, we use the Cyber Rodent robots, in which collision avoidance, recharging from battery pack, and "mating" by software reproduction are three major "extrinsic" rewards. We show in hardware experiments that the robots can find appropriate intrinsic rewards for the visual properties of battery packs and potential mating partners to promote approach behaviors.

6.1 Introduction

In application of reinforcement learning (Sutton and Barto, 1998) to real-world problems, the design of the reward function is critical for successful achievement of the task. Designing appropriate reward functions is a nontrivial, time-consuming process in practical applications. Although it appears straightforward to assign positive rewards to desired goal states and negative rewards to states to be avoided, finding a good balance between multiple rewards often needs careful tuning. Furthermore, if rewards are given only at isolated goal states, blind exploration of the state space takes a long time. Rewards at intermediate subgoals, or even along the trajectories leading to the goal, promote focused exploration, but appropriate design of such additional rewards usually requires prior knowledge of the task or trial and error by the experimenter.

In general, the reward functions in a reinforcement learning framework are categorized into two types: those directly representing the successful achievement of the task, which we call "extrinsic rewards," and those aimed for facilitating efficient and robust learning, which we call "intrinsic rewards." In this chapter, we consider how distributed autonomous robots, Cyber Rodents (Doya and Uchibe, 2005), can find appropriate intrinsic reward functions through evolution.

Neuromorphic and Brain-Based Robots, eds. Jeffrey L. Krichmar and Hiroaki Wagatsuma. Published by Cambridge University Press. © Cambridge University Press 2011.

Previous studies on intrinsic rewards proposed methods for realizing "curiosity" to promote exploration of novel states and actions, and for "shaping" to promote goal-directed search. Typical examples of the former are the exploratory bonuses (Främling, 2007), which set optimistic initial value functions (Wiewiora, 2003). While exploration bonuses just promote uniform scanning of the state space, recent studies called "intrinsically motivated reinforcement learning" (IMRL) aim at designing intrinsic rewards to guide robots to "interesting" parts of the state space. Barto and his colleagues (Barto et al., 2004; Singh et al., 2005; Stout et al., 2005) proposed an algorithm for intrinsically motivated reinforcement learning based on the theory of options (Sutton et al., 1999). Meeden et al. (2004) used the error of its own prediction as the intrinsic reward for a simulated robot to track a moving decoy robot. Oudeyer and his colleagues considered the progress of prediction learning as the intrinsic reward and demonstrated its effectiveness in behavioral development of Sony's AIBO robot learning (Oudeyer and Kaplan, 2004, 2007; Oudeyer et al., 2007). Takeuchi and colleagues also proposed the reduction of the prediction errors of the robot's internal model as the intrinsic reward (Takeuchi et al., 2006, 2007). Ng and colleagues showed that a shaping reward defined by the difference of a potential function does not affect the optimal policy (Ng et al., 1999). Singh and colleagues defined the "optimal reward function" as the one that maximizes a fitness function over a distribution of environments (Singh et al., 2009).

In most of the previous studies, the objective function was to maximize a weighted sum of extrinsic and intrinsic rewards. However, this makes optimization of the intrinsic reward difficult because maximization of the sum can result in maximization of only intrinsic rewards, leading to the failure of the task. Typical examples are excessive exploration to gather exploration bonuses and dwelling at subgoals with shaping rewards. To deal with this problem, Uchibe and Doya (2007) proposed the use of the constrained policy gradient reinforcement learning (CPGRL) in which the intrinsic rewards were maximized within the bounds specified by the extrinsic rewards. This enabled optimization of intrinsic rewards without compromising the main task goals specified by the extrinsic rewards.

In this chapter, we propose a method for autonomous agents to find appropriate intrinsic rewards by combining constrained reinforcement learning (Uchibe and Doya, 2007) and embodied evolution (Elfwing, 2007; Elfwing et al., 2008b). The agents have a fitness function and a fixed set of extrinsic rewards which specify the constraints for maintaining the fitness. Each agent learns its policy by the extrinsic and intrinsic rewards, and the intrinsic rewards are evolved by the fitness of the learned policy.

We test this framework in hardware experiments using a colony of Cyber Rodents (Doya and Uchibe, 2005), whose fitness depends on capturing battery packs for survival and successful copying of their program parameters, or "genes," by infrared communication for reproduction in software. Accordingly, positive extrinsic rewards are given for capturing a battery pack and for successful exchange of the the program parameters, or "mating," with another robot. In our previous study (Uchibe and Doya, 2008), the intrinsic reward was limited to a simple network with three weight parameters. In this study, the intrinsic reward function is given by a three-layer network with the vision sensor and the internal battery level as the inputs. The genes of an agent define the weights of the intrinsic reward network and are optimized by an embodied evolution scheme with multiple virtual agents in a physical robot (Elfwing et al., 2008b).

We first outline the general method of finding appropriate intrinsic reward functions by embodied evolution. We then explain our reinforcement learning method using an intrinsic reward function subject to the task constraints imposed as extrinsic reward functions. Next, we introduce the Cyber Rodent platform we use for our experiments and describe the implementation and result of the experiments.

6.2 Evolution of intrinsic reward

Here we propose a method for improving the intrinsic reward function by the framework of embodied evolution (Watson et al., 2002; Usui and Arita, 2003; Wischmann et al., 2007; Elfwing et al., 2008a, 2008b). We assume that there exist N_{robot} robots in the environment and they can physically interact with each other. Let X and U be a state space and an action space of the robot, respectively. At time step t, the j-th learning robot observes a state $x_t^j \in X$ and executes an action $u_t^j \in U$ with probability $\mu(u \mid x;\theta^j)$, which is parameterized by a policy parameter vector $\theta^j (j = 1, ..., N_{robot})$, where the superscript indicates the robot. We assume that each robot has its own intrinsic reward function $^I r(x,u;w^j)$ parameterized by an intrinsic reward vector w^j and $^E N$ extrinsic reward functions $^E r_i (x,u)(i = 1,...,^E N)$. It should be noted that the superscript is not necessary since all robots use the same extrinsic reward functions.

For a given θ^j, we define the long-term average rewards as

$$^I g\left(\theta^j, w^j\right) = \lim_{T\to\infty} \mathrm{E}_{\theta_j}\left[\frac{1}{T}\sum_{t=}^{T} {}^I r\left(x_t^j, u_t^j; w^j\right)\right] \text{ for } j = 1,...,N_{robot},$$

$$^E g_i\left(\theta^j\right) = \lim_{T\to\infty} \mathrm{E}_{\theta_j}\left[\frac{1}{T}\sum_{t=1}^{T} {}^E r_i\left(x_t^j, u_t^j\right)\right] \text{ for } i = 1,...,{}^E N,$$

(6.1)

where the expectation E_{θ_j} is taken over sequences of states and actions with state transition generated by the stochastic policy $\mu(u \mid x;\theta^j)$. It should be noted that the expectation is independent of the starting state theoretically under some conditions (for example, see Baxter and Bartlett, 2001; Konda and Tsitsiklis, 2003).

The goal of reinforcement learning here in each robot is to find a policy parameter vector θ^j that maximizes the long-term average intrinsic reward under the inequality constraints given by the average extrinsic rewards:

$$\max_{\theta} {}^I g\left(\theta^j, w^j\right), \text{ s.t. } {}^E g_i\left(\theta^j\right) \geq G_i^j \quad \left(i = 1,...,{}^E N\right)$$

(6.2)

where G_i^j is the minimal required average of the i-th extrinsic reward. This constrained optimization (Equation 6.2) is performed by each robot separately.

In contrast, the goal of evolution by a colony of robots is to find an intrinsic reward parameter w^j that promotes effective exploration. The performance of intrinsic reward is evaluated by a fitness value f^j, which is related to the set of extrinsic rewards Er_i^j. The goal of embodied evolution is to maximize the scalar fitness

$$\max_w \ f^j(w), \tag{6.3}$$

by changing w^j of the intrinsic reward function.

6.2.1   Improvement of intrinsic reward parameters

In order to optimize the intrinsic reward parameter vector formulated by Equation (6.2), we take the embodied evolution approach. Each robot has two types of populations: w_{self} and w_{other}.

$$w_{self}^j = \left\{ \left(w_1^j, f_1^j\right), \left(w_2^j, f_2^j\right), \dots, \left(w_{I_N}^j, f_{I_N}^j\right) \right\} \ \ w_{other}^j = \phi,$$

where ϕ denotes an empty set. Each robot evaluates a set of intrinsic reward parameter vectors $w_i^j (i = 1, \dots, {}^l N)$, in random order, by time-sharing: that is, taking control over the robot for a limited number of time steps.

The opportunity for a robot to change its intrinsic reward parameter vector is dependent on successful mating. Figure 6.1 illustrates the mating operation between two robots indexed by j and l. When two robots succeed in mating, the intrinsic reward parameter vector and fitness values are added to w_{other}^j. Figure 6.1 illustrates a mating process between j-th and l-th robots where the j-th and l-th robots adopt the intrinsic

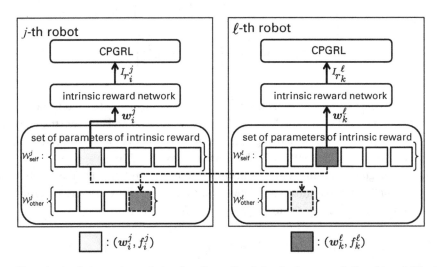

Figure 6.1   Data sharing between two robots when the mating behavior is successfully achieved. The j-th and l-th robots use the intrinsic reward parameterized by w_i^j and w_k^l respectively. After successful mating, the j-th robot receives w_k^l, and its fitness value f_k^l of the l-th robot, and vice versa.

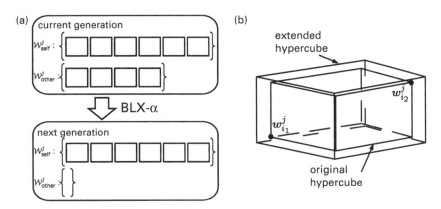

Figure 6.2 Evolutionary computation used in our method. (a) Generation alternation model. BLX-α is applied into $w^j = w^j_{self} \cup w^j_{other}$ to create a new w^j_{self}. w^j_{other} is set to an empty set after generation alternation. (b) Schematic illustration of the genetic operator based on the BLX-α. The center position of the original and extended hypercubes is given by $(w^j_{i_1} + w^j_{i_2})/2$.

reward parameterized by w^j_i and w^l_k, respectively. When a mating behavior has success-fully ended, w^j_{other} and w^l_{other} are updated by adding the corresponding pair of weights and fitness values as follows:

$$w^j_{other} \leftarrow w^j_{other} \cup \left\{\left(w^l_k, f^l_k\right)\right\}, \quad w^l_{other} \leftarrow w^l_{other} \cup \left\{\left(w^l_k, f^l_k\right)\right\},$$

After all intrinsic reward parameter vectors in w^j_{self} are evaluated, an evolutionary computation method named BLX-α (Eshelman and Schaffer, 1993) is applied into the set $w^j = w^j_{self} \cup w^j_{other}$ to create a new w^j_{self}, as shown in Figure 6.2(a). Suppose that w^j is an N_w dimensional vector. The BLX-α uniformly picks parameter values from points that lie on an interval that extends αI_m on either side of the interval $I_m = \left|w^j_{i_1,m} - w^j_{i_2,m}\right| (m = 1,\dots,N_w)$ between parents $w^j_{i_1}$ and $w^j_{i_2}$, where $w^j_{i*,m}$ is the m-th component of vector w^j_{i*}. The basic idea of the BLX-α is illustrated in Figure 6.2(b) in which a pair of $w^j_{i_1}$ and $w^j_{i_2}$ determines the original cube whose sides are parallel to axes of the coordinate system. The parameter α controls a trade-off between convergence and divergence in evolutionary processes. It has been shown that $\alpha = 0.5$ was a bal-anced relationship (Eshelman and Schaffer, 1993), and therefore BLX-0.5 is used in our implementation. Then, w^j is updated by the value which is randomly generated in the extended hypercube by using uniform distribution.

6.3 Constrained policy gradient reinforcement learning

Uchibe and Doya (2008) proposed Constrained Policy Gradient Reinforcement Learning (CPGRL) which solves the constrained problem (Equation 6.2). The superscript to denote the robot is omitted in this section since all robots use the same algorithm.

6.3.1   Gradient projection

Figure 6.3 illustrates the architecture of CPGRL and the intrinsic reward network. CPGRL consists of one stochastic policy, multiple gradient estimators, and a gradient projection module. Each gradient estimator generates an estimate of the long-term average reward and its estimated gradient with respect to the policy parameters. The gradient projection module computes a projection on to a feasible region, which is the set of points satisfying all the inequality constraints used in Equation (6.2). We first describe how to perform constrained optimization given policy gradients and then introduce our method to derive the gradients in the Section 6.3.2.

Let $\tilde{\nabla}^I g$ and $\tilde{\nabla}^I g_i (i = 1, ..., ^E N)$ denote the policy gradients for the intrinsic reward $^I r$ and extrinsic rewards $^E r_i$, respectively. Given the set of policy gradients and the estimates of the average rewards after the k-th episode, the policy parameters θ_k are updated by the gradient projection method as follows:

$$\theta_{k+1} = \theta_k + \Delta\theta_k$$

$$\Delta\theta_k = {}^I\alpha P\tilde{\nabla}^I g - {}^E\alpha d,$$

(6.4)

where $^I\alpha$ and $^E\alpha$ are the stepsize parameters, respectively. It should be noted that the matrix P projects $\tilde{\nabla}^I g$ into the subspace tangent to the active constraints while the vector d realizes a restoration move for the active constraints induced by the set of extrinsic rewards.

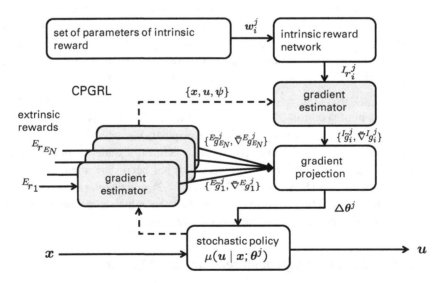

Figure 6.3   Learning architecture based on constrained policy gradient reinforcement learning. There exist $^E N + 1$ gradient estimators to estimate the policy gradients separately. The intrinsic reward network generates the intrinsic reward parameterized by w_i^j which is selected from a set of intrinsic reward parameters.

To compute P and d in general cases, the set of indices of the active inequality constraints is considered:

$$A = \left\{ i \middle| {}^{E}\tilde{g}_i - G_i \leq 0, i = 1, \ldots, {}^{E}N \right\},$$

where ${}^{E}\tilde{g}_i$ is an estimate of the average extrinsic reward (Equation 6.1). When A is an empty set, it means that the solution lies at the interior of the feasible region. In this case P and d are set to the identity matrix and zero vector, respectively. Hereafter we consider the case of $|A| > 0$ where $|A|$ denotes the number of active constraints. Then, we define

$$g_A = \left[{}^{E}\tilde{g}_{i_1} - G_{i_1} \; \cdots \; {}^{E}\tilde{g}_{i_{|A|}} - G_{i_{|A|}} \right]^{\mathrm{T}}$$
$$N_A = \left[\tilde{\nabla}^{E} g_{i_1} \cdots \tilde{\nabla}^{E} g_{i_{|A|}} \right]$$

where i_a, $a = 1, \ldots, |A|$ is an index to count the element in A. The projection matrix and restoration move are given by

$$P = I - N_A \left(N_A^T N_A \right)^{-1} N_A^T, \tag{6.5}$$

$$d = N_A \left(N_A^T N_A \right)^{-1} g_A \tag{6.6}$$

where I denotes the identity matrix. It should be noted that $Pd = 0$, meaning that d points to the direction of projection. Here, we should note that $N_A^T N_A$ in Equations (6.5) and (6.6) are not invertible if the set of active constraint gradients $\left\{ \tilde{\nabla}^{E} g_{i_j} \middle| j = 1, \ldots, |A| \right\}$ is linearly dependent. In addition, rank deficiency of $N_A^T N_A$ is sometimes detected due to the accuracy of numerical computation and/or biased samples. The pseudo-inverse of $N_A^T N_A$ should be used if it is not full-rank.

After the parameter update by Equation (6.4), if the projected update is zero, i.e. $P\tilde{\nabla}^{I} g = 0$, we check the convergence condition by the Lagrange multipliers,

$$\lambda = \left(N_A^T N_A \right)^{-1} N_A^T \tilde{\nabla}^{I} g.$$

If λ has no negative components, we have a solution and terminate. Otherwise, the active set is reevaluated by $A \leftarrow A \backslash \{r\}$ where $r = \mathrm{argmax}_{l \in A} \lambda_l$. After deleting one constraint from A, P and d are calculated again.

6.3.2   Estimate of policy gradients

There exist several methods to compute the gradient of the average reward. In the current implementation, we choose Konda's actor-critic method (Konda and Tsitsiklis, 2003). As opposed to the GPOMDP algorithm (Baxter and Bartlett, 2001), Konda's actor-critic requires an additional learning mechanism to approximate the state-action value function, but it can utilize the Markov property. Here, we briefly introduce the actor-critic algorithm to estimate the gradient of the average reward $^{E}r_i$, but it should be noted that the same algorithm is applied for the case of intrinsic reward.

For the given state and action, the function ψ is defined by

$$\psi(x,u) = \frac{\partial \ln \mu(u|x;\theta)}{\partial \theta}.$$

The robot interacts with the environment, producing a state, action, reward sequence. After receiving experiences, $(x_t, u_t, {}^{E}r_{i,t+1}, x_{t+}1, u_{t+1})$ an eligibility trace ψ is updated by

$$z_{t=1} = \beta z_t + \psi(x_t, u_t),$$

where $\beta \in [0,1]$ is a discount rate that controls the variance of the gradient estimate. Since z_t is independent of reward functions, z_t can be used for estimating gradients of different average rewards.

In the framework of policy gradient methods, the function ψ is used as a basis function vector in order to approximate the state-action value function:

$$^{E}Q_i\left(x_t, u; {}^{E}v_i\right) = {}^{E}v_i^{\mathrm{T}}\,\psi(x,u),$$

where $^{E}v_i$ is a parameter vector. The learning rule to train $^{E}v_i$ is given by the standard temporal difference method,

$$^{E}v_{i,t+1} = {}^{E}v_{i,t} + \alpha_Q\,{}^{E}\delta_{i,t}z_{t+1},$$

where α_Q and $^{E}\delta_{i,t}$ are the learning rate and the temporal difference error, respectively. For the sample $(x_t, u_t, {}^{E}r_{i,t+1}, x_{t+1}, u_{t+1})$, $^{E}\delta_{i,t}$ is calculated by

$$^{E}\delta_{i,t} = {}^{E}r_{i,t+1} - {}^{E}\tilde{g}_{i,t+1} + {}^{E}v_{i,t}^{\mathrm{T}}\left[\psi\left(x_{t+1}, u_{t+1,}\right) - \psi\left(x_t, u_t\right)\right],$$

where the estimate of the average reward is calculated by

$$^{E}\tilde{g}_{i,t+1} = {}^{E}\tilde{g}_{i,t} + \alpha_g\left({}^{E}r_{i,t+1} - {}^{E}\tilde{g}_{i,t}\right)$$

where α_g is a stepsize parameter. Then, all the gradients are updated in the same manner. For all $i = 1, \ldots, {}^{E}N$, the gradient of the long-term average reward is estimated by

$$\tilde{\nabla}^{E}g_{i,t+1} = \tilde{\nabla}^{E}g_{i,t} + \alpha_{pg}\left[{}^{E}Q_i\left(x_t, u_t\right)\psi\left(x_t, u_t\right) - \tilde{\nabla}^{E}g_{i,t}\right],$$

where α_{pg} is a stepsize parameter.

It should be noted that the parameters related to the intrinsic rewards such as $^l v$ and $\tilde{\nabla}^I g$ are set to zero when the intrinsic reward parameters are changed. Conversely, the parameters related to the policy and extrinsic rewards do not reset at all.

6.4 Cyber Rodent hardware

Before getting into the detail of experiments, our hardware system is explained briefly. Figure 6.4(a) shows the hardware of the Cyber Rodent (CR) (Doya and Uchibe, 2005). Its body is 22 cm in length and 1.75 kg in weight. The CR is endowed with a variety of sensory inputs, including an omnidirectional CMOS camera, an infrared (IR) range sensor, seven IR proximity sensors, gyros, and accelerometer. To represent an internal state, a three-color light-emitting diode (LED) (red, blue, and green) is mounted on the tail. The programs are coded in C on top of an embedded real-time operating system "eCos." In addition, the CR has an FPGA chip for real-time image processing, such as color blob detection.

Figure 6.4(b) shows a blue battery and a green battery (battery pack equipped with blue and green LED, respectively). Although there exist two types of battery packs, the CR cannot distinguish between them. The LED is lit if the battery is charged enough. Therefore, the CRs can find the charged battery by using visual information. It should be noted that the CR actually charges its own battery from the battery pack. The experimenters replace the discharged battery packs with new charged ones.

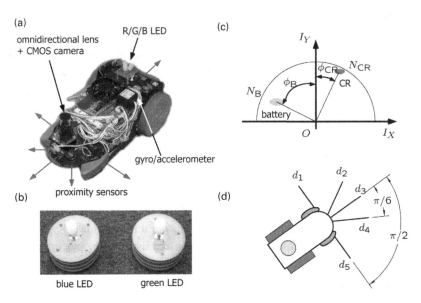

Figure 6.4 Our experimental system. (a) Hardware of the Cyber Rodent (CR). (b) Battery pack with blue/green LED. (c) Image coordinate system $O - I_x I_y$ and two angles ϕ_B and ϕ_{CR} to the nearest battery and CR are detected. (d) Five proximity sensors $d_1, \ldots, d_5$ mounted in front. Each proximity sensor measures a distance of up to 30 cm.

The motion system of the CR consists of two wheels that allow the CR to move at a velocity of 1.3 m/s, but the maximum velocity is limited to 0.2 m/s for safety in the experiments. Then, the action vector u is represented by $u = [u_l \; u_r]^T$ where u_l and u_r denote velocities of left and right wheels, respectively.

An image coordinate system $O - I_x I_y$ of the omnidirectional CMOS camera is shown in Figure 6.4(c). The battery pack is recognized as a color blob in the image, and the size of the blob N_B and an angle θ_B are utilized. In addition, another CR is also detected if the LED on the tail is turned on. As a result, the angle θ_{CR} and the size of the blob N_{CR} can be used to represent the relative position of another CR. Figure 6.4(d) shows the location of the five proximity sensors. The relative angle θ_D and distance d_{min} to the nearest obstacle are estimated from the readings of these proximity sensors (d_i, $i = 1, \ldots, 5$). In addition, each CR can measure its own battery level V which nonlinearly decreases according to the changes of the velocities of the wheels and increases when the CR catches the battery pack. These feature values are scaled to use them as inputs of feedforward neural networks. Since d_{min}, N_B, N_{CR} are scaled to [0,1] due to positivity the relative angles ϕ_d, ϕ_B, ϕ_{CR}, in radians between $[-\pi/2, \pi/2]$, are normalized between $[-1,1]$. As a result, the state vector x contains eight components

$$x = \begin{bmatrix} 1 \, d_o \, \phi_o \, N_B \, \phi_B \, N_{CR} \, \phi_{CR} \, V \end{bmatrix}^T, \tag{6.7}$$

where 1 is a bias component.

6.5   Experiments with the Cyber Rodents

We use the survival and mating task of the Cyber Rodents to test the proposed embodied evolution framework for finding intrinsic rewards. Figure 6.5 shows the experimental environment. There are three CRs (named as CR1, CR2, CR3; $N_{robot} = 3$), a number of battery packs, and four obstacles in a 6 m × 5 m field delimited by walls.

In this experiment, we use the following fitness function for optimization of the intrinsic reward function:

$$f^j = f^j_{battery} + f^j_{mating},$$

where
$f^j_{battery}$ is the number of obtained battery packs per three minutes, f^j_{mating} is the number of successful matings per three minutes to measure the running performance.

6.5.1   Stochastic policy

The CR must learn to find and approach the battery, move away from the obstacles, find other CRs, and so on. These behaviors are implemented in a stochastic policy $\mu(u \mid x; \theta)$ shown in Figure 6.6(a). This stochastic policy uses a two-dimensional

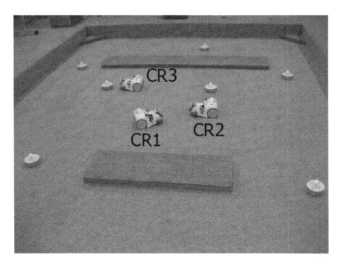

Figure 6.5   Embodied evolution in the real environment. There exist three Cyber Rodents (CR) and many battery packs. The size of the environment is 5 m × 4 m. Shaded rectangles are obstacles of which heights are about 0.05 m and they do not hide the battery packs from the CRs.

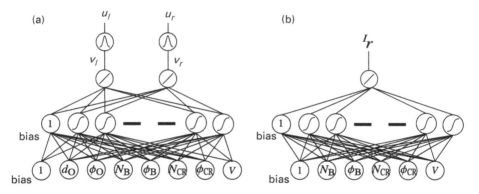

Figure 6.6   Two networks in the robot. (a) Stochastic policy $\mu(u|x;\theta)$ which consists of a Gaussian distribution and a three-layer feedforward neural neetwork (FNN). (b) Intrinsic reward $^1r(x,u;w)$ which is implemented by a three-layer FNN.

Gaussian distribution with mean v and covariance matrix Σ, and its mean vector v is calculated by a three-layer feedforward neural network (FNN) with 21 hidden nodes of sigmoidal activation function and two output nodes of linear activation function. More specifically, the outputs of FNN are velocities of left and right wheels ($v = [v_l, v_r]^T$) while the state vector (Equation 6.7) is sent to the input layer. The covariance matrix Σ is constant and it is initialized as a diagonal matrix diag[0.4 0.4]. All connection weights of FNN are represented in the policy parameter, which is trained by the CPGRL.

At each time step t the action u_t is chosen according to this stochastic policy. The CR is usually controlled by this network except when it catches the battery pack. During charging, the CR stops moving for three minutes. After recharging, the hand-coded behavior is executed to release the battery. Then, the CR moves around in the environment by the stochastic policy.

6.5.2   Reward functions

In this experiment, we prepare three extrinsic rewards as *biological* constraints. The first reward is for foraging behaviors defined by

$$^E r_1 = \begin{cases} 1-\dfrac{1}{1+\exp\left(10(V-0.5)\right)} & \text{if the CR catches the battery pack} \\ -0.1 & \text{if } V < \Theta v, \\ 0 & \text{otherwise,} \end{cases} \tag{6.8}$$

where Θ_v is a certain threshold. It should be noted that $^E r_i$ is explicitly dependent on the internal battery level V. When the CR catches the battery pack, a recharging behavior is executed automatically. The reward is for mating behaviors defined by

$$^E r_2 = \begin{cases} 1 & \text{if mating behavior is realized,} \\ 0 & \text{otherwise.} \end{cases}$$

Since successful mating behavior is essential to the survival of all sexually reproducing organisms, a mating behavior learned from this reward is important. The CR attempts to establish the IR communication link when another CR is detected. The last reward is for avoiding behaviors defined by

$$^E r_3 = \begin{cases} -1 & \text{if the CR makes a collision with the obstacles,} \\ 0 & \text{otherwise.} \end{cases}$$

A collision is estimated by the change of the reading from the accelerometer and the odometry of the wheels. The CR can distinguish between catching the battery pack and making a collision with obstacles by monitoring the internal battery level V. It should be noted that the CR should detect the environmental events described in the conditions of the extrinsic rewards by itself.

The intrinsic reward $^I r^j$ is realized by a three-layer FNN with 14 hidden nodes of sigmoidal activation function and a pure linear output node shown in Figure 6.6(b). The input consists of a part of the state vector (Equation 6.7), where features related to the obstacles are removed while the output is the intrinsic reward. This network is much more complicated than that of our previous studies (Uchibe and Doya, 2008).

6.5.3   Mating conditions

Success of mating behaviors is dependent on the performance on the CRs. If the constraints on $^{\varepsilon}r_1$ and $^{\varepsilon}r_3$ are satisfied, the red LED on the tail is turned on. As a result, another CR has a chance to find the CR that can mate with it. In Figure 6.5, CR1 and CR2 try to mate with each other. In addition, the LED of CR3 is turned off because the constraint on $^{\varepsilon}r_3$ is active due to a collision with the obstacle.

6.5.4   Other parameters

Since the most important parameters in the CPGRL are the threshold values G_i^j, we prepare three types of threshold values: T1:$G_1^j = 0.0$, $G_2^j = 0.2$, $G_3^j = 0.0$, T2:$G_1^j = 0.0$, $G_2^j = 0.5$, $G_3^j = 0.0$, and T3:$G_1^j = 0.2$, $G_2^j = 0.2$, $G_3^j = 0.0$. It is noted that the threshold G_2^j should have a small positive value to make this constraint meaningful because $\tilde{g}_2^j$, is always greater than or equal to zero. The settings T2 and T3 can be regarded as mating-oriented and foraging-oriented constraints respectively since the corresponding constraints are tighter than those of T1.

The number of intrinsic reward parameters is set to $^IN = 10$. The parameter vectors for the intrinsic rewards and stochastic policy are randomly initialized with a uniform probability distribution over the interval $[-1,1]$. To evaluate our embodied evolutionary system for finding intrinsic rewards statistically, we conducted five experimental runs. When the battery of the CR had run out and the CR could not continue to move around the field, the experimental run was interrupted by the experimenters. Since there are three settings of threshold values, $5 \times 3 = 15$ experimental runs are performed.

6.6   Experimental results

6.6.1   Improvement of fitness values

Fitness values were successfully improved by the proposed method shown in Figure 6.7. At first, we explain the results under the setting T1 in detail. Due to slow learning of the policy gradient algorithm, it took a long time to obtain avoiding behaviors as compared with our previous studies (Uchibe and Doya, 2004; Doya and Uchibe, 2005). Figure 6.7(a) shows the evolution of the fitness values used for optimizing the intrinsic reward parameters. It is shown that f reaches the relatively stable level of 6.48 ± 1.25 after five generations. In this sense, there were no improvements after five generations from a viewpoint of evolutionary computation, but the evolutionary process turns out to be more complicated than expected. Parts (a) and (c) of Figure 6.7 show that f_{battery} increased gradually while f_{mating} did not increase before five generations. It means that the CRs could learn battery foraging behaviors whereas successful mating rarely occurred. Interestingly, f_{battery} slowly decreased and f_{mating} increased after five generations.

Figure 6.7(d) shows the number of collisions with obstacles per three minutes. After the seventh generation, the CRs could learn avoiding behaviors. Since the stochastic

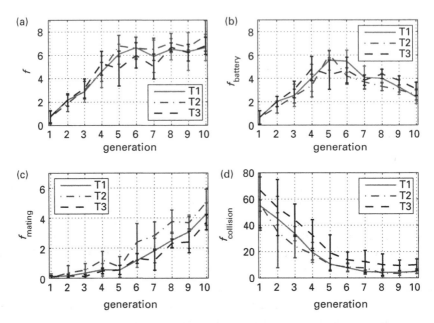

Figure 6.7 Evolution of the fitness values averaged over five runs and three CRs under the settings T1, T2 and T3. (a) $f = f_{battery} + f_{mating}$, (b) $f_{battery}$, (c) f_{mating}, and (d) $f_{collision}$. Each error bar represents the standard deviation.

policy sometimes produced an action that let the CR make collision with obstacles, $f_{collision}$ never converged to zero. Because the fitness function did not contain the term $f_{collision}$, this convergence was implicitly realized by embodied evolution.

Although a similar tendency was seen in the settings T2 and T3, they were slightly different. As can be seen from Figure 6.7(d), $f_{collision}$ of the setting T3 is larger than those of T1 and T2.

6.6.2   Obtained intrinsic rewards and fitness values

As discussed above, there was considerable difference in the learned behaviors although the fitness value was not improved after the fifth generation. In order to investigate the obtained intrinsic reward during evolution in more detail, we select one intrinsic reward parameter at the fifth generation, and let $^Ir(5)$ denote the intrinsic reward. To be able to visualize it, we divide the state space into nine distinct types. The top row of Figure 6.8 shows the intrinsic rewards when the battery of the robot is sufficiently charged (i.e. $V = 0.9$). Despite a large V, $^Ir(5)$ produces a large positive reward in the vicinity of $(\phi_{CR}, N_{CR}) = (0,1)$ shown in Figure 6.8(a). This peak is regarded as the desired state when the CR catches the battery pack, but it receives a small positive extrinsic reward calculated by Equation (6.8). When the CR sees another CR and the battery pack is not observed, $^Ir(5)$ generates a small positive reward in the vicinity of $(\phi_{CR}, N_{CR}) = (0,0)$ shown in Figure 6.8(b). It should be noted that N_{CR} approaches zero if the distance between two CRs becomes longer. Therefore, $^Ir(5)$ is not appropriate for learning mating behaviors. Figure 6.8(c) shows $^Ir(5)$

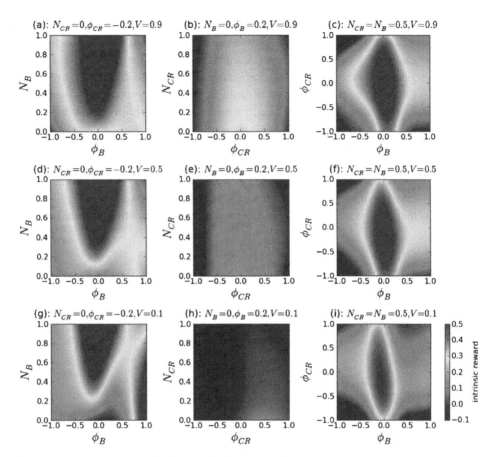

Figure 6.8 $^I r(5)$: an example of the intrinsic reward at the generation 5. Top row: The battery is sufficiently charged ($V = 0.9$). Middle row: The battery is sufficiently charged ($V = 0.5$). Bottom row: The CR needs to charge the battery immediately ($V = 0.1$). Left column: Only a battery pack is visible. Middle column: Only another CR is visible. Right column: Both the battery and another CR are visible.

when both the battery pack and another CR are observed. There exists a strong correlation between ϕ_b and the reward value while ϕ_{CR} does not affect the shape significantly.

The middle row of Figure 6.8 shows $^I r(5)$ with $V = 0.5$ and the shapes in the case of $V = 0.5$ are similar to those in the case of $V = 0.9$. The bottom row of Figure 6.8 shows the intrinsic rewards in the case of $V = 0.1$, that is, the CR has to charge its own battery immediately. If the CR observes the battery pack and the battery pack is invisible (see Figure 6.8g), there exist two peaks in the vicinities of $(\phi_B, N_B) = (0,1)$ and $(\phi_B, N_B) = (1,0)$. Although the former corresponds to the desired state, the latter is inappropriate in order to catch the battery pack. When the battery pack is not seen (see Figure 6.8h), $^I r(5)$ produces a small negative reward for $\phi_{CR} < 0$ so as to change the direction.

Then, we select one intrinsic reward parameter at the tenth generation, and let $^I r(10)$ denote the intrinsic reward. The top row of Figure 6.9 shows the intrinsic reward when the battery is sufficiently charged (i.e. $V = 0.9$). Figure 6.9(a) shows that $'r(10)$ generates a small negative reward when the CR sees the battery pack and another CR is not observed. It suggests that the CR learns to avoid the battery pack, and this is reasonable since the corresponding constraint is satisfied in this situation. Figure 6.9(b) represents that a large positive reward is given in the vicinity of $(\phi_{CR}, N_{CR}) = (1,0)$ which is the desired state for achieving mating behaviors. When both the battery pack and another CR are observed, Figure 6.9(c) shows there exists a strong correlation between ϕ_B as opposed to the case shown in Figure 6.8(c). It suggests that ϕ_B is not as important as ϕ_{CR} for exploration if V is sufficiently large.

The middle row of Figure 6.9 shows that $'r(10)$ with $V = 0.5$. In this, $'r(10)$ generates a small positive reward in the wide range of state space shown in Figure 6.9(d). It implies that $'r(10)$ is not helpful to find the battery pack in the environment. In fact, there exists

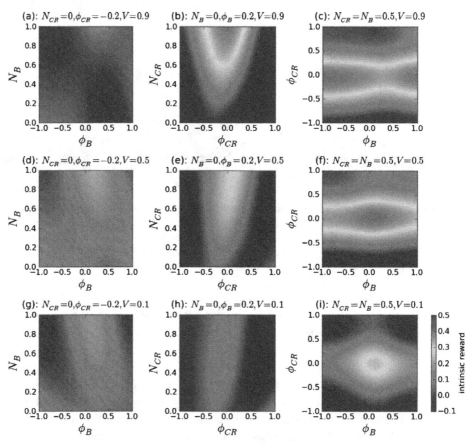

Figure 6.9 $'r(10)$: an example of the intrinsic reward at the generation 10. Top row: The battery is sufficiently charged ($V = 0.9$). Middle row: The battery is sufficiently charged ($V = 0.5$). Bottom row: The CR needs to charge the battery immediately ($V = 0.1$). Left column: Only a battery pack is visible. Middle column: Only another CR is visible. Right column: Both the battery and another CR are visible.

a correlation between ϕ_{CR} and the reward value shown in Figure 6.9(f). The shapes are similar between parts (b) and (e) of Figure 6.9.

The bottom row of Figure 6.9 shows $'r(10)$ in the case of $V = 0.1$, that is, the CR had to charge its own battery immediately. When the battery pack was not seen (see Figure 6.9h), $'r(10)$ produced a small negative reward for $\phi_{CR} > 0.4$ and the peak was observed in the vicinity of $(\phi_{CR}, N_{CR}) = (-0.1, 0.4)$. Figure 6.9(g) shows that $'r(10)$ generates a small positive value and has a maximum in the vicinity of $(\phi_B, N_B) = (0,1)$ when another CR is not observed, but its maximum value is smaller than that of Figure 6.9(b). This fact suggests that $'r(10)$ generates a large positive reward for searching another CR and a small positive reward for searching the battery pack, respectively. The reason for this is that the CR had many chances to find one of the battery packs because the number of them is greater than that of the CRs. In addition, a large supplementary reward related to the nearest battery pack prevented the CR from approaching it. In contrast, a successful mating behavior was not sensitive to the distance between two CRs because of the property of IR communication. In this case, watching another CR was regarded as an appropriate strategy for mating. Therefore, it is concluded that appropriate intrinsic rewards were obtained through embodied evolution.

6.6.3   Relation between the internal battery level and fitness values

We performed additional experiments to investigate how the internal battery level V affects the learning processes and five experimental runs were conducted. Figure 6.10(a) shows $f_{battery}$ with intrinsic rewards $'r(5)$ and $'r(10)$ when V was set to a fixed value. In other words, V remained unchanged even though the CR caught the battery pack. As can be seen from the figure, the CR trained by $'r(5)$ caught six battery packs per three minutes irrespective of the battery level. In contrast, V was correlated with $f_{battery}$ obtained by using $'r(10)$. The fact that $f_{battery}$ decreases as V increases suggests that the CR trained by $'r(10)$ tried to catch the battery pack if it was not necessary to charge its own battery.

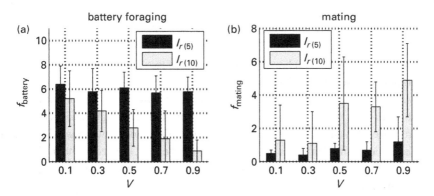

Figure 6.10   Comparison of fitness values between two intrinsic rewards. Black and gray bars represent the fitness values if the CR uses $'r(5)$ and $'r(10)$, respectively. Fitness values are averaged over five runs. Each error bar represents the standard deviation. (a) $f_{battery}$, (b) f_{mating}.

Figure 6.10(b) shows f_{mating} under the same condition. The CR trained by the intrinsic reward $'r(5)$ could not succeed in mating. However, the number of successful matings increases as V increases in the case of $'r(10)$. It should be noted that there was no significant difference between $'r(5)$ and $'r(10)$ from a viewpoint of fitness value f, as shown in Figure 6.7(a). Thus $'r(10)$ could be regarded as a good guiding reward after the CR learned a foraging behavior. However, the learned behaviors were also influenced by the constraints given by the extrinsic rewards and therefore we need more experiments and analysis. In fact if the constraints were not resolved by the CPGRL, learned behaviors were completely different even though the evolved reward function was used.

6.7   Conclusion

This chapter showed how a group of the real mobile robots named Cyber Rodents evolved the appropriate intrinsic reward function. By investigating the process on evolution, we found that the evolved intrinsic reward functions were dependent on the progress of learning. We have tested several hand-tuned reward functions in order to evaluate the efficiency of the evolved intrinsic rewards. The learning speed with the evolved intrinsic reward was similar to that with the intrinsic reward tuned by hand. If the intrinsic reward was not used, the CR failed to learn mating behaviors within 60 minutes as was suggested in our previous study (Uchibe and Doya, 2008).

It might be possible to seek an appropriate policy by directly optimizing the value function based on the evolutionary methods. Ideally speaking, extrinsic rewards are not required if an "optimal" intrinsic reward is given to the learning robots by the evolutionary computation. However, it is very difficult to find it from scratch because the evolutionary methods produce a lot of random (meaningless) functions and it is not practical to test them in the real environment. It is noted that maximization of the average of the intrinsic reward is meaningless from a viewpoint of experimenters because the CR without constraints just wandered in the environment. By introducing the constraints in the policy parameter space, the intrinsic reward is meaningful in policy improvement.

In our previous study (Doya and Uchibe, 2005), three issues were pointed out in embodied evolution: (1) how to estimate the other's (and own) fitness, (2) how to select the mating partner, and (3) how to mix the genes of two robots. The first point is simply realized by IR communication, but it should be realized via a nonverbal communication (Sato et al., 2008). The second point is implicitly solved by the framework of embodied evolution. In other words, the CR with good foraging and avoiding behaviors has many chances to mate with another, and it means that mating is made between good CRs. The BLX-α is applied to implement the third point. Since the search space of the intrinsic reward parameter vector w is relatively small, good values were found in the real experiments. More sophisticated methods should be developed to deal with a huge search space.

In our future work, we plan to address the following issues. It is, firstly, important to investigate the role of fitness function. Since the fitness function used in our experiment was tightly associated with the extrinsic rewards, the evolved intrinsic reward was task dependent. However, it is possible to utilize environmental structures and some properties of learning such as bias and variance to evaulate the intrinsic reward. Exploiting such information seems promising to improve the optimizing processes, and the evolved intrinsic reward is expected to be task independent such as exploration bonuses and progress of learning. Next, we will introduce a constraint to represent intrinsic reward functions. Our method evolved the intrinsic reward function, but it is possible to use it to evolve a potential function for policy-invariant shaping rewards (Ng *et al.*, 1999). Integrating the policy-invariant shaping reward with the CPGRL is one interesting topic.

References

Barto, A. G., Singh, S., and Chentanez, N. (2004). Intrinsically motivated learning of hierarchical collections of skills. In *Proceedings of the Third International Conference on Developmental Learning, ICDL 2004*. La Jolla, CA: UCSD Institute for Neural Computation, pp. 112–119.

Baxter, J. and Bartlett, P. L. (2001). Infinite-horizon gradient-based policy search. *Journal of Artificial Intelligence Research*, **15**, 319–350.

Doya, K. and Uchibe, E. (2005). The Cyber Rodent project: exploration of adaptive mechanisms for self-preservation and self-reproduction. *Adaptive Behavior*, **13**, 149–160.

Elfwing, S. (2007). *Embodied evolution of learning ability*. Ph.D. thesis, KTH School of Computer Science and Communication, Stockholm, Sweden.

Elfwing, S., Uchibe, E., Doya, K., and Christensen, H. I. (2008a). Co-evolution of rewards and meta-parameters in embodied evolution. In Sendhoff, B., Körner, E., Sporns, O., Ritter, H., and Doya, K. (eds.), *Creating Brain-Like Intelligence*. Berlin: Springer, pp. 278–302.

Elfwing, S., Uchibe, E., Doya, K., and Christensen, H. I. (2008b). Co-evolution of shaping rewards and meta-parameters in reinforcement learning. *Adaptive Behavior*, **16**(6), 400–412.

Eshelman, L. J. and Schaffer, J. D. (1993). Real-coded genetic algorithms and interval-schemata. In *Foundations of Genetic Algorithms*, Vol. 2. San Francisco, CA: Morgan Kaufmann, pp. 187–202.

Främling, K. (2007). Guiding exploration by pre-existing knowledge without modifying reward. *Neural Networks*, **20**(6), 736–747.

Konda, V. R. and Tsitsiklis, J. N. (2003). Actor-critic algorithms. *SIAM Journal on Control and Optimization*, **42**(4), 1143–1166.

Meeden, L. A., Marshall, J. B., and Blank, D. (2004). Self-motivated, task-independent reinforcement learning for robots. In *2004 AAAI Fall Symposium on Real-World Reinforcement Learning*. Menlo Park, CA: American Association for Artificial Intelligence.

Ng, A. Y., Harada, D., and Russel, S. (1999). Policy invariance under reward transformations: theory and application to reward shaping. In *Proceedings. of the 16th International Conference on Machine Learning*. International Machine Learning Society.

Oudeyer, P.-Y. and Kaplan, F. (2004). Intelligent adaptive curiosity: a source of self-development. In *Proceedings of the 4th International Workshop on Epigenetic Robotics*. Lund University Cognitive Studies 117. Lund, Sweden: Lund University, pp. 127–130.

Oudeyer, P.-Y. and Kaplan, F. (2007). What is intrinsic motivation? A typology of computational approaches. *Frontiers in Neurorobotics*, **1**(6), 1–14.

Oudeyer, P.-Y., Kaplan, F., and Hafner, V. (2007). Intrinsic motivation systems for autonomous mental development. *IEEE Transactions on Evolutionary Computation*, **11**(2), 265–286.

Sato, T., Uchibe, E., and Doya, K. (2008). Learning how, what, and whether to communicate: emergence of protocommunication in reinforcement learning agents. *Journal of Artificial Life and Robotics*, **12**, 70–74.

Singh, S., Barto, A. G., and Chentanez, N. (2005). Intrinsically motivated reinforcement learning. In Saul, L. K., Weiss, Y., and Bottou, L. (eds.), *Advances in Neural Information Processing Systems*, Vol. 17. Cambridge, MA: MIT Press, pp. 1281–1288.

Singh, S., Lewis, R., and Barto, A. G. (2009). Where do rewards come from? In *Proceedings of the Annual Conference of the Cognitive Science Society*, pp. 2601–2606.

Stout, A., Konidaris, G. D., and Barto, A. G. (2005). Intrinsically motivated reinforcement learning: a promising framework for developmental robot learning. In *Proceedings of the AAAI Spring Symposium Workshop on Developmental Robotics*.

Sutton, R. S. and Barto, A. G. (1998). *Reinforcement Learning*. Cambridge, MA: MIT Press/ Bradford Books.

Sutton, R. S., Precup, D., and Singh, S. (1999). Between MDPs and semi-MDPs: a framework for temporal abstraction in reinforcement learning. *Artificial Intelligence*, **112**, 181–211.

Takeuchi, J., Shouno, O., and Tsujino, H. (2006). Connectionist reinforcement learning with cursory intrinsic motivations and linear dependencies to multiple representations. In *Proceedings of International Joint Conference on Neural Networks*, pp. 54–61.

Takeuchi, J., Shouno, O., and Tsujino, H. (2007). Modular neural network for reinforcement learning with temporal intrinsic rewards. In *Proceedings of International Joint Conference on Neural Networks*, pp. 1151–1156.

Uchibe, E. and Doya, K. (2004). Competitive-cooperative-concurrent reinforcement learning with importance sampling. In Schaal, S., Ijspeert, A., Billard, A., *et al.* (eds.), *Proceedings of the Eighth International Conference on Simulation of Adaptive Behavior: From Animals to Animats 8*. Cambridge, MA: MIT Press, pp. 287–296.

Uchibe, E. and Doya, K. (2007). Constrained reinforcement learning from intrinsic and extrinsic rewards. In *Proceedings of 6th IEEE International Conference on Developmental Learning*, held London, UK, pp. 163–168.

Uchibe, E. and Doya, K. (2008). Finding intrinsic rewards by embodied evolution and constrained reinforcement learning. *Neural Networks*, **21**(10), 1447–1455.

Usui, Y. and Arita, T. (2003). Situated and embodied evolution in collective evolutionary robotics. In *Proceedings of the 8th International Symposium on Artificial Life and Robotics*, held Beppu, Japan, pp. 212–215.

Watson, R. A., Ficici, S. G., and Pollack, J. B. (2002). Embodied evolution: distributing an evolutionary algorithm in a population of robots. *Robotics and Autonomous Systems*, **39**, 1–18.

Wiewiora, E. (2003). Potential-based shaping and Q-value initialization are equivalent. *Journal of Artificial Intelligence Research*, **19**, 205–208.

Wischmann, S., Stamm, K., and Wörgötter, F. (2007). Embodied evolution and learning: the neglected timing of maturation. In *Advances in Artificial Life: 9th European Conference on Artificial Life*, held Lisbon, Portugal. Berlin: Springer, pp. 284–293.

7 A neuromorphically inspired architecture for cognitive robots

Mitch Wilkes, Erdem Erdemir, and Kazuhiko Kawamura

7.1 Introduction

After several decades of developmental research on intelligent robotics in our lab, we began to focus on the realization of mammalian adaptability functions for our upper-body humanoid robot ISAC (Intelligent Soft Arm Control) described in Kawamura *et al.* (2000, 2004). Currently, most engineering solutions used in robot designs do not have this level of learning and adaptation. Mammalian adaptability is highly desirable in a robot, because mammals are singularly adaptable goal-directed agents. Mammals learn from experiences with a distinctive degree of flexibility and richness that assures goal accomplishment by a very high proportion of individuals. Thus, in the future, robot capability will be substantially advanced once robots can actively seek goal-directed experiences and learn about new tasks under dynamic and challenging environments.

Seeking inspiration for how to achieve this goal, we look to the mammalian brain; in particular, to the structural and functional commonalities observed across mammalian species. From rodents to humans, mammals share many neural mechanisms and control processes relevant to adaptability. Mammals typically accomplish goals in a timely fashion, in situations from the familiar to the new and challenging. Moreover, mammals learn how to function effectively, with few innate capabilities and with little or no supervision of their learning. Albeit with many gaps in knowledge of what makes the human brain distinctively capable, enough seems to be known about the whole mammalian brain to inform architectural analysis and embodied modeling of mammalian brains.

Building upon humanoid robot research in our lab (Kawamura *et al.*, 2008) herein we describe the neuromorphically inspired cognitive architecture that we are implementing. Due to the size and complexity of the overall system, it is not practical to describe it all in detail here. Thus we focus on a more detailed discussion of our recent work on affordances and working memory. We describe cognitive models for affordance learning and report the results of learning task general knowledge from its experiences. From this we argue that, relative to prior approaches to goal-accomplishing robots (e.g. Fitzpatrick *et al.*, 2003; Stoytchev, 2005), the approach described in this chapter

Neuromorphic and Brain-Based Robots, eds. Jeffrey L. Krichmar and Hiroaki Wagatsuma. Published by Cambridge University Press. © Cambridge University Press 2011.

takes additional steps toward allowing robots to systematically learn how to integrate perception, action, task, and goal information from a relatively small number of experiences, so as to generate adaptive behaviors efficiently and flexibly. As such, we see the present findings as advancing the computational intelligence research agenda to realize mammalian adaptability within embodied artificial agents. A portion of the architecture, the working memory system, has also been implemented on a mobile robot. In the interests of illustrating the diversity of the approach, we also describe the application of the working memory system to a mobile robot for learning a visually guided navigation task.

7.2   Neuromorphically inspired cognitive architecture for a humanoid robot

"Cognition is a term referring to the mental processes involved in gaining knowledge and comprehension, including thinking, knowing, remembering, judging and problem solving. These are higher-level functions of the brain and encompass language, imagination, perception and planning" (About.com, 2011). Due to this broad definition, the task of developing a general cognitive architecture and subsequent computational models is extremely difficult. Nevertheless, cognitive architectures are designed to propose structural properties capturing key cognitive processes that exist in biological cognitive systems such as humans.

7.2.1   ISAC cognitive architecture

ISAC cognitive architecture was originally implemented as a multiagent based system to realize multilevel (e.g. reactive, routine, and deliberative) cognitive control functions (Kawamura *et al.*, 2008). The organization of ISAC's concurrently executing software modules mimics that of the mammalian brain in a number of ways, as illustrated in Figure 7.1. As shown, information about the external environment enters through the perceptual agents of the Perception-Action System. This information is stored in the Short Term Sensory Memory which makes it available to the Central Executive Agent (CEA). The CEA is composed of systems for goals and motivations, decision making, relational mapping, and internal rehearsal. A Working Memory (WM) System focuses attention onto the most relevant information and supports the decision making capability. Additionally, a Long Term Memory (LTM) contains what the robot already knows such as behaviors, etc. Finally, action on the external environment is accomplished by controlling the actuators through the Control Agents.

Key system components involving affordance learning are:

- *Relational mapping system*: Many brain regions, such as those within the hippocampus, perform statistical learning resulting in relational/associative organization of sensed experiences and procedural and declarative knowledge. ISAC has a set of relational mapping tools, geared toward the learning of affordance relations, that has a growing complement of statistical learning techniques.

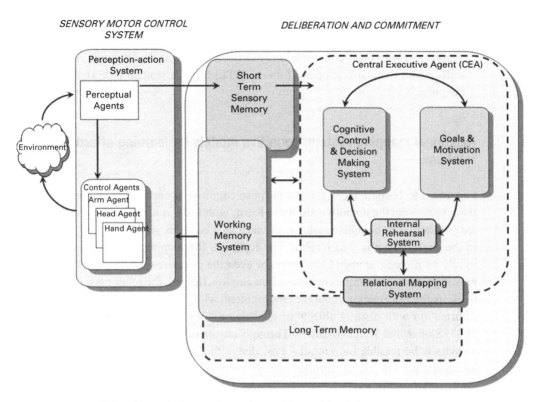

SENSORY MOTOR CONTROL SYSTEM

DELIBERATION AND COMMITMENT

Figure 7.1 ISAC (Intelligent Soft Arm Control) cognitive architecture.

- *Working memory system*: Dorsal–lateral prefrontal regions of the brain are thought to contain something akin to a scratchpad working memory, the content of which is biased both by emotional processes and by associations. ISAC similarly has a scratchpad working memory that emulates the registration, decay, and limited capacity of the brain's working memory. We have constructed a robotic working memory system whose implementation is supported by a software toolkit (Kawamura *et al.*, 2008). This particular module has also been implemented on a mobile robot and is reported herein.
- *Internal rehearsal system (IRS)*: To determine the importance of events, and to decide what to do in response, the human brain's prefrontal regions perform internal simulation of perception and action, both to revisit and to generalize from prior experiences, and to forecast likely outcomes of action alternatives (Hesslow, 2002). These capabilities are encapsulated in a distinct computational module called the internal rehearsal system.
- *Memory systems*: Organization of memory in the brain is quite different from the organization of data in a computer. Thus, we should not dismiss the possibility that the latter could resemble the former. ISAC memory structure is modular and currently divided into three components: short-term memory (STM), long-term memory (LTM), and the working memory system (WMS). Inspired by the work by Kanerva

(1988), we are also looking into sparse vector representation as a candidate unifying memory representation for ISAC memory systems. Such representation has much in common with other extensible array structures such as the Dynamic Array of the well-known Standard Template Library (STL) and the general data representation language XML.

7.3   Relational mapping system: cognitive models for learning affordance relations

For robots to become more general-purpose cognitive agents it will be necessary for them to possess the cognitive ability to learn, with little or no supervision, the knowledge required to complete tasks in the face of a complex stochastic nature of states in the environment in which robots are deployed. It is impractical in these situations to rely on preprogrammed knowledge, or even the preset reward functions that many existing robotic learning techniques often employ. Instead, the robot must mine statistical, spatial information about the environment, while simultaneously associating this information with distinct objects or goal-specific appraisals (Modayil and Kuipers, 2007; Stober and Kuipers, 2008). Through unsupervised statistical learning, it will eventually be feasible for a robot – provided with a set of goals, an action repertoire, and sufficient sensing capabilities – to develop its own ontology for comprehending (a) its situation, (b) its own functional capacities within that situation, and (c) the situation-based appraisals required to achieve goal-directed leverage of such capacities. Ultimately, what will be represented within the robot are task-specific relational goal-situation-action sets, namely, affordance relations, and the outcomes/evaluations associated with each set.

There are various methods for creating goal-situation-action sets and creating associations across such sets. Many of these methods also incorporate outcome information like an extra parameter or an indexing measure. In our lab we have investigated relational mapping techniques based on Gaussian mixture models (GMMs) (Calinon et al., 2007) and self-organizing maps (SOMs) (Kohonen, 1988). Each technique is fundamentally different in its instantiation, yet both provide similar functionality by creating goal-specific, general representations of situations, actions, and the outcomes achieved. These techniques statistically mine goal-relevant outcome knowledge from the agent's own experience. As a result, the representations formed are unique to the system that acquired this experience. Long-term memory is used as the experiential database that informs the formation of the relational maps. Long-term memory is ideally suited for this function because it already contains information related to specific goal-situation-action sets (Gordon et al., 2009). As they are detected, new situations elicit relational knowledge, which is used to drive action selection.

Using relational mapping in robotics is becoming more common. For example, Kawewong et al. (2008) applied self-organizing incremental neural networks (SOINN) (Shen and Hasegawa, 2005) to obtain spatial common patterns (SCP) for cognitive mapping to traverse mazes (see Kawewong et al., 2008, for details on SCP). Strosslin *et al.* (2005) used recurrent neural networks to represent navigation information related to location and action. These networks are trained from experience using Hebbian learning. Finally, the method described by Kuipers *et al.* (2004) uses the statistical-based SLAM method (Thrun *et al.*, 2005) to derive local maps, while hierarchical and topological information is simultaneously used to derive the relationships between local map features and actions. Like other work on relational mapping, the SLAM technique is primarily focused on localization and navigation of the external environment. By contrast, our work with relational maps focuses on localization and mapping of the internal decision space instantiated by the detection of external events in light of the system goals.

7.3.1 Internal rehearsal system

Neuroscience and computational neuroscience has recently made major advances in understanding at the systems level of mental rehearsal, which we call internal rehearsal from the point of view of robotics. Neuroscientists study how infants do physical activities, such as reaching, shaking, and holding, to explore the world, predict the outcomes of their activities, and develop motor skills (Gibson, 2000). As development proceeds, these activities become more controlled and goal oriented, which are the first steps towards creating affordance relations.

Recent findings in neuroscience showed that mental/internal rehearsal is as important as physical motor training. The ability to internally rehearse possible future steps of action in the mind is an important cognitive skill of the advanced human brain. Internal rehearsal is an active process during which the human internally simulates an action by activating an internal representation of an action within working memory, without any corresponding sensory input. In correlation with this, internal rehearsal is a "training method" by which the internal reproduction of a given act is repeated extensively with the intention of learning a new ability or improving performance (Pascual-Leone *et al.*, 1995; Gentili *et al.*, 2006; Allami *et al.*, 2008). It requires people to maintain and manipulate information (remembered past experiences) in their working memory and to be able to generalize, which in turn speeds up the learning process. Moreover, for tasks requiring embodied enactment that is both overt and skilled, mental rehearsal combined with physical practice has been found to facilitate the acquisition of the skill, yielding a more efficient and/or effective performance compared with physical practice alone (Pascual-Leone *et al.*, 1995).

It is known that humans are able to use sensory experiences in the absence of external stimuli, as illustrated by experimental results by, for example, Lee and Thompson (1982). It thus seems reasonable to assume the existence of an "inner sense" and internal rehearsal where sensory experiences and consequences of different behaviors may be anticipated.

The idea of the existence of such an inner sense (or model), however, does not necessarily go against the theory of embedded intelligence advocated by a number of researchers (e.g. Brooks, 1986; Clark, 1997) who de-emphasize the role of internal world models and instead emphasize the situated and embodied nature of intelligence.

An alternative to classical internal world models is the "simulation hypothesis" by Hesslow (2002) which accounts for the "inner world" in terms of internal simulation of perception and behavior. Our approach may be termed as a "grounded internal simulation" utilizing one type of internal representation of perception and behavior. Roy *et al.* (2004) used the term "mental model" to produce an internal model of the environment by projecting the external world through the robot's perceptual system onto its internal model. This internal model is constantly kept in synchronization with the physical environment as the robot executes tasks and continuously perceives the changes in the real world. This approach enables robots to make extensive use of their visualization abilities for spatial language understanding as well as assisting humans in various tasks. Our internal rehearsal model is similar to the inner world or the mental model proposed by Hesslow and Roy, respectively.

7.3.2   Design of the internal rehearsal system

Brain-inspired internal simulation research has now moved into the robotics field. For example, Shanahan (2006) proposed a cognitive architecture that combines internal simulation with Baars' Global Working Theory (1988) for a mobile robot. Shanahan's architecture diagram is a top-level diagram involving two sensorimotor loops: the reactive or first-order loop and the cognitive or higher-order loop. The first-order loop involves the sensory cortex (SC), motor cortex (MC), and basal ganglia (BG). This loop directly maps sensory input to motor actuation. The higher-order loop internally rehearses the decision from the first-order loop and changes the output of the system based on the observation of this rehearsal through the amygdala (Am) and surrounding emotional and memory system such as the limbic lobe in the brain.

In our architecture, the central executive agent (CEA) is responsible for the cognitive response, as shown in Figure 7.1. The internal rehearsal system (IRS) takes the working memory chunks as input along with the current internal and external state and attempts to rehearse the execution of any behaviors found in working memory. Once rehearsal is completed, the rehearsed result in the form of an augmented state representation is sent to the rule-based CEA within the cognitive control and decision making system. If IRS predicts failure on the task, CEA will suppress the arm agents, stopping the current behavior from being executed. If CEA can find a second behavior that can be used to complete the task, this information is sent to working memory, replacing the current behavior chunk. The arm agent begins performing the new action and IRS begins a new rehearsal.

7.3.3   Internal rehearsal to learn affordance relations

A promising approach we are currently focusing on to advance the robotic action selection mechanism is to train a robot so that it learns which situational features are most important to accomplish tasks across the broad range of changing circumstances. In our implementation, the affordance relations that connect situational features to behavioral repertoires are being used. As the robot learns to relate perceived situations to actions that help it achieve its goals, the robot is likely to perform more adeptly. For a robot to come to recognize affordance relations from its limited experiences, it needs to revisit and to reconsider its own experiences. Internal rehearsal was used to statistically estimate outcomes of possible actions, thereby increasing the efficiency and effectiveness with which the robot learns affordance relations on its own.

Experimental results 1: Collision detection

This subsection presents a case study on the task of reaching for a named object involving internal rehearsal as sense, memory, and planning are all required and the implementation is developed of an "inner sense" where sensory experiences and consequences of different behaviors may be anticipated.

The following experiment (Hall, 2007) is designed to evaluate how CEA and IRS work together. The experiment involves two percepts: Barney toy doll (target) and a Lego toy (obstacle) (Figure 7.2).

1. A task to reach-to-Barney is given to ISAC. ReachRight behavior is immediately placed by CEA and Barney into the working memory system as chunks.
2. Using the chunks, IRS will try to reach to the Barney with the right arm, but predicts a collision with the Lego toy.
3. CEA will suppress the arm agent based on this prediction from IRS.
4. CEA will use the episodic retrieval technique using key words and replace the behavior chunk ReachRight to ReachLeft.
5. IRS will reach to the Barney with the virtual left arm. This reach will be successful.
6. CEA will let the arm agent proceed to reach to the Barney using the left arm.

Collision detection techniques for IRS

The collision detection techniques used by the IRS involved virtual spheres around each joint of the arm that provide virtual force feedback. The approach is described in detail in Charoenseang (1999). The positions of the arms are computed from the measured joint angles of the arms of ISAC. The positions of objects in the robot's workspace are determined through vision. These spheres were designed to prevent both arms from colliding with an object or each other. The key to the spherical collision detection method is the distance from the center of one sphere to another. A virtual collision occurs when two spheres touch, and if a collision occurs with the right or left arm, the arm physically moves so that the colliding spheres no longer touch.

IRS uses this collision sphere concept in a different manner. Instead of using spheres around the elbow, the wrist, and the end effector, IRS models a detected object as a sphere as shown in Figure 7.2. A similar idea was used in obstacle avoidance for mobile robots by Vikenmark and Minguez (2006). In the next subsection we discuss how this method is used to predict whether a choice of action will lead to a collision.

Performance

When ISAC was given a command to reach to the Barney, CEA placed two chunks "ReachRight" and "Barney" into the working memory. Both the arm agent and IRS

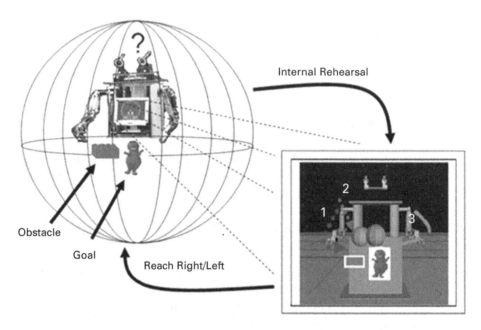

Figure 7.2   Concept of an internal rehearsal system "grounded simulation." The ISAC simulator displays a Barney doll and Lego toy as spheres and gives its decision.

began to process these chunks. IRS completed the computation within 3.2 seconds and sent its results to the CEA. At the same time, the activator agent sent a motion command to the right arm agent to perform the reaching motion. The right arm agent would take 11 seconds to perform this type of reach if no obstacle existed.

When IRS finished, it found a collision and sent the specific time when the collision would have occurred if it had kept executing the reaching behavior to CEA. The left image in Figure 7.3 shows the trajectories of the right arm collision points during the rehearsal. CEA took this result and determined that it did not reach to the Barney. CEA then suppressed the arm agent and prevented the right arm from further action.

CEA then decided to use the left arm and replaced the working memory chunks with "ReachLeft" and "Barney." IRS and the activator agent were once again initiated, and IRS internally rehearsed the reach skill and determined no collision with the Lego toy as shown in the right image in Figure 7.3. Both the wrist and end-effector points entered the Barney percept sphere on the sixteenth step out of the total of 69 interpolation steps. CEA determines this as a success and did not impede the activator agent, thus allowing ISAC to reach to Barney using the left arm. Figure 7.4 illustrates the entire rehearsal process.

Experimental results 2: Internal rehearsal using affordance relations

This experiment introduces a new approach for robots to learn general affordance relations from their experience. Our approach is based on the following two issues:

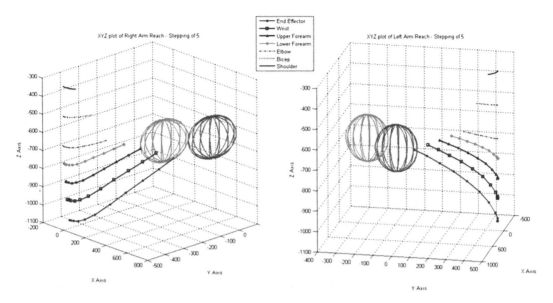

Figure 7.3 The ISAC simulator uses Internal Rehearsal System to create trajectories for the right arm and the left arm. The light gray sphere (left) represents the Lego toy and the darker gray sphere represents the Barney toy. These spheres are used in the collision detection algorithm.

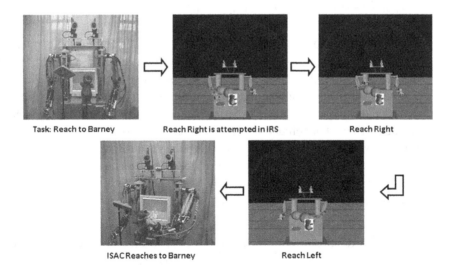

Figure 7.4 ISAC created an inner world and represented the objects as spheres. It uses these spheres to detect collisions and gave a decision to use one of its hands to reach an object.

1. The affordances are modeled as statistical relations among actions, object properties, and the effects of actions on objects, in the context of a goal that specifies preferred effects and outcomes.
2. The robot engages in internal rehearsal by playing out virtual scenarios grounded in, yet different from, actual experiences to exploit the general-knowledge potential of actual experiences.

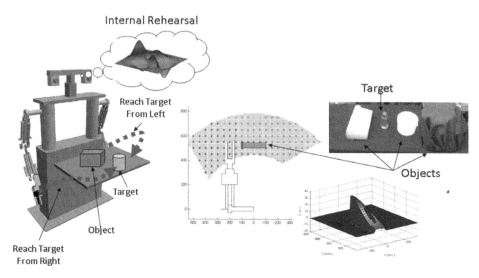

Figure 7.5   The ISAC simulator and internal rehearsal using impedance surfaces (Erdemir *et al.*, 2008a) (© 2008 IEEE).

The experimental results on traversability affordance learning using ISAC are shown in Figure 7.5 (Erdemir *et al.*, 2008a, 2008b).

Experimental method

In this experiment, a different shape of gripper was mounted on each robot arm, as depicted in Figure 7.6. Objects of varying shapes were then presented in the workspace. The heights and edges of objects were determined using simple stereo vision and edge detection techniques. A human experimenter provided the information whether an arm reached the target or collided with an obstacle. The reason why a human experimenter was involved in this experiment was to keep the vision algorithm as simple as possible and get rid of complicated vision-based collision detection algorithms. The experimenter's information was used to build GMMs and for the estimation maximization algorithm. The experiment can be summarized in four steps:

1. The first step of the experiment was to generate collision data during the babbling stage. ISAC attempted to reach to a number of goal objects placed by a human trainer throughout the workspace. Since ISAC had no prior knowledge of collision, it naively plotted paths (using internal rehearsal) and attempted the shortest path from the starting position to each goal position (Ulutas *et al.*, 2008). If the arm collided with an obstacle, the point at which the collision occurred was recorded (shown as gray squares in Figure 7.5) and the attempt to reach to the goal was terminated.
2. The second step was to summarize and start to generalize the likelihoods of collisions in different regions of space for each arm by using GMM submodels (Calinon *et al.*, 2007; the GMM Toolbox is available at http://lasa.epfl.ch/sourcecode/index.php).

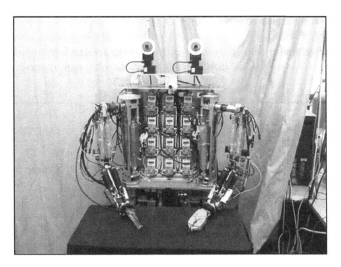

Figure 7.6   ISAC (Intelligent Soft Arm Control) humanoid robot (© 2008 IEEE).

3. The third step involved visually discriminating the edges of the otherwise completely unfamiliar objects and fusing these edge data with the collision data, to create the virtual-high impedance Gaussian surfaces.
4. The final step of the experiment involved the internal rehearsal system (IRS). This step creates a Gaussian surface for the current environment comprising unfamiliar objects in a novel configuration. Using these surfaces, IRS evaluates the limits of its kinematics to project whether or not it can traverse the environment with one of its arms and reach the designated goal object without collision. This internal rehearsal allows ISAC to make decisions on possible actions it can take such as:
   • "collision with the left arm, so will use right arm to reach"
   • "collision with the right arm, so will use left arm to reach"
   • "collision with the both arms, so will not do anything" and
   • "no collision with either arm, so will use one of the arms to reach."

Performance

These outcomes of the IRS were evaluated for adequacy and for optimality by a human experimenter observing the performance of the system. One hundred test scenarios were presented to the system and the IRS had to come up with solutions. Eight of these scenarios were randomly selected from the 100 and are shown in Table 7.1, where each row of the table describes one scenario, the IRS result, and the comments of a human experimenter or observer. We have also seen the very similar results in real experiments using ISAC. For all trials, ISAC exhibited adequate performance; that is, ISAC chose a course of action that would not result in a collision. Of the trials 8% resulted in suboptimal actions; that is, there was a collision-free action ISAC could have taken but ISAC did not discover the action. In the table, the plus sign represents the target, and

Table 7.1. Internal rehearsal experiment results. (© 2008 IEEE)

The plus sign represents the target and the other objects (rectangle, cylinder, triangle, and the block arc) represent the impediment objects. In every trial, ISAC tries to reach the plus sign by traversing through obstacles.

Trial #	The environment	IRS output	The human experimenter
1		It can only reach from left, use left arm	Correct
2		It can only reach to object from right, use right arm	Correct
3		It can not reach to object, stop	Correct
4		It can reach to target using both arms, select one	Correct
5		It can only reach to object from right, use right arm	Correct, but it can reach from left also

Table 7.1. (*cont.*)

Trial #	The environment	IRS output	The human experimenter
6	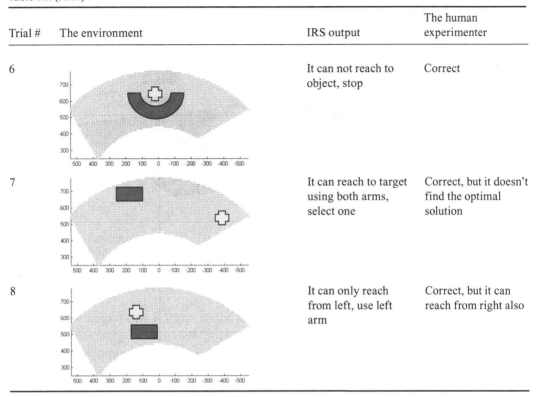	It can not reach to object, stop	Correct
7		It can reach to target using both arms, select one	Correct, but it doesn't find the optimal solution
8		It can only reach from left, use left arm	Correct, but it can reach from right also

the other objects, rectangle, cylinder, triangle, and the block arc represent objects that form obstacles to reaching the target.

During the experiments, we discovered an interesting result: the impact of the shape of the gripper on collision probability and the formation of impedance surfaces as shown in Figure 7.7. In simulation, the shape of the gripper was an intrinsic part of the simulation and it had no effect on experiments. In the real-world experiment, we found that since we did not predefine the exact gripper shape for each arm, additional collision data were gathered near the edges of the obstacles. These data were found to follow a Gaussian distribution. We therefore added an additional term to the collision probability to represent different grippers used. For example, given an object, first the edges were found and the impedance surface was calculated around this object as a conditional probability of collision occurrence by combining of GMM submodels and the Gaussian distribution of the specific hand. This in turn yielded the result that ISAC was willing to move the arm with the smaller gripper closer to an obstacle than the other arm. This shows that ISAC is beginning to learn how to use each gripper distinctively (Erdemir *et al.*, 2008a).

We analyzed ISAC's performance on traversability affordances giving attention to the correctness of the decisions that it made during the reaching task. For example, when ISAC gave a decision that it could not reach to the target by either

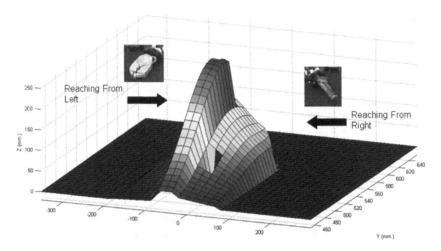

Figure 7.7   The impedance surface created for an object located at (0, 550). The impedance surface does not allow the left hand to reach the object, but ISAC can reach the object using its right hand (Erdemir *et al.*, 2008a) (© 2008 IEEE).

hand, but reached the target by one of its hands when it was forced by suppressing IRS, this was counted as a wrong decision. When ISAC gave a decision that it could reach the target but could not reach after the trial, we counted this also a wrong decision.

7.4   Working memory system

Complex robots are typically bombarded with a large number of stimuli, especially when the robot has a sufficiently sophisticated visual system. In these cases of large numbers of stimuli impinging on the robot, attention to the stimulus (i.e. knowing what to pay attention to and what to ignore) is vital. The limited capacity property of a working memory system provides focus for the robot to search for appropriate actions in order to accomplish the given tasks. In fact, the key point faced by the working memory system that is utilized in this proposed robot architecture is the determination of which chunks[1] of information should be actively retained in the working memory, and which may be safely discarded, for the critical task success. Therefore, it may be appropriate to make use of a working memory model for the developmental problem of learning the proper stimuli in order to trigger an action: the response. A straightforward approach for a critical selection mechanism would be to write procedures or methods that could be used to determine which chunks are essential for a particular task. In the proposed architecture, more general and adaptive learning methods are pursued.

---

[1] In this context, the term "chunks" is used to refer to the memory items that are utilized by the working memory.

The working memory model that is used in this architecture facilitates an adaptive mechanism that intelligently updates the contents of the memory by *learning* from *experience* (Phillips and Noelle, 2005). A toolkit, WMtk, for implementing this model is presented in Phillips and Noelle (2005) and Skubic *et al.* (2004). We should note that in this section, words such as "doing," "acting," or "selecting" may appear in descriptions of the role of working memory, and these are not the usual terms for describing working memory function, especially in the biological literature. Here we take a more engineering-oriented point of view in which overall functionality is examined rather than focusing on specific biological details. In the sense that a working memory system learns to act as a sort of gate or selector for which information should be retained and which should be discarded, these engineering-oriented terms are appropriate.

The WMtk (Skubic *et al.*, 2004) essentially implements the computational model of working memory updating, which is grounded in interactions between the prefrontal cortex and the dopamine system and utilizes a neural network version of the temporal difference (TD) learning algorithm. It contains classes and methods for constructing a working memory system to select working memory contents. The toolkit is very flexible and configurable, such that it lets the designer adjust several parameters, such as the working memory size, learning rate, exploration rate, and so on. Moreover, the WMtk requires several user-defined functions to determine how the reward of the current time step is going to be produced, or how the contents of the working memory will be released when no longer needed for the system. Even though the basis of the WMtk relies on established reinforcement learning techniques, the most distinctive feature of the toolkit is that it is not limited to selecting one item out of a small fixed discrete set of items, as most of the traditional reinforcement learning systems select. The toolkit explores every possible combination of collection of chunks, which can be fit within the limited capacity of the working memory. The combination of chunks which provides the highest estimate value of the future reward is selected and the chunk in this combination is retained in the working memory. This feature of the WMtk can be very useful in robotic applications. The robot is not limited to only one single item to consider. For instance, in many applications a landmark location is represented by only one percept. However, a landmark location may be represented as a combination of percepts, which may help the efficiency of the robot's localization process. In addition, this would also help to increase the number of unique landmark locations in the navigation path of the robot.

A specific case, which briefly demonstrates the working principles of the WMtk, is shown in Figure 7.8. Four chunks are provided as an input vector along with the state and reward signals. The working memory system will then assess the value of these various chunks given the current system state and/or the state of the environment. The center component represents the WMtk itself as well as the chunks that are held in the working memory store. The interpretations of the chunks for our system are also depicted. In this case, depending on the state and reward criteria, WMtk decides to hold on to chunk3 from the input chunk vector and chunk7'which is already held in the working memory from the previous time steps. Details of the WMtk design principles can be found in Skubic *et al.* (2004).

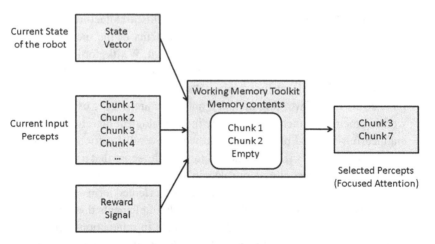

Figure 7.8   An example which demonstrates WMtk's working principles.

7.4.1   The cognitive structure: the perceptual system and the working memory structure combined

Our mobile robot is a Pioneer 2AT with a consumer grade digital video camera mounted on it pointing forward and slightly downward. It uses a robust image segmentation method based on very high-dimensional color histograms. The visual system has been described elsewhere (Wilkes *et al.*, 2005; Hunter *et al.*, 2008; Wang *et al.*, 2009) and will not be described here. In the examples described herein, the robot's vision system had been trained via supervised learning on the main percepts in the robot's environment. All that is necessary for our purposes here is to know that the result is an image that has been segmented into these percepts. After the segmented image has been obtained, the final stage of the perceptual system is to produce inputs for the working memory system, referred to as "chunks," in order for the robot to acquire sensory–motor associations to guide its actions. The input chunks for the working memory system are the locations and some other properties that describe moderately large regions, or "blobs," produced by the segmentation process. Each blob represents a specific cluster, or percept, in the feature space, but it also represents a somewhat large grouping, or clustering, of pixels in the image space. This simultaneous clustering in both the feature space and the image space is usually indicative of a meaningful percept, whereas percepts that tend to show up only as scattered very small spots in the segmented image are regarded as substantially less meaningful in this work. A typical segmentation result is given in Figure 7.9.

Since this architecture is applied to a mobile robot platform, the connected-component labeling algorithm is only applied to the lower half of the entire image. It is assumed that the objects that appear in the upper half contain many distracting percepts from distant objects. Also, distant objects experience greater variability in lighting conditions. This also helps to reduce the number of inputs for the working memory system to consider, as well as to improve the performance of the perceptual system.

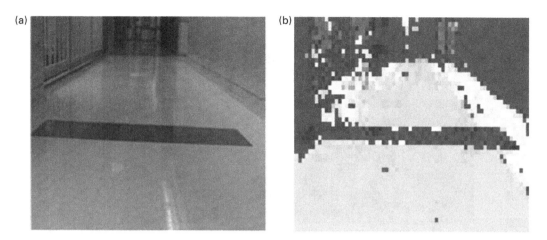

Figure 7.9   A typical segmentation result of the system. (a) The environment. (b) The segmentation result.

The next section describes the environment where the robot will be operating. The remainder of Section 7.4 describes a sequence of learning tasks that build upon one another. The learning is accomplished by way of the learning mechanisms built into the WMtk for the purposes of focusing attention onto the most salient percepts for accomplishing the task. In the first task the robot learns the meanings of the percepts relative to motion. In the second, the robot learns which percepts are most important for identifying a landmark location, and in the third the robot learns a more complex navigation task. This demonstrates the ability of a working memory system to facilitate learning complex tasks.

7.4.2   Environment for vision-guided navigation

The navigation takes place in the hall outside of the Intelligent Robotics Laboratory in Featheringill Hall at Vanderbilt University. The hallway has yellow floor tiles in the center with white tiles along the edges near the wall. The hall also has periodically located black tiles across the center of the hall forming a decorative stripe. The walls consist of wood panels, light blue painted wall sections, and a light blue railing. There are also brick columns and blue floor tiles at the ends of the hall. The hallway is shown in Figure 7.10.

7.4.3   Learn percepts for motion

In order for a robot to navigate safely, it has to move in open space. Therefore, the first step is to learn the percepts that will yield an open path for navigation through the robot's own interaction with the world.

Once meaningful blobs or percepts are obtained from the images acquired from the camera, the robot needs to learn the association of the percepts with the task of

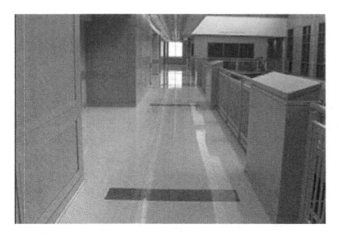

Figure 7.10   The navigation environment.

motion. In other words, the robot needs to determine whether the percepts represent an obstacle or an open space, since the robot does not have any prior information about these percepts. In order to have such association in this task, the reward criterion for the working memory (WM) system is selected to be the distance traveled by the robot, since percepts that are in the open space allow the robot to move further. At each time step, the robot is allowed to move five meters. The WM size parameter is set to 1 in order to assess the percepts individually. Therefore, the WM can only select one of the available input chunks at each time step. At first, the robot captures an image, performs segmentation, and locates the percepts in the image. Initially, since there is no reward information (i.e. no displacement is made by the robot), the WM randomly chooses one of the available chunks. Next, the robot directs itself toward the selected chunk and proceeds forward for five meters or until sonar sensor indicates an obstacle, which forces the robot to stop. The distance taken by the robot is returned as a reward for the WM system and associated with the selected chunk previously. If the robot moved for five meters then it will receive the maximum amount of reward, if not, it will receive a partial reward which is the distance it traveled. The same procedure is taken, starting from the first step, multiple times, which allows the WM system to intelligently update its internal parameters associated with each available chunk in the environment, depending on the reward received at each episode.

Figure 7.11 shows the plot of the cumulative reward weight associations for each percept versus the number trials. The percepts that are detected decrease in value until around episodes 50–70 where the dominant percept, labeled as "YellowFloor," begins to grow in a linear fashion. All percepts that are not encountered often do not change much or at all from the initial value. Note that only percepts that are located at the lower half of the image are presented to the working memory. Therefore, some of the percepts are encountered rarely during the motion of the robot, even though they are still in the long-term memory of the robot. After "YellowFloor" percept is determined to be the dominant percept associated with open path, it is blocked at the ninetieth

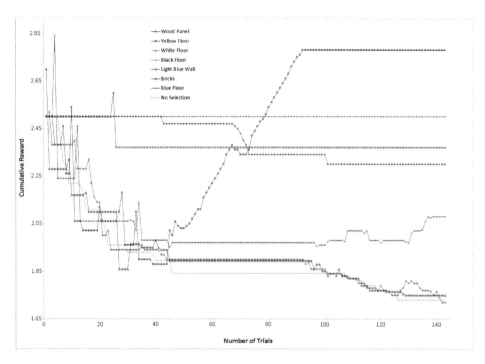

Figure 7.11 Plot for the reward weights for each percept for each trial. Percept "YellowFloor" blocked at episode 90. "BlackFloor" percept seems to be the second option for the open path.

episode to observe how the remaining percepts will be affected in working memory. The blocking of the dominant percept allows for further development of the other percepts, clearly showing a second best option for the open path. Note that the percept labeled "BlackFloor" begins to rise and other percepts representing less motion, such as the "WoodPanel," are further decreased.

7.4.4   Learning a landmark location

In a navigation task, landmarks are essential, in the sense that the robot might take an action on a specific landmark. In the first stage, the robot learned which percept will provide the open path to move safely. Now, it must learn about landmark locations in order to localize itself in the environment. In this stage, the black floor tiles are found to be convenient as landmark locations. This time, the WM size parameter is set to values of 1, 2, and 3 to determine which percept or combinations of percepts should be selected for recognizing a landmark location.

A set of training images is acquired from the environment to represent landmark and non-landmark locations, as seen in Figure 7.12. The images are labeled as either a landmark image (i.e. the image contains percepts that may be used as a landmark) or a non-landmark image (i.e. no landmark percepts are present). As mentioned in the previous paragraph, the presence of a black floor tile in the foreground is an indication of a

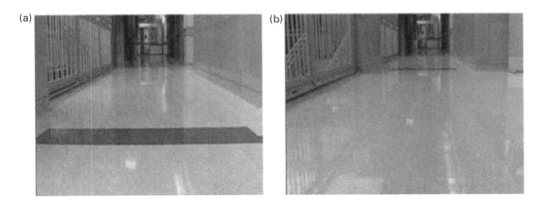

Figure 7.12   (a) A landmark image. (b) A non-landmark image.

landmark; however, the robot is not given this information directly. It must learn which percept(s) indicate a landmark. The number of landmark and non-landmark images is equal in the collected set of images. The training images from the set are selected randomly and processed in order to obtain the chunks for the WM system. Each percept that is available in the image is presented twice to the WM, once as a chunk that indicates the presence of a landmark and once as a chunk indicating no landmark present, in order to consider all the possibilities for a percept. Once the WM has selected a set of chunks, the selected chunks are examined to see how many indicate the presence of a landmark and how many indicate no landmark is present. Whichever achieves a majority is chosen as the decision on the presence of a landmark. A tie vote is interpreted as a choice of no landmark. If the choice is correct the reward is 1, otherwise it is 0. Each of the WM sizes is trained for both 1000 and 5000 episodes.

The task of learning the landmark location converges quickly in all cases. Table 7.2 shows the correct landmark detection percentages. Examination of the log files of the choices made during training shows a consistent tendency towards percept "BlackFloor_L" (BlackFloor indicating landmark). The WM has shown that it can learn which percepts identify landmark locations quickly and with high accuracy.

7.4.5   Learning a vision-guided navigation task

At this point, the robot knows which percepts yield open space, as well as which percepts are considered to be landmark points. Now the question becomes how the robot can learn to associate a sequence of percepts for open space along with the percepts for landmark points in order to reach a goal position. Once this is achieved, the robot can learn a navigation task and accomplish the task successfully with the aid of its knowledge.

In this final stage, the robot needs to learn a navigation task by utilizing the previously learned behavior for finding the open path, as well as the landmark percept it has learned. It has to associate actions with the sequence of landmarks seen along the

Table 7.2. Percentage of landmark classification

Working memory size	1000 trials (%)	5000 trials (%)
1	98.10	99.52
2	95.50	97.42
3	98.00	99.38

navigation. The objective of the robot is to navigate along the hallway until it reaches the third landmark. Additionally, it should also remember (i.e. exhibit a delayed response) a contingent situation that will change the task completely into a new one. If it sees a contingent percept (i.e. a green ball) along the navigation path, it has to hold on to it until it reaches the last landmark and then come back to its initial position. The delayed response task is widely used in cognitive neuroscience in order to evaluate the properties of working memory (O'Reilly *et al.*, 1999; Hunter *et al.*, 2008). If no green ball is detected along the navigation path, the robot is required to learn to stop at the third landmark. The robot makes a decision, moves with a small distance increment and stops. The time required for this cycle is referred to as one time step. This procedure continues until the navigation is complete. The procedure for experiment 3 is as follows.

Initially, the robot captures an image and segments the percepts in the environment. A list of possible actions, such as "move," "stop," and "turn around" will be presented as input chunks to the working memory. The WM system will be rewarded or punished by the possible actions chosen by the robot along the navigation path. These three action chunks are always provided to the WM in the input chunk vector at each time step.

In addition to the action chunks, the WM is presented with the percepts detected in the environment. However, only "YellowFloor," "BlackFloor," and "GreenBall" percepts are presented, if they are detected by the perceptual system. Since the task requires only remembering the "GreenBall" chunk, the other percepts are treated as distractors, that is to say, the system has to learn that the "YellowFloor" and "BlackFloor" percepts are not important as contingent percepts.

Finally, the WM is also presented with a "Nothing" chunk, meaning that the system does not make any selection. Therefore, the maximum number of chunks that can be presented to the working memory is seven (i.e. "move," "stop," "turn around," "YellowFloor," "BlackFloor," "GreenBall," and "Nothing").

The working memory size is set to two. One slot is dedicated only for an action chunk and the other one is dedicated only for a percept chunk. Thus, the WM is required to *learn* to select an action chunk as well as a percept chunk.

Once the candidate input chunk vector is presented to working memory, a decision is made by the system. The robot either moves, stops, or turns around depending on the action selection made by the working memory at each time step. Furthermore, if a "GreenBall" percept is detected, the WM is expected to remember the "GreenBall" chunk in its second output slot.

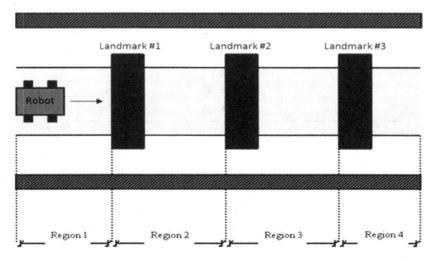

Figure 7.13   The navigation path.

The learning criteria faced by the working memory are not trivial; indeed, they are challenging. The robot needs to learn a considerable amount of information from a large combinatorial chunk space. Thus, the training is performed in a simulation environment and all the possible chunks are presented to the robot at each time step, except the "GreenBall." This chunk is presented only once, randomly at a particular region. The navigation path is depicted in Figure 7.13. The robot is trained for each region (i.e. each of the states from 1 to 4) of the navigation path and a reward value (+1 for positive reward and −1 for negative) is given for correct action and percept choice. Each region represents a state for the WM system. However, in order to speed up the learning, the training state is switched from one to another, only if a set number of positive rewards (defined as the positive reward threshold, PRT) are received in a row at each state. That is, the choices for a particular state must be correctly chosen PRT times in a row before the next state may be trained. For instance, assume that the PRT is 10. A *successful trial* (progress through all the states 1 to 4) is defined as not receiving any negative reward. Therefore, the system must receive 40 positive rewards (10 for each region) in a row in order for the trial to be considered as successful.

Figure 7.14 shows the learning curve of the system, as a plot of successful trials over a sliding 25 point averaging window for 10 000 trials (performed off-line in simulation) and for PRT = 10 and PRT = 20. Table 7.3 shows the number of successful trials for different choices of PRT.

These numbers are not unreasonable, considering the fact that we are imposing a very strict rule that is receiving multiple positive rewards in a row for each region. If at any time step of the training the system fails to choose the correct chunk combination, the whole trial is considered to be an unsuccessful trial. In all of the cases, there is a positive learning trend. As the PRT is increases, the system makes fewer mistakes overall and the speed of the training is significantly increased in terms of episodes.

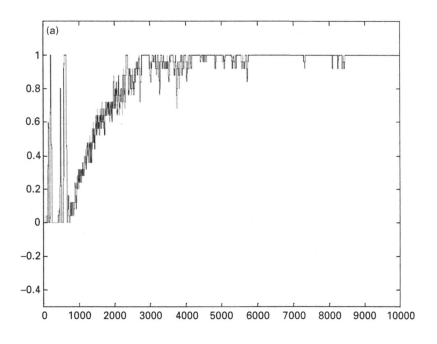

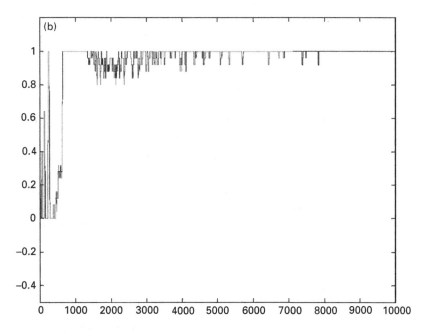

Figure 7.14   Learning curves. (a) PRT = 10, (b) PRT = 20.

Table 7.3. Number of successful trials for 10 000 trials and for different positive reward thresholds

Positive reward threshold	Successful trials (out of 10 000)	Percentage of successful trials
1	7591	75.91
7	8275	82.75
10	8502	85.02
20	9330	93.30

The robot successfully navigated in the hallway and it came back to its initial position when a green ball percept was presented. The robot chose the correct actions in the action selection slot and chose the "Nothing" percept, meaning that no percept is held in the working memory. However, once the contingent percept is presented along the navigation, the robot remembered the contingent percept ("GreenBall") in the percept selection slot of the WM at each time step. Thus, the robot has successfully learned a complex task based on previously learned fundamental behaviors.

7.5   Conclusions

The field of cognitive robotics is attracting an increasing number of researchers from not only robotics and computer science, but from other disciplines such as developmental psychology and neuroscience, as evidenced from other chapters in this volume. This chapter outlined our recent effort to develop a robotic cognitive architecture in which a number of cognitive control loops are running in parallel. Contributions include the implementation of a reflective module called the internal rehearsal system that can internally rehearse the action to help improve task performance, and the use of affordance relations to learn and execute new tasks. Collectively, these cognitive models are expected to realize a certain level of adaptivity in goal accomplishment and decision making for our ISAC humanoid robot. Results of experiments conducted so far are encouraging. The results presented here show the effectiveness of internal rehearsal in enabling a robot to solve task scenarios for which it was not specifically trained. Other results presented show the value of a working memory system for learning complex navigation tasks. We are hoping that our continuous efforts to develop computational cognitive models will further contribute to the field of cognitive robotics.

Acknowledgments
The authors would like to thank Flo Wahidi, Carl Frankel, Mert Tugcu, and Jonathan Hunter in the Center for Intelligent Systems. This work was supported in part under NSF grant EIA0325641, "ITR: A Biologically Inspired Adaptive Working Memory System for Efficient Robot Control and Learning."

References

About.com (2011). Psychology. Online: http://psychology.about.com/od/cindex/g/def_cognition.htm

Allami, N., Paulignan, Y., Brovelli, A., and Boussaoud, D. (2008). Visuo-motor learning with combination of different rates of motor imagery and physical practice. *Experimental Brain Research*, **184**, 105–113.

Baars, B. J. (1988). *A Cognitive Theory of Consciousness*. Cambridge, UK: Cambridge University Press.

Brooks, R. A. (1986). A robust layered control system for a mobile robot. *IEEE Journal of Robotics and Automation*, **2**, 14–23.

Calinon, S., Guenter, F., and Billard, A. (2007). On learning, representing, and generalizing a task in a humanoid robot. *IEEE Transactions on Systems, Man, and Cybernetics*, Part B, **37**(2), 286–298.

Charoenseang, S. (1999). A PC-based virtual reality system for dual-arm humanoid robot control. Ph.D. Dissertation, Vanderbilt University, Nashville, TN.

Clark, A. (1997). *Being There: Putting Brains, Body, and World Together Again*. Cambridge, MA: MIT Press.

Erdemir, E., Frankel, C.B., Thornton, S., Ulutas, B., and Kawamura, K. (2008a). A robot rehearses internally and learns an affordance relation. In *Proceedings of IEEE International Conference on Development and Learning*.

Erdemir, E., Frankel, C. B., Kawamura, K., *et al.* (2008b). Towards a cognitive robot that uses internal rehearsal to learn affordance relations. In *Proceedings of the IEEE/RSJ International Conference on Intelligent Robots and Systems*, pp. 2016–2021.

Fitzpatrick, P., Metta, G., Natale, L., Rao, S., and Sandini, G. (2003). Learning about objects through action – initial steps towards artificial cognition. In *Proceedings of the IEEE/RSJ International Conference on Intelligent Robots and Systems*, Vol. 3, pp. 3140–3145.

Gentili, R., Papaxanthis, C., and Pozzo, T. (2006). Improvement and generalization of arm motor performance through motor imagery practice. *Neuroscience*, **137**, 761–772.

Gibson, E. (2000). Perceptual learning in development: Some basic concepts. *Ecological Psychology*, **12**(4), 295–302.

Gordon, S. M., Frankel, C. B., and Kawamura, K. (2009). Neuromorphically inspired self-organizing episodic memory for embedded agents. In *Proceedings of 2009 IEEE Symposium Series on Computational Intelligence*.

Hall, J. (2007). Internal rehearsal for a cognitive robot using collision detection. M.S. Thesis, Vanderbilt University, Nashville, TN.

Hesslow, G. (2002). Conscious thought as simulation of behavior and perception. *Trends in Cognitive Science*, **6**, 242–247.

Hunter, J. E., Wilkes, D. M., Levin, D.T., Heaton, C., and Saylor, M. M. (2008). Autonomous segmentation of human action for behaviour analysis. In *Proceedings of the 7th IEEE International Conference on Development and Learning (ICDL)*, held in Monterey, CA, pp. 250–255.

Kanerva, P. (1988). *Sparse Distributed Memory*. Cambridge, MA: MIT Press.

Kawamura, K., Peters, R. A., II, Wilkes, D. M., Alford, W. A., and Rogers, T. E. (2000). ISAC: foundations in human-humanoid interaction. *IEEE Intelligent Systems and Their Applications*, **15**, 38–45.

Kawamura, K., Peters, R. A., II, Bodenheimer, R., *et al.* (2004). Multiagent-based cognitive robot architecture and its realization. *International Journal of Humanoid Robotics*, **1**(1), 65–93.

Kawamura, K., Gordon, S. M., Ratanaswasd, P., Erdemir, E., and Hall, J. F. (2008). Implementation of cognitive control for a humanoid robot. *International Journal of Humanoid Robotics*, **5**(3), 1–40.

Kawewong, A., Honda, Y., Tsuboyama, M., and Hasegawa, O. (2008). A common neural-pattern based reasoning for mobile robot cognitive mapping. In *Proceedings of the INNS-NNN Symposia*. Springer Online, pp. 32–39.

Kohonen, T. (1988). *Self-Organization and Associative Memory*. New York: Springer-Verlag.

Kuipers, B., Modayil, J., Beeson, P., Macmahon, M., and Savelli, F. (2004). Local metrical and global topological maps in the hybrid spatial semantic hierarchy. In *Proceedings of the IEEE International Conference on Robotics and Automation*.

Lee, D.N. and Thompson, J. A. I. (1982). Vision in action: the control of locomotion. In Ingle, D., Gooddale, M. A., and Mansfield, R. J. W. (eds.), *Analysis of Visual Behavior*. Cambridge, MA: MIT Press.

Modayil, J. and Kuipers, B. (2007). Autonomous development of a grounded object ontology by a learning robot. In *Proceedings of the 22nd Conference on Artificial Intelligence*, Vol. 2. AAAI Press, pp. 1095–1101.

O'Reilly, R., Braver, T., and Cohen, J. (1999). A biologically based computational model of working memory. In Miyake, A. and Shah, P. (eds.), *Models of Working Memory: Mechanisms of Active Maintenance and Executive Control*. Cambridge, UK: Cambridge University Press, pp. 375–411.

Pascual-Leone, A., Nguyet, D., Cohen, L. G., *et al.* (1995). Modulation of muscle responses evoked by transcranial magnetic stimulation during the acquisition of new fine motor skills. *Journal of Neurophysiology*, **74**, 1037–1045.

Phillips, J. L. and Noelle, D. C. (2005). A biologically inspired working memory framework for robots. In *Proceedings of the 27th Annual Meeting of the Cognitive Science Society*, held in Stresa, Italy.

Roy, D., Hsiao, K. and Mavridis, N. (2004). Mental imagery for a conversational robot. *IEEE Transactions on Systems, Man, and Cybernetics*, Part B, **34**(3), 1374–1383.

Shanahan, M.P. (2006). A cognitive architecture that combines internal simulation with a global workspace. *Consciousness and Cognition*, **15**, 433–449.

Shen, F. and Hasegawa, O. (2005). An incremental network for online unsupervised classification and topology learning. *Neural Networks*, **19**(1), pp. 90–106.

Skubic, M., Noelle, D., Wilkes, M., Kawamura, K., and Keller, J. M. (2004). A biologically inspired adaptive working memory for robots. *Proceedings of the 2004 AAAI Symposium Series Workshop on Cognitive Science and Robotics*, held in Washington, D.C., pp. 68–75.

Stoytchev, A. (2005). Toward learning the binding affordances of objects: a behavior-grounded approach. *Proceedings of the AAAI Symposium on Developmental Robotics*, held at Stanford University, pp. 17–22.

Strosslin, T., Sheynikhovich, D., Chavariaga, R., and Gerstner, W. (2005). Robust self-localization and navigation based on hippocampal place cells. *Neural Networks*, **18**(9), 1125–1140.

Thrun, S., Burgard, W., and Fox, D. (2005). *Probabilistic Robotics*. Cambridge MA: MIT Press.

Ulutas, B., Erdemir, E., and Kawamura, K. (2008). Application of a hybrid controller with non-contact impedance to a humanoid robot. Proceedings of the *10th IEEE International Workshop on Variable Structure Systems*, pp. 378–383.

Vikenmark, D. and Minguez, J. (2006). Reactive obstacle avoidance for mobile robots that operate in confined 3D workspaces. In *IEEE Mediterranean Electro-technical Conference, MELECON*, pp. 1246–1251.

Wang, X., Tugcu, M., Hunter, J. E., and Wilkes, D. M. (2009). Exploration of configural representation in landmark learning using working memory toolkit. *Pattern Recognition Letters*, **30**(1), 66–79.

Wilkes, D. M., Tugcu, M., Hunter, J. E., and Noelle, D. (2005). Working memory and perception. *Proceedings of 14th Annual IEEE International Workshop on Robot and Human Interactive Communication (RO-MAN 2005)*, pp. 686–691.

8 Autonomous visuomotor development for neuromorphic robots

Zhengping Ji, Juyang Weng, and Danil Prokhorov

8.1 Introduction

It has been a huge challenge to program autonomous robots for unstructured and new environments. Various modules are difficult to program and so is the coordination among modules and motors. Existing neuroanatomical studies have suggested that the brain uses similar mechanisms to coordinate the different sensor modalities (e.g. visual and auditory) and the different motor modalities (e.g. arms, legs, and the vocal tract). Via sensorimotor interactions with the robot's internal and external environments, autonomous mental development (AMD) in this chapter models the brain as not only an information processor (e.g. brain regions and their interconnections), but also the causality for its development (e.g. why each region does what it does). The mechanisms of AMD suggest that the function of each brain region is not preset statically before birth by the genome, but is instead the emergent consequence of its interconnections with other brain regions through the lifetime experience. The experience of interactions not only greatly shapes what each region does, but also how different regions cooperate. The latter seems harder to program than a static function. As a general-purpose model of sensorimotor systems, this chapter describes the developmental program for the visuomotor system of a developmental robot. Based on the brain-inspired mechanisms, the developmental program enables a network to wire itself and to adapt "on the fly" using bottom-up signals from sensors and top-down signals from externally supervised or self-supervised acting activities. These simple mechanisms are sufficient for the neuromorphic Where What Network 1 (WWN-1) to demonstrate small-scale but practical-grade performance for the two highly intertwined problems of vision – attention and recognition – in the presence of complex backgrounds.

8.1.1 Developmental robotics

A robot for unstructured and new environments needs to see, hear, touch, move, manipulate, speak, and perform many other tasks. Conventionally, these robotic functions are hand programmed, each by a different set of techniques. In contrast, there have been no known neuroscience studies that prove the existence of a holistically

Neuromorphic and Brain-Based Robots, eds. Jeffrey L. Krichmar and Hiroaki Wagatsuma. Published by Cambridge University Press. © Cambridge University Press 2011.

aware central controller inside the biological brain. The genomic equivalence principle (e.g. Purves *et al.*, 2004), dramatically demonstrated by mammal cloning, has shown that the genome in the nucleus of any somatic cell (i.e. any cell that forms the body) carries the complete genetic information for normal development (in typical ecological environments) from a single cell to an adult body having 100 trillion cells. This suggests that the basic units of the brain development (and learning) are cells. Based on its genetic and cellular properties, each cell interacts with other cells during its development, including mitosis, differentiation, migration, growth of dendrites and axons, connection, synaptic adaptation, and response generation. Many cells autonomously interact to form tissues, organs, and cortex (e.g. Purves *et al.*, 2004; Sur and Rubenstein, 2005). Thus, for the developmental program (DP) of a developmental agent, we focus on cell mechanisms. Other brain-like properties and capabilities are emergent.

A major characteristic of autonomous mental development is that the DP is not task specific. By task nonspecificity, we mean that the same DP should enable the robot to learn an open number of tasks. One may ask: "If I want my robot to perform only one task $f(O, A, B)$ – pick up an object O from position A and deliver it to position B – why do I need to use a task-nonspecific developmental program?" As discussed in Weng (2009), this is a muddy task measured by factors in five categories. For example, it requires a rich set of capabilities, from dealing with open and new environments, to finding object O from the complex backgrounds at position A, to reaching and grasping the object, to avoiding various obstacles along the way from position A to position B, to identifying the position B, and to placing the object properly in the environment of B. There has been no existing robot software that can deal with this task reliably in open urban environments.

Facing the great challenges from many such robotic tasks, the work of AMD outlined in Weng *et al.* (2001) aims to learn the skills for such and many other tasks using a unified, task-nonspecific DP – not only individual skills themselves, but also recalling the required skills at various task contexts.

It is important to note that by the term *autonomous mental development*, we mean that a robot autonomously develops, regulated by a sensor-effector specific but task-nonspecific DP. By contrast, the term *developmental robotics* has been used in a larger sense, where techniques may involve some task-specific nature, to simulate some aspects of child learning, as surveyed by Lungarella *et al.* (2003) and Asada *et al.* (2009). Here, the word "developmental" in "developmental robotics" was inherited from *developmental psychology*. However, the authors argue that developmental robotics should move toward autonomous mental development.

The general-purpose DP is able to develop a sensorimotor pathway that links many receptors and many effectors. These receptors can be in the retina for vision, in the cochlea for audition, and in the skin for touch. The effectors can be in the arms for pointing and object manipulation, in the vocal tract for talking and language-based communication, and in the legs for walking and navigation.

We are not able to experimentally demonstrate a solution to all these grand challenge capabilities at this point. Here, we take robotic vision as an example of a sensory modality. The other sensory modalities, such as audition and touch (range sensors) follow the same principles. For motor modalities, we consider two effectors and their behavior coordination: a simple arm and a simple vocal tract. We will train the arm for generating only "where" information and train the vocal tract for generating only "what" information, but their behaviors are coordinated based on their experience, taught or practiced. The same effectors should be able to be taught for other information needed for each effector and the required coordination: for example, object distance information for the arm and object orientation information for the arm and the vocal tract. In other words, our principled system example below is sensor and effector specific after training, but not task specific (e.g. not just for recognizing a particular set of objects).

We argue that the perceptual, cognitive, and behavioral skills required by the above tasks require extensive developmental experience – teaching, learning, and practice. In the following, we focus on the developmental program for an early version of a visuomotor system, called Where What Network 1 (WWN-1) (Ji *et al.*, 2008), as a principled system example.

Suppose that the WWN-1 has a camera, which takes images from the environment. The environment may have an object of interest in a complex background. The WWN-1 has two types of robotic effectors. One is a "where" effector (i.e. a simple arm), which tells the location of the object of interest. Although we will use pixel position as the output of the "where" effector, the WWN-1 is able to learn an appropriate representation in the real-world two-dimensional coordinate system. The other effector is a "what" effector (i.e. a simple vocal tract), which tells the type of the attended object, so that the robot can "speak" about the type of the object it is looking at.

8.1.2   Biological architectures

The primate visual pathways have been extensively investigated in neuroscience: branching primarily from the visual cortex area V2, two primary pathways exist, called the dorsal pathway and the ventral pathway, respectively. The dorsal stream begins with V1, through V2, the dorsomedial area and MT (also known as V5), to the posterior parietal cortex. The control of attention employment is believed to mostly take place in the dorsal pathway, sometimes called the "where" pathway after the work by Mishkin *et al.* (1983). The ventral stream begins from V1, through V2, V4, and to the inferior temporal cortex. The ventral stream, also called the "what" pathway after the work by Mishkin *et al.* (1983), is mainly associated with the recognition and identification of visual stimuli.

Attention and recognition are known as a tightly intertwined problem for general scenes. Without attention, recognition cannot do well; recognition requires attended spatial areas for the further processing. Without recognition, attention is limited; attention not only needs bottom-up saliency-based cues, but also top-down target-dependent signals.

The successful modeling of the "where" and "what" pathway involves the integration of bottom-up and top-down cues, such as to provide coherent control signals for the focus of attention, and the interplay between attentional tuning and object recognition. Studies in psychology, physiology, and neuroscience provided computational models for attention (both bottom-up and top-down) and its perspective of object recognition capabilities.

Bottom-up attention

Bottom-up attention, also called saliency-based attention, uses different properties of sensory inputs: for example, color, shape, and illuminance to extract saliency. The first explicit computational model of bottom-up attention was proposed by Koch and Ullman (1985), in which a "saliency map" was used to encode stimuli saliency at every location in the visual scene. More recently, Itti *et al.* (1998) integrated color, intensity, and orientation as basic features, and extracted intensity information in six scales for attention control. Backer *et al.* (2001) applied a similar strategy to an active vision system, called NAVIS (Neural Active VISion), emphasizing the visual attention selection in a dynamic visual scene. Instead of directly using some low-level features like orientation and intensity, they accommodated additional processing to find middle-level features, for example symmetry and eccentricity, to build the feature map.

In contrast to the above bottom-up attention models, our alternative view about the brain's bottom-up attention is that sensory bottom-up saliency is an emergent phenomenon of combined mechanisms – matching between the neuronal input and the neuronal weight vector of the best matched neuron plus the competition (via lateral inhibition) among neurons in the same cortical area. More attended features recruit more neurons, which result in statistically better matches in the feature match, as described in the lobe component analysis (LCA) model for a general purpose cortical area by Weng and Luciw (2009). For example, if the brain attended to yellow flowers more often than attending to green grass when both were present in the past, "yellow flower" neurons match better than "green grass" neurons when there is no top-down bias (although this is very rare). Thus, the top-matched "yellow flower" neuron wins in bottom-up competition. Therefore, in our WWN-1 cortical model, the DP does not statically specify which features are salient – bottom-up saliency is an emergent phenomenon from the experience of WWN-1.

Top-down attention

Volitional shifts of attention are also thought to be performed top-down, through spatially defined weighting of the various feature maps. Early top-down attention models selected the conspicuous positions (bottom-up) regardless of being occupied by objects or not, and then the candidate positions were used to transform (i.e. position-based top-down control) the input image into the master map for further recognition. Olshausen *et al.* (1993) proposed an appearance-kept shift model from a given attention control to achieve position and scale transformation for the assumed succeeding master object map. A top-down attention model was later discussed by Tsotsos *et al.* (1995), who implemented attention selection using a combination of a bottom-up feature extraction scheme and a top-down selective tuning scheme, also for the assumed succeeding master object map. A more extreme view was expressed by the "scanpath theory" of Stark and Choi (1996), in which the control of eye movements was almost exclusively under top-down control. Mozer and Sitton (1998) proposed a model called MORSEL, to combine the object recognition and attention, in which attention was shown to help recognition. A top-down, knowledge-based recognition component, presented by a hierarchical knowledge tree, was introduced by Schill *et al.* (2001), where object classes were defined by several critical points and the corresponding eye movement commands that maximized the information gain. Rao and Ballard (2005) described an approach allowing a pair of cooperating neural networks to estimate object identity and object transformations, respectively.

Aforementioned top-down mechanisms assume that the attention control in terms of location and size ("where") is already given. The above top-down models are about how the attended patch in the retina is translated and scaled to a hypothetically assumed internal *master map* for object recognition. This can be called *attention-guided recognition*.

However, the original top-down attention problem is still open in the direction from "what" to "where": how object type information ("what") is originated and how such a *type-based* attention signal is integrated into the object localization subsystem ("where"). This problem has hardly been addressed computationally so far for general objects. In engineering, there have been very rich algorithms that explicitly search over the entire input image for a particular class of object (e.g. human faces) by Moghaddam and Pentland (1995); Yang *et al.* (2002); Viola and Jones (2004).

Our model does not assume that there is an internal master map. There seems no evidence for its existence. From the above discussion about the way neurons migrate and determine their roles through experience, there is no need to have an internal master map to enable the entire network work as desired. In WWN-1, the top-down signal ("where" or "what") is originated from the corresponding ("where" or "what") motor output, taught by the teacher (environment). When emerging at any time, such top-down attention information has developed top-down wiring to take effect in the earlier layers – boost the pre-action potential of targeted neurons (for the matched location or type) to have an increased pre-action potential in the competition. The neurons that actually win and fire are those that not only match well with the bottom-up inputs (objective evidence) but also match well with the top-down inputs (subjective goal). In other words, our cortical model is different from all the above appearance-kept shift models. Our model does not keep the visual appearance from one layer to the next. Instead, the winner's response provides sufficient information about the bottom-up input (matching a firing neuron with the bottom-up weight vector) and the top-down input (matching a firing neuron with the top-down weight vector). Using this unified mechanism, recognition and attention (bottom-up and top-down) are accomplished in every layer using the aforementioned cortical model LCA (Weng and Luciw, 2009), instead of appearance shift only in earlier layers and recognition only after a hypothetically assumed internal master map.

In summary, top-down attention in our model is a developed *internal action* as originally proposed by the self-aware and self-effecting (SASE) architecture model by Weng (2007).

8.1.3　Biological visuomotor systems

As discussed above, the most striking concept of the developmental architecture of WWN-1 is that we do not assume the existence of an appearance-kept master object map. The extensive back-projections from the motor areas to earlier cortical areas, reported in existing neuroanatomical studies such as those reviewed by Felleman and Van Essen (1991), seem to be consistent with the scheme here. In WWN-1, the "where" motor is an area that is truly type invariant, but not exactly so in any internal map. Likewise, the "what" motor area is an area that is truly location invariant, but not exactly so in any internal map. These motor properties gave advantages for interactive development as external environment (e.g. teacher) can directly observe and shape the motor responses but not the "skull-closed" internal representations. By "skull-closed" we mean that all the internal parts of the network, except its input and output ports that are meant for direct interactions with the environment, are not accessible to the environment during "living" – training and testing. This is analogous to the skull of the human brain, which closes all internal parts of the brain to the external environment. If a trainer interactively examines what is in the "skull" and interactively changes some parameters inside the "skull" during training, he violates the "skull-closed" condition. The goal of using the "closed-skull" concept is to guarantee that the development inside the skull is fully autonomous after the "birth." The "skull-closed" concept is also important to distinguish external actions (e.g. move hands) and internal actions (e.g. attention).

It is important to note that although traditional neural networks use emergent representation, they were not shown to emerge top-down attention for dealing with general objects in complex backgrounds as internal actions.

The following technical characteristics make such work technically novel and challenging:

1. Develop both attention and recognition as ubiquitous internal actions.
2. Integrate bottom-up and top-down attention as concurrent information streams.
3. Enable supervised and unsupervised learning in any order suited for development.
4. Local-to-global invariance from early to later processing, through multiscale receptive fields.
5. In-place learning: each neuron adapts "in-place" through interactions with its environment and it does not need an extra dedicated learner (e.g. to compute partial derivatives). The WWN-1 uses the top-k mechanisms (i.e. selects the largest k neurons) to simulate in-place competition among neurons in the same layer, which is not in-place per se but is still local and computationally more efficient as it avoids iterations with a layer.

As this is a very challenging design and understanding task, we concentrate on (a) the network design issue: how such a network can be designed so that attention and recognition can assist each other; (b) how to understand a series of theoretical, conceptual, and algorithmic issues that arise from such a network.

To verify the mechanisms that are required for both design and understanding, in the experimental results presented, we limit the complexity of the cognitive behaviors to be learned:

1. We do not deal with different sizes of the object. This requires more areas each having different sizes of receptive fields.
2. Although the network is meant to deal with a variety of within-class object variations, we use the same foreground object but with different backgrounds in testing. Larger within-class variation is the subject for future studies.
3. We assume that there is a single object in the input image.

However, they should be considered the limitations of the agent, not the limitation to a particular task. For example, the network can in principle deal with any number of object patterns (to appear in Luciw and Weng, 2010) and any object location of the input image (to appear in Ji and Weng, 2010) in general unknown backgrounds.

Regardless of these limitations, as far as we know, this was the first general-purpose where–what system for attending and recognizing objects from complex backgrounds, when its earlier version appeared in Ji *et al.* (2008).

In what follows, we first explain the structure of the proposed WWN-1. Key components of the model are presented in Sections 8.3, 8.4, 8.5, addressing local receptive field, cortical activation, and lateral connections, respectively. Section 8.6 provides the algorithm of weight adaptation in the proposed network. Experimental results are reported in Section 8.7 and concluding remarks are provided in Section 8.8. Section 8.9 discusses the related implications.

8.2   Network overview

Structurally, WWN-1 is a set of connected two-dimensional cortical layers, each containing a set of neurons, arranged in a multilevel hierarchy. The number of levels of neurons is determined by the size of local receptive fields and staggered distance, discussed in Section 8.3. An example of the network is shown in Figure 8.1. Its network architecture and parameters will be used in our experiments discussed in Section 8.7. We use a moderate size of network, so that there are not enough neurons to memorize every object view at every pixel location. Thus, every neuron must deal with one or multiple objects at multiple pixel locations.

The network operates at discrete times $t = 0,1,\ldots$, where the external sensors are considered to be at the bottom (layer 0) and the external motors at the top. Neurons are interconnected with non-negative weights. It is not good to consider lateral inhibition as a negative number in axons, as lateral inhibition can be realized by interneurons that release GABA which is inhibitory, making a neuron less likely to fire. For each neuron i in a layer l, there are four weight vectors, corresponding to four different neuronal fields, as illustrated in Figure 8.2:

1. bottom-up weight vector $\mathbf{w}_{bi}$ that links connections from its local input field in the previous level;
2. top-down weight vector $\mathbf{w}_{ti}$ that links connections from its effector field, either local or global, in the next level;

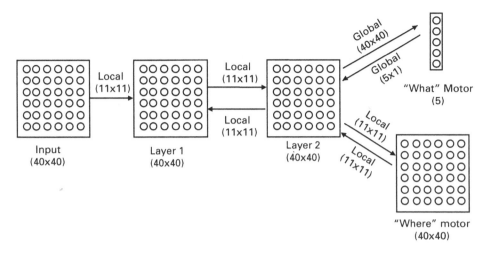

Figure 8.1   Implemented architecture of the Where What Network 1. The network is connected by dense interlayer connections in two directions, bottom-up and top-down, such that every neuron has both input field (from the previous layer) and effector field (from the next layer), the size of which is specified next to the corresponding line. A neuron is placed at a 2D position in a layer, forming a neuronal grid with $n \times n$ neurons.

3. lateral weight vector $\mathbf{w}_{hi}$ that links inhibitory connections from neurons in the same layer (large range);

4. lateral weight vector $\mathbf{w}_{ei}$ that links excitatory connections from neurons in the same layer (small range).

All excitatory inputs are simulated as neuronal inputs. However, in our simulation, we found that simulating inhibitory inputs as negative inputs caused undesirable oscillations and, consequently, did not allow winner neurons to emerge quickly. Instead, we use the top-k mechanisms to simulate the relationships among neurons that are connected by inhibitory connections. That is, the top-k mechanisms sort out the winner neurons explicitly within each network update as a single pass.

It is important to note that it is *not* a conventional feedforward network which uses feedback links (e.g. error backpropagation) only during learning. All the above links are active during operation, which includes learning and response generation. As discussed in Weng et al. (2001), an autonomous mental development system must learn while performing. There is not a separate learning phase for the brain at all.

The process of biological development includes two stages: prenatal development and postnatal development. The former uses spontaneous (cortex internally originated) sensory and motor signals. In our WWN-1, we used Gaussian profile centered at different locations as the initial weights for different neurons in the same layer. The latter stage uses real-world sensory and motor experience, while the robot autonomously learns and performs via active interactions with their environments including human teachers. In our experiments, we used real-world images and desired motor signals to train the network. As the network learns while performing, the trainer can impose the

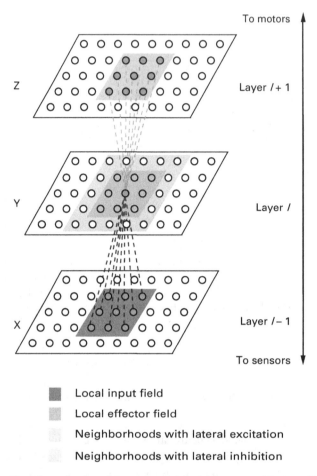

To motors

Z

Layer $l + 1$

Y

Layer l

X

Layer $l - 1$

To sensors

▮ Local input field

▢ Local effector field

▢ Neighborhoods with lateral excitation

▢ Neighborhoods with lateral inhibition

Figure 8.2   Neural connections. Neurons are placed (given a position) on different layers in an end-to-end hierarchy – from sensors to motors. A neuron has feedforward, horizontal, and feedback projections to it. Only the connections from and to a centered cell are shown, but all the other neurons in the feature layer have the same default connections.

desired motor signals on the corresponding motor ends at the correct time. While such supervisory signal is absent, the network self-generates its motor signals from the network learned so far. Therefore, in principle, training and performing can be interleaved in the way that the human teacher likes.

8.3   Hierarchical receptive fields

The receptive field of a neuron (Hubel and Wiesel, 1962) is the perceived area in an input array (image in this case). For a hierarchical neural structure, small, simple receptive fields in an early cortex will be gradually combined to form large, complex receptive fields in a later cortex. WWN-1 utilizes square, staggered receptive fields

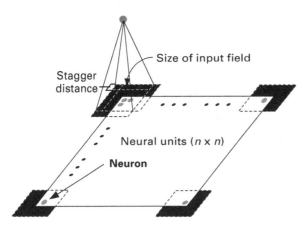

Figure 8.3   The input field boundaries and the organization scheme for neurons in a layer. When the local input field falls out of the input neuronal plane, the corresponding inputs are zeros (black areas in the figure).

to provide a structural basis for local attention. Attention selection needs to suppress neuronal responses whose receptive fields fall out of the attended receptive field. Each neuron receives its input from a restricted region in the previous layer: that is, the local input field. Figure 8.3 shows the organization of square input fields in a layer consisting of $n \times n$ neural units. Wherever a connection falls outside of the neuronal plane, the input is always 0. Let S_l and d_l be the number of neurons and staggered distance in the current layer l. The total number of input fields, namely the number of neurons in the next layer, is thus determined by:

$$S_{l+1} = \left(\frac{\sqrt{S_l}}{d_l} \right)^2 . \tag{8.1}$$

For $n \times n$ neurons shown in Figure 8.3, therefore, there are $n \times n$ neurons in the next layer, when the staggered distance is set to be 1.

The overlapped square input fields allow the network to obtain alternative receptive fields at multiple scales and positions. Figure 8.4 shows how the receptive fields increase from one layer to the next until the entire input is covered with a single receptive field. This representation provides information for receptive fields at different locations and with different sizes.

8.4   Cortical activation

The cortical activation of layer 1 is computed the same way as described in Weng *et al.* (2008), except that local connections are applied here. The preresponse y_i is determined by

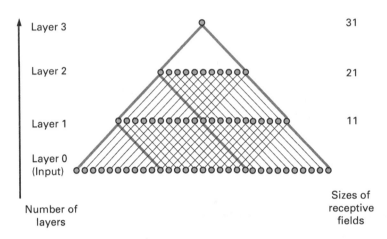

Figure 8.4   A 1D illustration of receptive fields in different scales of WWN-1. The size of the receptive field in a particular layer is 10 larger than its previous layer in this diagram (shown at the right), whereas the size of input field is set to be 11 at each layer.

$$y_i = (1 - \alpha^{(l)}) \frac{\mathbf{w_{b_i}}(t) \cdot \mathbf{x}_i(t)}{\left\| \mathbf{w_{b_i}}(t) \right\| \left\| \mathbf{x}_i(t) \right\|} + \alpha^{(l)} \frac{\mathbf{w_{t_i}}(t) \cdot \mathbf{y}_i(t)}{\left\| \mathbf{w_{t_i}}(t) \right\| \left\| \mathbf{y}_i(t) \right\|}$$

where $\mathbf{x}_i$ is the local bottom-up input and $\mathbf{y}_i$ is the local or global top-down input (i.e. neural responses from the next layer) of neuron i. $\alpha^{(1)}(0 \leq \alpha^{(1)} \leq 1, l = 1)$ denotes a layer-dependent weight that controls the maximum contribution by the top-down versus the bottom-up. The length normalization of $\mathbf{x}_i$ and $\mathbf{y}_i$ ensures that the bottom-up part and top-down part are equally scaled. Layer 2 of WWN-1, however, receives the top-down projections from both "where" motor layer and "what" motor layer (Figure 8.5). Thus, the preresponse y_i of the neuron i is determined by

$$y_i = (1 - \alpha^{(l)}) \frac{\mathbf{w_{b_i}}(t) \cdot \mathbf{x}_i(t)}{\left\| \mathbf{w_{b_i}}(t) \right\| \left\| \mathbf{x}_i(t) \right\|} + \alpha^{(l)} \left((1 - \gamma^{(l)}) \frac{\mathbf{w_{t_{1_i}}}(t) \cdot \mathbf{y}_{1_i}(t)}{\left\| \mathbf{w_{t_{1_i}}}(t) \right\| \left\| \mathbf{y}_{1_i}(t) \right\|} + \gamma^{(l)} \frac{\mathbf{w_{t_{2_i}}}(t) \cdot \mathbf{y}_{2_i}(t)}{\left\| \mathbf{w_{t_{2_i}}}(t) \right\| \left\| \mathbf{y}_{2_i}(t) \right\|} \right)$$

where $\mathbf{w_{t_{1_i}}}$ and $\mathbf{w_{t_{2_i}}}$ are top-down weights received from "where" and "what" motors, respectively, and y_{1i} and y_{2i} are the top-down inputs from the "where" motor and "what" motor, respectively, and $\gamma^{(1)}(0 \leq \gamma^{(1)} \leq 1, l = 2)$ is the layer-dependent weight that controls the maximum contribution by the "what" motor.

In WWN-1, bottom-up attention is a natural consequence of experience of interactions (winning in competition). No internal object master map is required. Its internal representations, for example neuronal weights, are developed through the regulation of

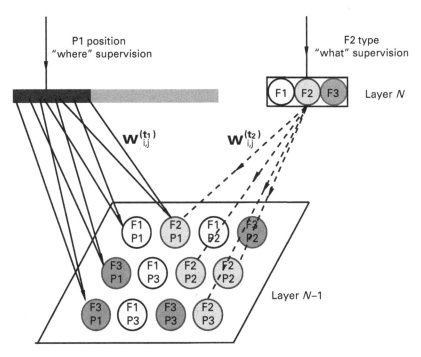

Figure 8.5   Top-down connections supervise the learning of motor-specific features in layer 2.

cell-centered computations in the two-way information flows. By contrast, instead of a complicated selection of spatial-oriented or object-dependent feature pools in traditional views, the top-down mechanisms of motor-specific controls are conducted in the WWN-1 to develop position-based and object-based attentions concurrently. This tight integration not only allows different alternative sources of top-down attention control to use the same network mechanisms, but also opens the door toward future self-generated autonomous attention (e.g. through the introduction of novelty-driven mechanisms in motor behaviors).

8.5   Neuron competition

Lateral inhibition is a mechanism of competition among neurons in the same layer. The output of neuron A is used to inhibit the output of neuron B, which shares a part of the input field with A, totally or partially. As an example shown in Figure 8.6, the neighborhood of lateral inhibition contains $(2h - 1) \times (2h - 1)$ neurons, because neurons i and $i - h$ do not share any input field at all. We realize that the net effect of lateral inhibition is (a) for the strongly responding neurons to effectively suppress weakly responding neurons, and (b) for the weakly responding neurons to less effectively suppress strongly responding neurons. Since each neuron needs the output of other neurons in the same layer and they also need the output from this neuron, a direct

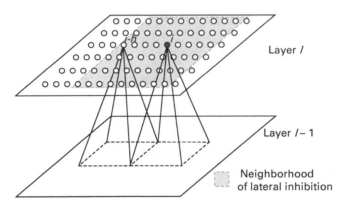

Figure 8.6   The neuron i has a $(2h-1) \times (2h-1)$ neighborhood of lateral inhibition, while neuron i and neuron $i-h$ did not share any input fields.

computation will require iterations, which is time consuming. To avoid iterations, we use the following local top-k mechanism.

For any neuron i in the layer l, we sort all the preresponses from neurons centered at positions inside the input field of neuron i. After sorting, they are in order: $y_1 \geq y_2 \geq \ldots \geq y_m$. The preresponses of top-k responding neurons are scaled with non-zero factors. All other neurons in the neighborhood have zero responses. The response of neuron i is then

$$\bar{y}_i = \begin{cases} y_i \left(y_i - y_{k+1} \right) \big/ \left(y_1 - y_{k+1} \right) & \text{if } 1 \leq i \leq k, \\ 0 & \text{otherwise.} \end{cases}$$

In other words, if the preresponse of neuron i is the local top-k, then this response is the same as its preresponse. Otherwise, its response is lower than its preresponse, to simulate lateral inhibition. A larger k gives more information about the position of the input in relation to the top-k winning neurons. However, an overly large k will violate the sparse-coding principle (i.e. neurons should be selective in responding so that different neurons detect different features). In our experiments, k is set at 5% of the number of neurons in the local input field. Sparse coding, as discussed by Olshausen and Field (1996), as a result of lateral inhibition, is stimulated by the local top-k rule. It allows relatively few winning neurons to fire in order to disregard the distraction from irrelevant feature detectors.

8.6   Weight adaptation

After the layer responses have been computed, the connection weights of each neuron are updated if the neuron has a non-zero response. Both bottom-up and top-down weights adapt according to the same biologically motivated mechanism: the Hebb rule. For a neuron i with a non-zero response (along with its 3×3 neighboring neurons), the weights are updated using the neuron's own internal temporally scheduled plasticity:

$$\mathbf{w}_{\mathbf{b}_i}(t+1) = (1 - \Phi(n_i))\mathbf{w}_{\mathbf{b}_i}(t) + \Phi(n_i)\bar{y}_i.x_i(t)$$
$$\mathbf{w}_{\mathbf{t}_i}(t+1) = (1 - \Phi(n_i))\mathbf{w}_{\mathbf{t}_i}(t) + \Phi(n_i)\bar{y}_i.z_i(t)$$

The 3×3 updating rule is to model the lateral excitation on the short-range neighboring neurons, in order to achieve a smooth representation across the layer.

The scheduled plasticity is determined by

$$\Phi(n_i) = \frac{1 + \mu(n_i)}{n_i},$$

where n_i is the number of updates that the neuron has gone through, and $\mu(n_i)$ is a plasticity scheduling function defined as

$$\mu(n_i) = \begin{cases} 0 & \text{if } n_i \leq t_1, \\ c \times (n_i - t_1)/(t_2 - t_1) & \text{if } t_1 \leq n_i \leq t_2 \\ c + (n_i - t_2)/r & \text{if } t_2 \leq n_i, \end{cases}$$

where the plasticity parameters $t_1 = 20$, $t_2 = 200$, $c = 2$, $r = 2000$ in our implementation.

Finally, the neuron age n_i is incremented: $n_i \rightarrow n_i+1$. All neurons that do not fire (i.e. zero-response neurons) keep their weight vector and age unchanged as the long-term memory for the current context.

8.7   Experiments

Figure 8.1 above showed a specific set of resource parameters and the architecture implemented in our experiment, where $\alpha^{(1)} = 0.3$, $\alpha^{(2)} = 0.7$ and $\gamma^{(2)} = 0.5$ for the training process. The images of objects are normalized in size to 20 rows and 20 columns. One of five different object types is placed at one of five different positions in a 40 × 40 background image. The background images are randomly selected from a collection of natural images[1]. Each object–position combination is presented with 20 backgrounds, such that there are 5 (objects) × 5 (positions) × 20 (backgrounds) = 500 samples in total. A set of data examples is shown in Figure 8.7.

8.7.1   Development of layer 1

We develop the bottom-up weights in layer 1 first. In this, 500 000 of 40 × 40-pixel image patches were randomly selected from the 13 natural images (no object presence),

---

[1] From www.cis.hut.fi/projects/ica/data/images/ via Helsinki University of Technology.

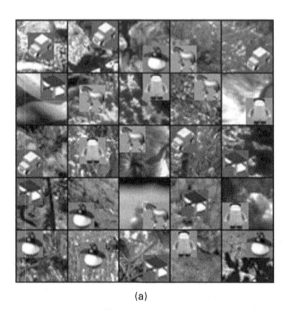

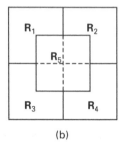

(b)

(a)

Figure 8.7   (a) Twenty-five examples of images used in the experiment, containing five objects defined by "what" motors: "car," "horse," "penguin," "person," and "table." When an object such as "car" appears in the image, the corresponding neuron in "what" motor is set to be 1 and all others to be 0. (b) Five regions defined by "where" motors. When an object appears in one region, such as R_1, all the "where" motors in R_1 are set to be 1 and others set to be 0. The "what" and "where" motors supervise the learning of neuron weights in previous layers, through the top-down connections described in Figure 8.5.

learned through the cell-centered learning algorithm described in Sections 8.3–8.6, without supervision on motors ($\alpha^{(1)} = 0$ and $\alpha^{(2)} = 0$). The developed bottom-up synaptic weights of all neurons in layer 1 are shown as image patches in Figure 8.8, each perceiving a local input field with size 11×11. Many of the developed features resemble the orientation selective cells that were observed in V1 area, as discussed in Hubel and Wiesel (1959) and Olshausen and Field (1997).

8.7.2   Recognition through attention

It is important to note that a developmental system should never stop learning. The network always performs an open-ended learning as outlined in Weng *et al.* (2001). We can "freeze" the network for testing, but the network should be able to continuously learn forever and should try to learn as fast as possible. The dual optimality of LCA in Weng and Luciw (2009) is for quickest learning. After the development of V1 weights, the network fully developed all its weights (both bottom-up and top-down) in V1 and other cortical areas, perceiving images containing objects in five defined positions.

With each update using a training image and coupled motors, the network is evaluated by all available stimuli for object recognition. We set $\gamma^{(2)} = 0$ to disable the top-down

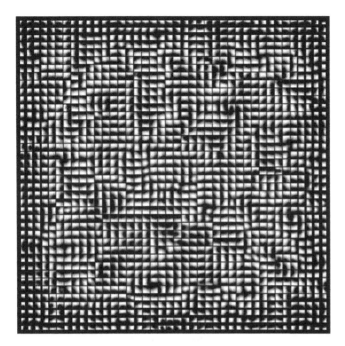

Figure 8.8   Bottom-up weights of 40 × 40 neurons in the developed layer 1. Each small image patch (40 × 40 pixels) presents a bottom-up weight of one neuron in the grid plane.

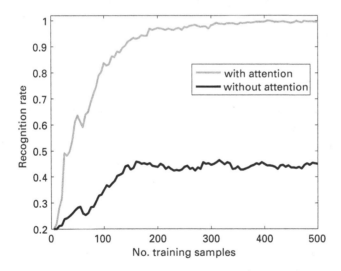

Figure 8.9   Recognition rate with incremental learning, using one frame of training images at a time.

supervision from the "what" pathway, but still supervised the attended region of "where" motors, using 11 × 11 local effector fields to guide the agent's attention. As shown in Figure 8.9, approximately 25% of samples are sufficient to achieve a 90% recognition rate. However, the recognition rate is only about 45% if the attention motor is not

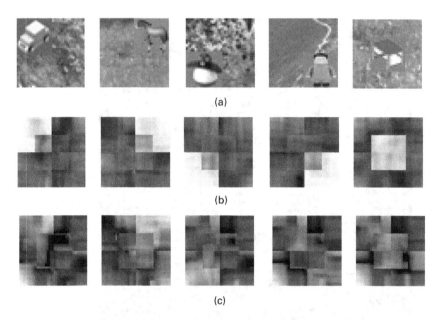

Figure 8.10   (a) Examples of image stimuli disjoint from training. (b) Responses of attention ("where") motors when the network was supervised through "what" motors. (c) Responses of attention ("where") motor when "what" supervision is not available.

available (all zeros) during the testing. This shows how top-down "where" supervision helps the recognition of "what" information and demonstrates the capability of recognition through attention.

8.7.3   Attention through recognition

To examine the effect of top-down "what" supervision in identifying where the object is, we tested images with disjoint backgrounds from training. The attention results from five examples are shown in Figure 8.10, where the network presented better attention capability with the assistance of "what" supervision. This shows how top-down "what" supervision helps location finding of "where".

8.7.4   Motor-specific features

The bottom-up weights of "what" and "where" motors are shown in Figure 8.11. Part (a) of Figure 8.11 shows that each "what" motor detects the corresponding features at different locations (i.e. position invariance for "what" motors). Part (b) of Figure 8.11 indicates that each "where" motor's bottom-up weight vector gives the average pattern in its input field across different objects. They are selective in the sense that each neuron pays attention to a specific "where" area, and fires across different objects for object invariance.

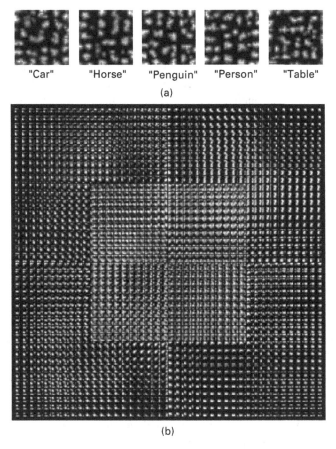

"Car"   "Horse"   "Penguin"   "Person"   "Table"

(a)

(b)

Figure 8.11 (a) Bottom-up weights of five "what" motors. Via top-down teaching signals, each "what" motor (e.g. "car") pools the corresponding type-specific feature at different locations, presenting the location invariance. (b) Bottom-up weights of 40 × 40 "where" motors. Via top-down teaching signals, each "where" motor averages location-specific patterns (e.g. layer-2 firing responses in upper-left corner) across multiple objects, presenting the type invariance.

8.8 Conclusion

In this chapter, we describe a neuromorphic developmental architecture to model robotic attention and recognition interactively via a Y-shaped structure that spans from sensors all the way to motors in both directions. The proposed WWN-1 contains local feature detectors at every layer. When two kinds of motor layers are connected with layer 2, top-down connections from one motor layer help the output from another motor layer in an interesting way. Specifically,

1. When the "what" motor is on during stimuli presentation (e.g. when the robot wants to find a type of object), the features that are (learned to be) associated with this particular object are boosted from top-down attention (i.e. expectation). These boosted

object-specific features relatively suppress the features that respond to background. Such suppression enables the "where" motors to report locations where features are boosted.

2. Conversely, when the "where" motor is on during stimuli presentation (e.g. when the robot wants to recognize the object at a particular location), the features that are (learned to be) associated with this "where" motor are boosted from top-down attention (i.e. here covert attention instead of overt eye saccade). These boosted features corresponding to the attended object suppress the features that respond to background. Such suppression leads to a significant boost in foreground recognition rate with presented natural background (from 45% to 100% in the experiment). Both the bottom-up and top-down attention mechanisms have been integrated in the top-k spatial competition rule, as it takes into account both bottom-up feature inputs and top-down context inputs (e.g. expectation, goal, etc.).

8.9   Discussion

Lately, the "where"–"what" theory has been enriched through functional magnetic resonance imaging (fMRI) studies (e.g. Aguirre and D'Esposito, 1997). The posterior parietal and premotor areas are more active in tasks demanding position information while the lingual and fusiform gyri demonstrated greater activity during tasks demanding appearance information. It appears that every pathway deals with exactly "how" to generate the "bridge" representation between the sensory end and the motor end. For example, as the arm deals with not just pointing and reaching, but also manipulation, the dorsal pathway must contain the lobe components for all the manipulation needs. As the vocal tract speaks not just "what" information about the object, the ventral pathway must contain the lobe components for all the language needs.

With the traditional approach, the programmer starts with a given robotic task. He/she would handcraft what features each of the two hidden layers (modules) detects and what states each layer (module) has. He/she would handcraft explicit rules to select (coordinate in general) internally generated incompatible actions (e.g. different actions from the same motor area). The developmental visuomotor example here does not start with any task. The current sensory and motor contexts provide information for the desired behaviors. As we can see, what each layer does and how different layers coordinate all depend on developmental learning experience. For example, typically multiple actions pop up at each motor area. The motor area of WWN-1 picks up the one with the highest response as the most probable one. No explicit, task-specific, action-coordination rules are required.

The principles of the developmental networks here are intended to serve for the "brain" of future real robots with more sophisticated behaviors. Experimental results for arbitrary pixel locations (<1.6 pixel error) with general object contours were obtained after WWN-1 was first published in Ji *et al.* (2008) and subsequently appeared in Ji and Weng (2010). Network mechanisms for dealing with multiple objects of interest appear in Luciw and Weng (2010). Note that it is intractably expensive for a convolutional network to deal with pixel-level location precision, as discussed in Weng *et al.* (1997). Like the cortex, WWN-1 does not use shift-invariant filters (e.g. with convolutional networks) so that the limited neuronal resource is optimally used for all cases, whether the motor end requires shift-invariance or not. The simulated robot driven by WWN-1 here has only two hidden "brain" areas and only two motor areas. WWN-1 does not have enough earlier areas to deal with all the sizes of receptive fields. It also does not have enough later areas in WWN-1 to cope with all the sizes of effective fields where many muscles can fire together for actions such as walking, dancing, singing, and somersaulting. It is not difficult to transform this system to a real robot demonstration. However, deployments in robot applications will require more areas in the "brain" model and more teaching and practice. For more effective teaching, in addition, the neuromodulatory system is required (e.g. the dopamine and other systems) and a more powerful learning mode – communicative learning (Weng, 2004) – is required.

It is true that given the same environmental setting, sometimes different behaviors are needed by different tasks. This task-dependent setting will be dealt with by a more mature developmental robot through its task memory, either external (e.g. computer hardware) or internal (e.g. recalling the task when multiple actions pop up). This is an interesting future research topic.

References

Aguirre, G. K. and D'Esposito, M. (1997). Environmental knowledge is subserved by separable dorsal/ventral neural areas. *Journal of Neuroscience*, **17**(7), 2512–2518.

Asada, M., Hosoda, K., Kuniyoshi, Y., *et al.* (2009). Cognitive developmental robotics: a survey. *IEEE Transactions on Autonomous Mental Development*, **1**(1), 12–34.

Backer, G., Mertsching, B., and Bollmann, M. (2001). Data- and model-driven gaze control for an active-vision system. *IEEE Transactions on Pattern Analysis and Machine Intelligence*, **23**(12), 1415–1429.

Felleman, D. J. and Van Essen, D. C. (1991). Distributed hierarchical processing in the primate cerebral cortex. *Cerebral Cortex*, **1**, 1–47.

Hubel, D. H. and Wiesel, T. N. (1959). Receptive fields of single neurons in the cat's striate cortex. *Journal of Physiology*, **148**, 574–591.

Hubel, D. H. and Wiesel, T. N. (1962). Receptive fields, binocular interaction and functional architecture in the cat's visual cortex. *Journal of Physiology*, **160**(1), 107–155.

Itti, L., Koch, C., and Niebur, E. (1998). A model of saliency-based visual attention for rapid scene analysis. *IEEE Transactions on Pattern Analysis and Machine Intelligence*, **20**(11), 1254–1259.

Ji, Z. and Weng, J. (2010). WWN-2: a biologically inspired neural network for concurrent visual attention and recognition. In *Proceedings of the IEEE International Joint Conference on Neural Networks*, pp. 1–8.

Ji, Z., Weng, J., and Prokhorov, D. (2008). Where-What Network 1: "Where" and "What" assist each other through top-down connections. In *Proceedings of the IEEE International Conference on Development and Learning*, pp. 61–66.

Koch, C. and Ullman, S. (1985). Shifts in selective visual attention: towards the underlying neural circuitry. *Human Neurobiology*, **4**, 219–227.

Luciw, M. and Weng, J. (2010). Where What Network 3: developmental top-down attention with multiple meaningful foregrounds. In *Proceedings of the IEEE International Joint Conference on Neural Networks*, pp. 1–8.

Lungarella, M., Metta, G., Pfeifer, R., and Sandini, G. (2003). Developmental robotics: a survey. *Connection Science*, **15**(4), 151–190.

Mishkin, M., Unterleider, L. G., and Macko, K. A. (1983). Object vision and space vision: two cortical pathways. *Trends in Neuroscience*, **6**, 414–417.

Moghaddam, B. and Pentland, A. (1995) (June). Maximum likelihood detection of faces and hands. In *Proceedings of the Workshop on Automatic Face- and Gesture-Recognition*, pp. 122–128.

Mozer, M. and Sitton, M. (1998). Computational modeling of spatial attention. In Pashler, H. (ed.), *Attention*. London: UCL Press, pp. 341–393.

Olshausen, B. A. and Field, D. J. (1996). Emergence of simple-cell receptive field properties by learning a sparse code for natural images. *Nature*, **381** (June 13), 607–609.

Olshausen, B. A. and Field, D. J. (1997). Sparse coding with an overcomplete basis set: a strategy used by V1? *Vision Research*, **37**(23), 3311–3325.

Olshausen, B. A., Anderson, C. H., and Van Essen, D. C. (1993). A neurobiological model of visual attention and invariant pattern recognition based on dynamic routing of information. *Journal of Neuroscience*, **13**(11), 4700–4719.

Purves, W. K., Sadava, D., Orians, G. H., and Heller, H. C. (2004). *Life: The Science of Biology*. 7th edn. Sunderland, MA: Sinauer.

Rao, R. P. N. and Ballard, D. H. (2005). Probabilistic models of attention based on iconic representations and predictive coding. In Itti, L., Rees, G., and Tsotsos, J. (eds.), *Neurobiology of Attention*. New York: Academic Press, pp. 553–561.

Schill, K., Umkehrer, E., Beinlich, S., Krieger, G., and Zetzsche, C. (2001). Scene analysis with saccadic eye movements: top-down and bottom-up modeling. *Journal of Electronic Imaging*, **10**(1), 152–160.

Stark, L. W. and Choi, Y. S. (1996). Experimental metaphysics: the scanpath as an epistemological mechanism. In Zangemeister, W. H., Stiehl, H. S., and Freska, C. (eds.), *Visual Attention and Cognition*. Amsterdam: Elsevier Science, pp. 3–96.

Sur, M. and Rubenstein, J. L. R. (2005). Patterning and plasticity of the cerebral cortex. *Science*, **310**, 805–810.

Tsotsos, J. K., Culhane, S. M., Wai, W. Y. K., *et al.* (1995). Modeling visual attention via selective tuning. *Artificial Intelligence*, **78**, 507–545.

Viola, P. and Jones, M. J. (2004). Robust real-time face detection. *International Journal of Computer Vision*, **57**(2), 137–154.

Weng, J. (2004). Developmental robotics: theory and experiments. *International Journal of Humanoid Robotics*, **1**(2), 199–235.

Weng, J. (2007). On developmental mental architectures. *Neurocomputing*, **70**(13–15), 2303–2323.

Weng, J. (2009). Task muddiness, intelligence metrics, and the necessity of autonomous mental development. *Minds and Machines*, **19**(1), 93–115.

Weng, J. and Luciw, M. (2009). Dually optimal neuronal layers: lobe component analysis. *IEEE Transactions on Autonomous Mental Development*, **1**(1), 68–85.

Weng, J., Ahuja, N., and Huang, T. S. (1997). Learning recognition and segmentation using the Cresceptron. *International Journal of Computer Vision*, **25**(2), 109–143.

Weng, J., McClelland, J., Pentland, A., *et al.* (2001). Autonomous mental development by robots and animals. *Science*, **291**(5504), 599–600.

Weng, J., Luwang, T., Lu, H., and Xue, X. (2008). Multilayer in-place learning networks for modeling functional layers in the laminar cortex. *Neural Networks*, **21**, 150–159.

Yang, M., Kriegman, D. J., and Ahuja, N. (2002). Detecting faces in images: a survey. *IEEE Transactions on Pattern Analysis and Machine Intelligence*, **24**, 34–58.

9 Brain-inspired robots for autistic training and care

Emilia I. Barakova and Loe Feijs

An increasing number of projects worldwide are investigating the possibility of including robots in assessment and therapy practices for individuals with autism. There are two major reasons for considering this possibility: the special interest of autistic people in robots and electronic tools, and the rapid developments in multi-disciplinary studies on the nature of social interaction and on autism as atypical social behavior.

Several branches of the social sciences and neurosciences, which aim to understand the social brain, advocate the perspective that social behaviors (e.g. shared attention, turn taking, and imitation) have evolved as an additional functionality of a general sensorimotor system for action. The basic feature of this system is the existence of a common representation between perception for action and the action itself. An extended social brain system facilitates processing of emotional stimuli, empathy, and perspective taking.

This chapter will describe a research line that builds on this perspective and incorporates theories from social sciences and neurosciences. Within this perspective, movement is modeled or generated as a basic behavior that will further determine some aspects of social interaction. Typical and atypical (as seen when observing persons with autism) movement patterns are simulated in the robot's sensorimotor system for action, as the difference is assumed to be caused by processing that takes place in the superior temporal sulcus and parietal areas of the brain. As a result, these different movement patterns emerge in the robot simulation. These patterns can be used in games for behavioral training of autistic people with robots and other tools with sensorimotor features.

The difference in movement patterns between typical and autistic persons has been investigated through considering goal-directed movements. Motor imitation is the most studied social behavior that is associated with goal-directed movements. We believe that there is a relationship between autistic people finding it difficult to imitate and their goal-directed movement patterns. Our research is focused on creating social games that promote imitation and other social behavior in autistic people. We are investigating different robotic systems that will measure and give feedback on motor imitation and social behavioral patterns of autistic people.

Neuromorphic and Brain-Based Robots, eds. Jeffrey L. Krichmar and Hiroaki Wagatsuma. Published by Cambridge University Press. © Cambridge University Press 2011.

Much robot imitation is inspired by the studies on motor imitation and on detecting motor intentions: that is, intentions directed towards inanimate objects. A more general "social perception" system processes emotionally rich facial expressions, body postures, and actions of others, and then triggers appropriate emotional responses. The recognition of emotional movements is the next level in our research on incorporating human social movements and responses within behavioral training of children with autism.

This chapter is organized as follows. In Section 9.1, we introduce the findings regarding the atypical motor behavior of people with autism that possibly contributes to the known shortcomings in their social behavior, as expressed in imitation and emotional movement behaviors. We introduce the most plausible theories for neurological causes of the atypical autistic behavior and propose a neural model that simulates typical and autistic behavior followed by a simulation of grasping behavior on a robot. In Section 9.2, we explain how social skills can be enhanced by training motor behaviors through games and playful interaction scenarios. We also outline how to include robots that express basic motor and interaction behaviors for training social skills. Section 9.3 introduces the robotic platforms used in the experiments with autistic children that will be presented in Section 9.5. Section 9.4 introduces Laban movement analysis, a method that is needed for qualitative evaluation of human movement behaviors and for the generation of expressive (qualitatively distinctive) behaviors of robots. Section 9.5 features several game scenarios and Section 9.6 puts the work in perspective.

9.1 Enhancement of social skills with robots

9.1.1 Action, imitation, and social behavior

The ability to understand and respond to other persons' actions is a core component of social behavior. In this respect, goal-oriented grasping, imitation of actions, and expression of emotional attitude in the action have been studied extensively through animal and human experiments. Across the spectrum of autism-related disorders, in which impairments in social development are typical, the cognitive functions that are embodied by action appear to be the most affected (Williams, 2008). While communication skills based on gestures, facial expressions, and eye movements are underdeveloped by autistic people, those abilities that are less dependent upon integration with actions, such as certain sensory, mathematical, and mnemonic abilities, may be enhanced. Therefore, the mechanisms that underpin different movement behaviors, such as goal-oriented action, imitation, self–other matching, and motor expression of emotional attitude through physical behavior, are fundamental to our understanding of autism.

After thorough analysis of the existing literature, Leary and Hill (1996) pointed out that the importance of motor impairment in autism has been overlooked. Others (Damasio and Maurer, 1978; Vilensky *et al.*, 1981; Bauman, 1992; Manjiviona and Prior, 1995; Teitelbaum *et al.*, 1998) indicated that the motor functions of people with autism differ or are impaired. Leary and Hill (1996) provided an explanatory analysis of the bibliography on movement impairments in autism, aiming to show how some of the socially referenced characteristics of autism might be based on neurological symptoms of movement disturbance. Moreover, the authors argued that the application of social context to the observed behaviors may divert attention from neurological explanations for the same behaviors. They proposed that a shift in focus to a movement perspective may provide new insights, which could result in the development of useful tools for future diagnosis and rehabilitation.

The most characteristic abnormal motor behaviors exhibited by people with autism are as follows. First, there are repetitive and stereotypical movements of the body, limbs, and fingers. Second, people with autism exhibit unusual gait patterns such as poorly coordinated limb movements and shortened steps, as well as "toe walking" (Damasio and Maurer, 1978; Vilensky et al., 1981). Third, poor performance of motor imitation tasks and the failure to use gestures for communicative purposes have been found in many studies that compare autistic and typical behavior (for a review see Smith and Bryson, 1994).

In this chapter we focus on the last group of motor abnormalities. Studies on visuomotor priming consider actions, especially goal-oriented actions such as grasping, as inseparable from sensing, seeing, and recognizing these actions by others (Gallese et al., 1996; Rizzolatti et al., 2002). During observation of graspable objects and tools, an individual's motor cortical areas have been shown to code the object in terms of one or more potential actions with these objects (Murata et al., 1997; Rizzolatti and Luppino, 2001). Craighero et al. (2002) suggested that motor preparation not only involves premotor cortical areas, but also evokes a representation of the prepared action in visual terms, located in the posterior parietal region and superior temporal sulcus. Because of the motor involvement during observation of actions and objects, actions are internally simulated by the observer, as shown by different studies from neurosciences, such as those based on single cell recordings (Gallese et al., 1996; Umiltá et al., 2001; Rizzolatti et al., 2002); brain imaging methods (Janerod, 2001; Rizzolatti et al., 2001, 2002; Decety, 2002); and transcranial magnetic stimulation (Fadiga et al., 1995; Strafella and Paus, 2000). In addition, behavioral methods such as transfer paradigms (Vogt, 1995, 1996; Hecht et al., 2001) and stimulus-response compatibility paradigms (Smith and Bryson, 1994) have shown concordant results.

The above-mentioned studies identify a mirror neuron system that comprises three main cortical areas in the brain: the premotor cortex (F5), the inferior parietal lobule (PF), and the superior temporal sulcus (STS). This system creates an affordance to implement goal-oriented tasks first, such as grasping, and has further evolved to dynamically represent the sensory and motor correlation of an action in the same brain structure. In this way, perceiving and performing an action exploit the same representation: that is, the action of the conspecific represented in the acting agent. Correspondingly, the mirror neuron system can facilitate imitation functionality as a natural addition to the goal-oriented actions. Because individuals with autism have difficulty communicating socially and understanding the emotions and intentions of others, the hypothesis that people with autism have a dysfunctional mirror neuron system has received a lot of attention in the literature, following a number of studies that reported weak mirror neuron system responses in individuals with autism. Such a straightforward explanation that a system of three brain areas could embody all the causes of abnormal action preparation, action understanding, and action imitation is very tempting, especially if one aims at a computational model that can be implemented on a robot. However, there is recent counter-evidence about the dysfunctional mirror neuron system in autism. Dinstein and colleagues (2010) showed that mirror system areas of individuals with autism not only responded strongly during movement observation, but did so in a movement-selective manner such that different movements exhibited unique neural responses. The mirror system responses of individuals with autism were, therefore, equivalent to those for controls. It will be most interesting to monitor future research into the mirror system hypothesis.

Dinstain and colleagues support the theory that noisy neural responses may cause the environment to be perceived as inconsistent and confused, making it difficult for the child to cope with the outside world, and driving him or her to develop autistic behavioral symptoms in response. Both the opponents and the supporters of the contribution of the mirror neuron system to the specificity of the autistic behavior (see, for instance, Iacoboni and Dapretto, 2006) agree that there is a much larger system that is involved in action preparation, understanding, and imitation. We base our experiments on the understanding that the perception, execution, and imitation of actions are at the core of the autistic behavior. In particular, we simulate the effect of cue delay by multisensory integration on the global behavior, which is not in contradiction with either of the mentioned theories.

Motor imitation represents one of the earliest forms of reciprocal interaction observed between infant and caregiver (Nadel, 2004). It is foundational for an infant's emerging ability to detect the correspondence between self and others (Meltzoff and Moore, 1997). The early opportunity for an infant to detect similarities with others leads to later understanding of other's intentional behavior and to the development of a theory of mind. The system for social interaction also embodies emotional aspects of the imitative or reciprocal behaviors. The studies of human emotion that are related to observable human behavior in terms of postures and movement (e.g. Emery and Amaral, 2000; Rotshtein *et al.*, 2001; Adolphs, 2002; De Gelder, 2006) place the amygdala at the core of a network of emotional brain structures. The amygdala and STS are directly connected and involved in the recognition of emotional body language. The amygdala decodes the affective relevance of sensory inputs and initiates affective behaviors via its connections to the motor systems (Emery and Amaral, 2000). To extend the already suggested network to an even more complex neural structure that involves brain structures and mechanisms that relate to emotional processing is a challenging task. Instead we propose to include the resonance theory (common coding principle) of behaviors that include emotional content as an addition to the typical movement which is involved in imitation or other reciprocal social behaviors.

The role of the social interaction system therefore extends from motor control (for instance in goal-directed grasping) to imitation that is the basis for developing social communication skills, such as theory of mind, empathy, and emotional body language.

The different motor behavior of people with autism may lead to differences in motor learning, which we are going to explore further.

9.1.2   Simulation of grasping behavior by autistic and typical people

After a thorough analysis of the bibliography on movement impairment in autism, Leary and Hill (1996) outlined how deficits in movement preparation and execution could lead to many of the behaviors exhibited by individuals with autism. Difficulties in planning and executing simple discrete movements can lead to problems in learning to coordinate diverse muscle groups into a unitary movement pattern. Moreover, when a person is unable to respond to another's action in a timely fashion, he or she will miss the positive reinforcement associated with interpersonal interaction.

Behavioral evidence of human perception and action indicates that organisms make use of multisensory stimulation. Under normal circumstances, multisensory stimulation leads to enhanced perceptions of, and facilitates responses to, objects in the environment (e.g. Sumby and Pollack, 1954; Stein *et al.*, 1989; Bolognini *et al.*, 2005). However, literature shows that imprecise grasping or other motor or executive dysfunctions observed in autistic patients are caused by a disturbance in a dynamic mechanism that involves multisensory processing and integration. This can be caused by discrepancies between stimuli that are normally concordant. In these circumstances, multisensory stimulation actually leads to inaccurate perceptions and responses regarding location, identity, and timing. Temporal binding, for instance, is identified as a dynamic mechanism that is disrupted and likely implicated in the perceptual and higher-order deficits observed in autism (Brock *et al.*, 2002). In other studies, atypical processing is specifically associated with enhanced sensory processing or discrimination in various modalities (Mottron and Burack, 2001; O'Riordan *et al.*, 2001). Some studies argue for a broader neurological problem such as an executive function deficit in the coordination of sources of information from different modalities (Ozonoff *et al.*, 1994; Russo *et al.*, 2007).

All these works suggest that the dynamic aspects of integration of multisensory input influence the formation of coherent perception, planning, and coordination of action. Even more concrete, many studies assume that simple motor planning is intact, but the use of externally guided visual feedback is diminished, affecting the quality of motor performance and postural stability, and resulting in the lack of effective sequencing of actions (Masterton and Biederman, 1983; Smith and Bryson, 1994; Stone *et al.*, 1997; Gepner *et al.*, 2001). Therefore, perceptually challenging tasks that require smooth integration of visual with vestibular–proprioceptive information may be particularly difficult to perform and could result in poor quality of motor performance on complex tasks.

We test this assumption by simulating the dynamic mechanism of temporal multisensory integration to investigate how the atypical formation of coherent perception might influence the coordination of action, and compare the results with experimental studies by typical and autistic patients. Temporal multisensory integration has previously been discussed in the context of autism (Brock *et al.*, 2002; Iarocci and McDonald,

2006) in attempts to obtain a clear understanding of the underlying biological mechanism of interaction and to simulate it in the robotics setting (Barakova and Lourens, 2005; Barakova and Chonnaparamutt, 2009). Masterton and Biederman (1983), in particular, have shown by studying grasping that a proper interplay between integration of distal (visual) and proximal (proprioceptive) cues is essential.

For the purpose of simulating grasping behavior on robots we simulate the integration of these cues first. We expect that by varying the parameters for the two sensory cues that give formative feedback on the grasping behaviors, we can approximate autistic and typical behavior. Emulating typical and autistic behaviors on robots and gaining sufficient understanding of the differences will make it possible to include these in behavioral training of autistic people through games and training scenarios. In particular, many studies conclude that people with autism rely more on proprioceptive than on visual sensory feedback. By designing appropriate game scenarios, we can try to motivate them to use visual cues more often by letting them play games that include reaching and also imitation movements that depend on the visual feedback and not on proprioception.

This section will feature three experiments, after a brief introduction of the model. The first experiment shows how integration of robots' visual and proprioceptive cues simulates grasping behavior. The impact of delays in each of the sensory modalities is then investigated. The experiments are made with a simulated "e-puck" robot, and aim to find the proper parameters for experiments with the physical robot, and to examine the abruptness of the changes that delays in different cues will cause. The second experiment shows the effect of changes in the robot's heading direction with tuned weighting parameters of the neural field model in the cases of no delay, delay for the visual cue, and delay for the proprioceptive cue. This experiment shows how closely a dynamic neural field (DNF) model can approximate grasping by humans. Lastly, the parameters of the DNF model found in these experiments and the effects of the delay of sensory cues on the integration are used in the third experiment with an e-puck robot.

Dynamic neural field model for generation of human-like movements

The integration process that causes the movement behavior is a dynamic temporal mechanism. Proper modeling of dynamic (temporal) integration mechanisms requires a dynamic neural model. Erlhagen and Schöner (2002), Iossifidis and Steinhage (2001), and Schöner *et al.* (1995) have adapted the dynamic neural field (DNF) model of Amari (1977) for controlling mobile robots and robot manipulators and producing close-to-human behavior.

The DNF model has been proposed as a mathematical model for neural processing (Amari, 1977; Schöner *et al.*, 1995; Erlhagen and Schöner, 2002). The main characteristics of this model are its inherent properties for stimulus enhancement and cooperative and competitive interactions within and across stimulus–response representations.

Erlhagen and Schöner (2002) formalized the extension of the theoretical model to the dynamic field theory of motor programming, explaining how it could be used for robotics and behavioral-modeling applications. The DNF model has been used in robotics for navigation and manipulation of objects (Iossifidis and Steinhage, 2001; Schauer and Gross, 2004; Faubel and Schöner, 2006), multimodal integration (Sauser and Billard, 2006), and imitation (Steinhage, 2000). Applications feature biologically convincing methods that can optimize more than one behavioral goal, contradictory sensory information, or sensorimotor tasks that require common representation. Thelen *et al.* (2001) have modeled the dynamics of movement planning by integrating the visual input and motor memory to generate the decision for the direction of reaching.

A feature of the model that is interesting for us is that it possesses dynamic properties useful for multisensory and sensorimotor integration. We suggest that the dynamic characteristics of the model can be used for investigating the temporal aspects of multimodal integration. The temporal window for integration is shown to have an impact on multisensory interaction, so we investigate the possibilities for its adaptation within the neural field model and its impact on the computational outcomes. The presentation of the sensory cues within the DNF model is in the form of Gaussian distributions. We tune the variance of these distributions according to the experimental findings, and experiment with the delay in the presentation of each cue in accordance with the realistic times of sensory processing of different modalities, while, of course, following the restrictions of the experimental platform.

Integration of robots' visual and proprioceptive cues simulates grasping behavior

At the period the experimental work was performed, we only had available a mobile robot that lacked the structure of a human arm. Therefore, the action of the robot was defined as turning towards and approaching an object that is intended to be grasped. Our experiments were therefore restricted to a two-dimensional task of reaching a target.

On the basis of earlier findings (Van Beers *et al.*, 1998; Barakova and Lourens, 2005), it was established that two complementary sensory cues, namely proprioception and vision, are necessary and sufficient for reaching, as well as for precision gripping by the robot. Unbalance of the same two cues may cause the different grasping observed in autistic people, as explained in the previous sections. In this experiment, we assume that the robot always sees the target at a fixed direction that is located at some distance in front of it. Then, the robot has to move from the initial position by turning to the target's direction and moving to the target. The proprioceptive or self-motion information is the angular deviation of the head direction of the robot from the initial position. Vision data are used for spotting the landmark or goal direction. The parameters of DNF were tuned empirically, taking the suggestions from human experiments (Van Beers *et al.*, 1998) into account.

Our hypothesis was that a delay in the activation corresponding to each of the sensory cues may cause or contribute to imprecise motor behavior. In the underlying system for action, the integration between the visual and proprioceptive information takes place in the parietal area, before the intention for the action has taken place. With the following experiment we tested the impact of the delay in the activation caused by each of the sensory modalities. We experimented with different delay intervals.

To test the effect of cue delay on the sensory integration, each cue signal was delayed by a different time interval when a goal-finding task was performed. Several tests were made with a simulated robot that performs target-following tasks. In each test, after the robot determined a heading direction, the target was moved so that the heading direction of the robot changed by different angles. Figure 9.1 depicts trajectories with changes of the heading direction corresponding to 5, 15, and 25 degrees and 15, 30, and

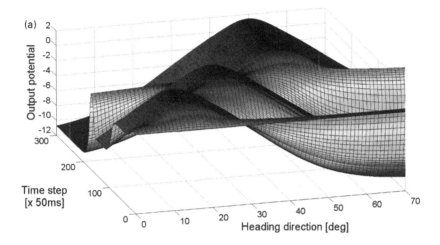

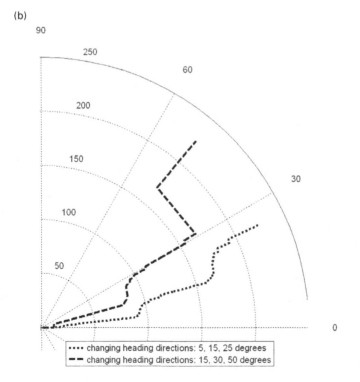

Figure 9.1   (a) The output potential with heading direction changing with 15–30–50 degrees. (b) The trajectories of the robot in polar coordinates with heading direction changing correspondingly with 5–15–25, and 15–30–50 degrees.

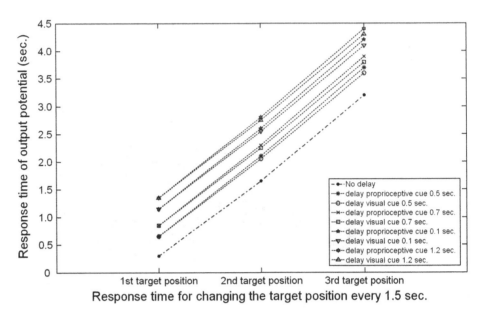

Figure 9.2   Response time of output potential: without delay and with the delay of each cue.

50 degrees with no introduced sensory delays. Figure 9.1(a) shows the output potential of the second trajectory, and Figure 9.1(b) shows the two trajectories in polar coordinates. Polar coordinate representation was chosen because it corresponds to the actual movement of the robot from its egocentric perspective.

Several trials were made to compare the effect of changing heading direction with no cue delay, with a delay in the proprioceptive cue, and with a delay in the visual cue. Figure 9.2 shows the response time for the robot to decide the direction of the movement. The visual cue delay has a more significant effect on response time than the proprioceptive cue. To obtain further information on the delay effect for each cue, the experiment of changing heading direction was carried out for three successive steps. In every experiment, a delay in proprioceptive cue had less of an effect for generating the new heading direction. With equal cue delays, and with the neural field parameters constant for both cues, the experiments differed in the abruptness of changes in heading direction.

Effects of cue delays on grasping

With the second experiment we tested whether the DNF model correctly approximates the dominance of proprioceptive over visual information for autistic people. Autistic subjects were reported to use visual information in order to determine the location of the target slot; however, they relied on proprioceptive information for reaching.

A grasping of an object in a two-coordinate plane was simulated. The sensory models of the visual and the proprioceptive cues are based on the findings of Van Beers and colleagues (1998). Three objects were located in random positions in space. We

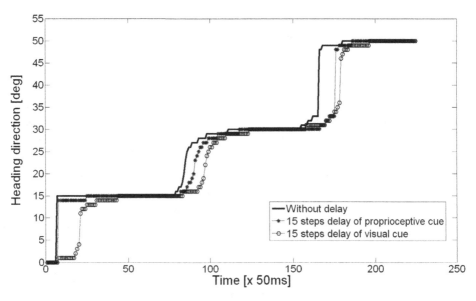

Figure 9.3   Heading direction of the e-puck robot with and without delay when changing the target direction from 0 to 15 to 30 to 50 degrees. The three lines depict the change of heading direction after sensory integration without cue delays, and with a delay of 15 steps for each cue.

assume that when a subject has to grasp an object, he/she has to turn in the direction of the object. This means that the object is always located in front of the subject at the moment of grasping. This assumption is used to design the robot simulation. Figure 9.3 shows the results of the simulation. For proximal grasping, the proprioceptive cue has more effect on the output potential than the visual cue. As shown in Figure 9.2, with the same delay time, the output potential takes relatively longer to be generated in the case of a delay for the proprioceptive cue.

Experimental data from Van Beers *et al.* (1998) show that the precision of movement is affected differently in terms of depth and azimuth motion by the visual and proprioceptive cues. The proprioceptive cue is more precise when the depth (distant goal) is targeted, and vision is more accurate in proximal (moment to moment) movements. To simulate this effect, the Gaussian ratio and amplitude of both cues were tuned to correspond to the variances in movement accuracy as found by Van Beers *et al.* (1998). Figure 9.3 shows the change of heading direction of the robot with tuned weighting parameters of the neural field model in the cases of no delay, delay for the visual cue, and delay for the proprioceptive cue. This result is in agreement with the experimental studies (Van Beers *et al.*, 1998), and shows that the DNF model correctly approximates the precision of movement when the parameters for the two cues are directly borrowed from experiments with humans.

Modeling grasping behaviors of autistic and typical people by a robot.

For the third experiment, an e-puck mobile robot was used (www.e-puck.org). The robot is equipped with infrared sensors that were used to obtain the information about the turning angle of the robot, which we will refer to as proprioceptive information. The obstacle-free space determined the possible direction of the robot for the next moment-to-moment movement. Vision was used to determine the target direction of the robot.

In the robot experiment, we can assume that proprioceptive or visual information has been delayed so the simulated movement will depend on the nondelayed cue. The influence of each sensory cue on the output behavior was tested after the experimental scenario was simplified by using only one obstacle in the arena. With this simplification, the influence of any artifact on the outcome of the experiment is excluded. In the absence of sensory cue delays, the robot can avoid the obstacle and reach the target. When delay was applied to the proprioceptive or to the visual input, the robot took different trajectories. Depending on the distance of the obstacle and the speed of the robot, changing the delays had different effects. Figure 9.4 shows three sample trajectories of the robot: without delay, with delay for the proprioceptive sensory cue, and with delay for the visual cue.

Proprioceptive cue delay resulted in a collision between the robot and the obstacle. With a visual cue delay, the robot started to move in an arbitrary direction until the visual input was received, but nevertheless avoided the obstacle.

This result could be compared with autistic and typical behaviors. When both cues are integrated in time, a typical movement behavior occurs. When the visual cue is delayed (i.e. the robot relies more on the proprioceptive information), the proximal obstacle is avoided, but the handling of reaching the distant object is interrupted. This may resemble the inability of autistic people to combine simple movements with a global complex behavior (as suggested by Masterton and Biederman, 1983; Smith and Bryson, 1994; Stone et al., 1997).

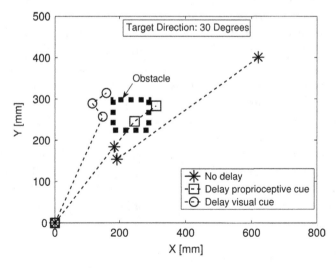

Figure 9.4   Robot trajectories from sample experiments with no delay, proprioceptive cue delay, and visual cue delay.

Behavioral training with robot grasping

We made the following steps towards practical implementation of the insights gained from the above experiments. We applied the dynamic neural field (DNF) model (Amari, 1977; Schöner *et al.*, 1995; Erlhagen and Schöner, 2002) to multimodal interaction of sensory cues obtained from a mobile robot in order to show the impact of different temporal aspects of the integration on the precision of movements. For further user tests, we put forward the hypothesis that temporally uncoordinated sensory integration might be a reason for the poor motor skills of persons with autism.

Even if this assumption is too simplistic an approximation of grasping behavior by autistic people, the simulation gives a fair approximation of the actual autistic behavior. Using these results we can incorporate the behaviors in a humanoid robot or prepare games with the i-blocks platform, both featured in Section 9.3, and use them in games that aim to train for better usage or integration of the visual cue.

The DNF model ensures human-like decision making and smooth motions when different external stimuli are present. However, unreliable sensory information can result in totally different behavioral solutions when the robot starts from the same starting point in the same arena. Unrepeatable behavior may be caused by detection failure of the sensors or imprecise tuning of the parameters of the DNF model. This results in the robot either departing from the natural path or colliding with an obstacle. To fulfill our ambition of simulating the sensory integration process of autistic people, we are currently appling a two-dimensional DNF on the humanoid robot NAO (www. aldebaran-robotics.com/eng). The NAO robot can be involved in giving active feedback (coaching) on the behavior of the autistic child and a comment (reflection) on its own behavior, if it is parameterized as autistic-like behavior.

9.2 Social skill enhancement with robot-mediated games

We explore the hypothesis that social skill training in autism should have as a basic component the training of motor skills. As can be further elaborated from the reasoning in the previous section, the training of goal-oriented movements, such as grasping of an object, imitation of a movement, and permitting turn taking, facilitates social interaction on a motor level. The social interaction context requires that the behaviors are not taken in isolation but are included in realistic scenarios.

Teaching social movement patterns can take many forms. Since our research is directed at children, we choose to design game scenarios. The most obvious value of games is enjoyment and sharing of social experiences with others (Vygotsky, 1966). In addition, play is widely used as a preferred educational activity for young children to acquire a variety of skills for life, such as motor coordination and social and cognitive skills (Rauterberg, 2004).

Malone and Lepper (1987) have pointed out the importance of intrinsic motivation in games. Intrinsically motivating activities are those in which people will engage for no reward other than the interest and enjoyment that accompanies them. They identified factors such as challenge, curiosity, control, fantasy, competition, cooperation, and recognition. Note that the first four of these are individual factors whereas the other three are interpersonal factors.

Whereas traditional game design aims at creating a balanced mix of the seven factors identified by Malone and Lepper (1987), assuming they all make a positive contribution to the attractiveness of the game, the role of the factors in this balance is probably different for children with autism. For the individual factors, they could cope with even more demanding challenges. But the interpersonal factors are likely to be more taxing and at the same time contributing less to the intrinsic motivation.

In addition, children with autism feel comfortable with structure and clearly defined rules, which gives another incentive to use games to stimulate social interaction between them. The most important forms of play that link motor and social development are as follows.

• *Object play.* Children with autism spectrum disorder explore objects less often and less thoroughly than their peers. Promoting early object-directed play is important for development of meaningful perceptual representation and later of functional, symbolic, and social play (Van Berckelaer-Onnes, 2003).
• *Functional play.* Functional play relates to the ability to use an object in accordance with a socially designed function. Shortcomings in the functional use of objects may result from the motor difficulties addressed in Sections 9.1 and 9.2, and from the inability of a child to relate to people. Other people play a vital role in showing children how to use objects properly in a context of joint attention and imitation.
• *Peer or social play.* Social play is especially challenging to children with autism, because of their difficulties with imitation, sharing toys, taking turns, and understanding emotional expressions. Several reviews of imitation in autism indicated that most but not all studies illustrate an early lack of imitation and later problems in imitation on demand (Stein *et al.*, 1989; Smith and Bryson, 1994). Imitation by others, however, is effective in establishing social contact in autism (Nadel *et al.*, 2006).

All the above-mentioned forms of play relate to physical play (Bekker *et al.*, 2010) and are based on the motor activities of the players. We add a new dimension to the play with physical objects that will promote social skills and the relevant motor skills, by using play objects that are able to behave: that is, they have sensors and actuators and can express some intelligent behaviors. We refer to such play objects as robots, although some of them (like the i-cube platform) could be classified as tangible interaction tools. In the next sections, we introduce the robotic platforms we used and elaborate on how play with robots can contribute to the behavioral training of children with autism.

9.3   Robotic platforms for grasping, imitation, and social interaction games

Physical play (Bekker *et al.*, 2010) is based on the motor activities of the players. Robots have controlled and repetitive movements, which are features that are understood by and are appealing to autistic children. Robots therefore raise the children's interest in nonverbal social communication, expressed via movement and postures. In addition, robots are intellectually challenging, and can stimulate the curiosity of autistic children. Encouraging play using a robotic toy may foster individual development up to the child's potential (Marti *et al.*, 2009).

Visuomotor priming by robots has shown to be beneficial for people with autism (Pierno *et al.*, 2008). In general, a movement behavior that is performed multiple times by a human actor would be perceived differently each time by people with autism, whereas for a typically developing person this is perceived as the same behavior. Because of this we proposed involving robotic co-players in the games, since robots can perform the same movement multiple times in the same way or in a precisely controlled new way. In addition it has been shown that autistic children have affinity with robots and they find it easier, less intimidating, and even fascinating to have a robot for a play partner or a mediator of play.

In most of the studies that use robots in games with autistic children, the robot is used as a play partner, and in some as a mediator of play (Robins *et al.*, 2004; Barakova and Lourens, 2010). We suggest that the robot has to encourage social interaction in various ways, by explaining or demonstrating the rules of social interaction, or by being a tool in a game that requires collaboration, persuading the children subconsciously towards associative or collaborative play (Barakova *et al.*, 2007, 2009). For these purposes, we first simulate simple robot behaviors such as grasping, pointing, and waving for the expression of goal-oriented and social behaviors. The simulations are based on a bio-inspired neural model of social interaction, which makes it possible to easily approximate autistic or typical motor behavior on the basis of changing the model parameters (Barakova and Chonaparamutt, 2009). In addition we develop games and tools to measure or perceive the children's body language by a robot or a tangible tool. We include these robots and tangibles in games and play scenarios that include motor imitation, turn taking, and emotional interaction, and will eventually facilitate the enhancement of the children's social skills.

To trigger more advanced forms of social play, we develop physical objects that have their own means of stimulating social interaction. These include: sensors so that the objects can record the changes in the surrounding world; some learning or adaptation mechanism that will facilitate decision making and ensure a level of autonomy; and actuators so that the objects can express behavior. A physical object with such features is in a broad sense a robot independently of its shape or means of behavior. We aim at a higher level of autonomy than the currently available robots have. The difference in this new level of autonomy is in the robot's ability to interpret human movement behavior and to behave in such a way that is understandable to humans. Specifically, we aim at designing robots that can themselves express emotional behaviors, as well as understand emotional expressions in other agents. In this section, we give an overview of the robot platforms used in our experiments. In the conducted experiments, three platforms with different degrees of complexity have been used (in increasing degree of complexity): i-blocks, a multiagent platform of interactive blocks; e-puck, a wheeled mobile robot; and NAO, a humanoid robot.

9.3.1   The i-blocks – a multiagent platform of interactive blocks

We developed a multiagent platform of interactive blocks (Alers and Barakova, 2009; Barakova *et al.*, 2007, 2009), where the blocks can be classified either as robotic entities, since they can sense the environment and react on it by expressing different behaviors, or as tangibles, since they are embodied objects with sensors and actuators, which invite interaction with users through simple and natural physical interaction metaphors (Figure 9.5a). The blocks emit colored light and interact when positioned in each other's vicinity. Depending on the algorithm that is loaded on each block at any one moment, they express a different set of local interaction behaviors that cause emergent collective behaviors.

The blocks can be used to make constructions with regular forms and precise positioning. The fascination of autistic children for patterns and regularity makes the blocks an appealing toy for them. The emergently changing behavior of the i-blocks stimulates their explorative behavior (Barakova *et al.*, 2007). We have chosen blocks with cubic shape and a size that can easily be grasped by a child, but still big enough to prevent a single child from "occupying" all the blocks. This may encourage other children to join them in building patterns together or at least make the child allow others, such as another child or a caregiver, to add to his/her construction.

The overall behavior of the system depends on local interactions, and therefore forms an embodied multiagent system (Barakova *et al.*, 2007). The complexity of the emerging behaviors depends on the complexity of the individual behaviors of the blocks. The technical details of the first stage of the development of this platform are described in Alers and Barakova (2009). In a further development of the platform, a built-in accelerometer is used to record the children's hand movements and to facilitate a number of imitation games. The complexity of the internal organization of the blocks is similar to that of commercial minirobots, with sensors, microcontroller, and controllable light-emitting diodes (LEDs); so we define them as robotic agents, whose motor behavior is expressed not through motion, but through changing color and intensity of light (Figure 9.5b).

We distinguish between the platform and the specific games. By platform we mean the hardware, including form, sensors, actuators, microcontroller, and the programming environment, which allows different behaviors to be simulated. By game we mean the specified rules as coded by the embedded program to make the blocks behave, together with the explanation of the rules to the players. The game/platform distinction makes it easier to develop several games and compare different games on the same platform.

The blocks were specially designed to fit the play habits and the patterns of thinking of autistic children. Initial user tests (as reported in Barakova *et al.*, 2007; Barakova and Lourens, 2010) have shown that children find them very engaging and enjoyable. In general, the advantages of these blocks are: (1) direct manipulations of tangible objects can be registered exactly, and multimodal feedback can be provided; (2) i-blocks are suitable for training goal-directed actions such as grasping and object manipulation; (3) i-blocks are relatively simple and reliable technological tools and can easily be connected to computers, robots, and other media.

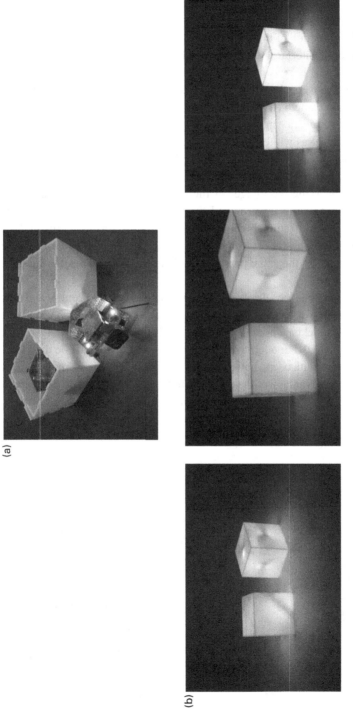

Figure 9.5 The developed multiagent system of interactive blocks (i-blocks): (a) internals of the block platform and (b) three examples of emergent light patterns when the blocks are put in each other's vicinity.

9.3.2   The e-puck mobile robot

The e-puck robot (www.e-puck.org) is a small mobile robot measuring 70 mm in diameter and 55 mm in height (Figure 9.6). It is equipped with infrared distance sensors that are located around the body at 10, 45, 90, 270, 315 and 350 degrees with respect to the heading direction of the robot. The robot was controlled by a personal computer using a Bluetooth interface (www.bluetooth.org). A rectangular arena was constructed for the robot which measured about 100 cm × 70 cm. The arena was fenced by cardboard walls which were about 10 cm high. The robot's movements were filmed by a Logitech QuickCam camera (www.logitech.com) suspended about 160 cm above the floor of the arena. The camera captured the entire arena using 320 × 240 pixels at 10 Hz. The floor of the arena was white. The robot was fitted with a black cap for maximal contrast so that tracking the robot while it moved was easy. All image processing and tracking of the location of the robot was done using RoboRealm software (www.roborealm. com). Processing the images of the camera included correcting for radial distortion. The tracking software provided the approximate location of the center of the robot in each camera frame. Furthermore, the tracking software provided a measure of the movement of the robot. Processing of the images and tracking the robot was done in real-time by the same personal computer that ran the software for controlling the e-puck robot.

This robot has the advantage that it is relatively easy to control and many ideas can be easily tested. For instance, the integration of proprioceptive and visual information using the DNF model for a humanoid robot would need a computationally more expensive two-dimensional DNF model, while the parameter tuning would be the same. For the actual experiments with users, however, the two-dimensional DNF model can be simplified.

Another advantage of the e-puck robot is its abstract shape. We conduct experiments where only the effect of movement on the children has to be evaluated. This includes testing the ability of autistic and typically developing children to classify emotional expressiveness of movements.

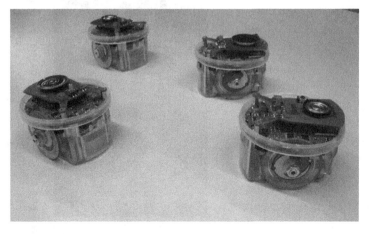

Figure 9.6   Four e-puck robots.

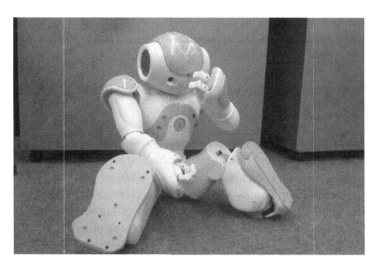

Figure 9.7   NAO robot.

9.3.3   The humanoid robot, NAO

The commercially available humanoid robot NAO (www.aldebaran-robotics.com/eng) is illustrated in Figure 9.7. The robot has 25 degrees of freedom (DOF), five in each leg and arm, and one in each hand. Further, it has two DOF in its head and one in the pelvis. The platform contains two color cameras with a maximum resolution of 640×480 pixels at a speed of 30 frames per second. The platform contains an embedded AMD Geode 500 MHz processor (www.amd.com) and is shipped with an embedded Linux distribution. A software library called NaoQi is used to control the robot. This is an easy-to-use C++ interface to the robot's sensors and actuators. Due to this library, it is relatively easy to control the robot's actuators and make use of advanced routines that let the robot move and talk using text-to-speech conversion.

The advantage of the humanoid robot is that it can interact with humans on both a physical and a social level. Since autistic people find humans intimidating, many successful experiments have shown that robots are less threatening to autistic children. Human-like interaction can also be trained in such a robot. Current developments in robotics allow robots to be programmed by demonstration and imitation. Therefore, NAO can, with certain restrictions, learn to imitate behaviors in seemingly natural interactions. Since autistic people like predictability and being in control, the repetitive and simplified movements of NAO can be beneficial for training. Pierno *et al.* (2008) have shown that interaction with robots has an effect on visuomotor priming processes, and that priming by a robot has a better effect on autistic persons than priming by a human.[1] This is because an

---

[1] Pierno *et al.* (2008) have shown that people with autism respond better on visuomotor priming by a robot than typically developing people through the following experiment. Participants were requested to observe either a human or a robotic arm model performing a reach-to-grasp action towards a spherical object. Subsequently, the observers were asked to perform the same action towards the same object. As a result the children with autism learned faster when primed by a robotic but not by a human arm movement. The opposite pattern was found for typical children.

autistic person will interpret the details of the same human action as novel, and experiments with humanoid robots can be constant or changed in a controlled manner.

9.4   Laban movement analysis for emotional dialog between robots and humans

In addition to social interaction conveyed by instrumental movements, emotional body language plays an important role in evaluating play behaviors with humans and robots. Making a robot understand or express emotional body language requires an appropriate description framework. Laban movement analysis (LMA) is a method for describing the expressive (qualitative) features of the movements and posture. It was created by Rudolf Von Laban, a dance theorist, as a practical method for recording all forms of human motion. While Laban first refers to his notation, as well as to other systems, as choreography, for its final form he introduced the term kinetography and initially published it as "Schrifttanz" (written dance or script-dance) (Laban and Lawrence, 1947).

Laban movement analysis emphasizes the processes underlying motor actions rather than the resultant motor action. Using the motion determinants that a body takes in space, LMA makes it possible to differentiate expressive and emotional actions. For instance, the difference between punching someone in anger and reaching for a glass is slight in terms of body organization – both rely on extension of the arm. However, the strength of the movement, the control of the movement, and the timing of the movement are all very different. This example shows how the three qualities, namely weight, flow, and time, respectively, help characterize the emotional load of movements.

LMA was used to evaluate fighting behaviors of rats (Fourod and Pellis, 2003), to diagnose autistic patients (Dott, 1995), to explain the differences in sexual behavior in Japanese macaques (Vasey *et al.*, 2006), and to analyze the quality of movement by recovering stroke patients (Mottron and Burack, 2001). We use LMA for the description of the kinematic and nonkinematic movements made by human subjects that perform emotional actions. The reliability of the nonkinematic measures in LMA has been validated in previous studies (Fourod and Whishaw, 2006; Vasey *et al.*, 2006). We focus on effort (Laban and Lawrence, 1947) or dynamics, in an attempt to understand the more subtle characteristics about the way a movement is performed with respect to intention. LMA emphasizes how internal feelings and intentions govern the patterning of movement throughout the whole body. It provides a complex understanding of intention.

Similar to the common coding/mirroring paradigm, LMA is useful in describing the interaction in the physical world which is caused by physical robots that move or perceive movements of humans and other agents (robots). Therefore using LMA has many possibilities: to design a robot that understands the emotional state of a human player and responds in an adequate manner; to design robot behaviors that imitate, enhance, or counteract an emotional state of a person; to design socially believable robotic (embodied) characters that provoke social interaction; and to create constantly adapting interaction based on movement or emotional understanding of a robot.

In order to identify the contribution of body movements to the recognition of emotion, it is important to have a clear and suitable description of these movements. However, LMA does not provide a straightforward way of assigning quantitative measures to movement qualities: instead, it provides descriptors for the content of human body movements in terms of the following categories: Body, Space, Effort, and Relationship. For instance, the Effort category relates to the dynamic and expressive characteristics of the movement. It comprises four movement qualities: weight, space (not to be confused with the Space category), time, and flow. Each quality represents a continuum between opposite polarities: weight varies between strength and lightness, space varies between direct and indirect, time varies between sudden and sustained, and flow varies between bound and free. Effort qualities usually appear in combinations called "states" or "drives." When two motion qualities are combined, it is called the inner attitude or incomplete effort. They are suitable for expressing mental states. When three motion qualities are combined, they form externalized drives.

According to Fourod and Pellis (2003), the Laban Effort parameters can be translated into low-level movement parameters such as curvature, velocity, and acceleration. We have shown (Barakova and Lourans, 2010) that this relation is reciprocal: that is, if the factors that are the components of the Passion drive (i.e. time, weight, and flow) are combined, it is possible to make a judgment about the emotional load of the movement.

Connecting the Laban factors to emotional states is a two-stage process. First, the correct correspondence between the Laban factors and emotions has to be established. Camurri *et al.* (2002) and Fagerberg *et al.* (2003) have independently used LMA to classify dance gestures in terms of basic emotions: anger, fear, grief, and joy. Their analysis overlaps for three of these emotions, namely anger, fear, and joy (happiness). We use the coding that corresponds to the relation between Laban movement qualities and emotions as introduced by Camurri *et al.* (2002).

Second, since we work with partially subjective parameters, a classification method that can deal with a sufficient degree of uncertainty has to be deployed. For this purpose we used variations of neural classifiers for both analysis and synthesis of emotional movement.

For the purpose of mediation of play between children, a robot that can engage in reciprocal social interaction through movement was used. In particular, we are designing behaviors to support collective games for the humanoid robot NAO. The game scenarios that are constructed on the basis of this interactive behavior aim to help children with autism learn to recognize emotional movements from a robot partner and to produce similar movements.

Recognition of emotional behaviors is a challenging task by itself. A performer and certified Laban movement analyst was asked to enact waving behaviors with different emotional coloring, namely angry, happy, sad, and polite. The waving was chosen for several reasons. First, it is a behavior that is used exclusively in a social context. Second, it can relatively easily be tracked by a single camera. Third, several emotional

(a)

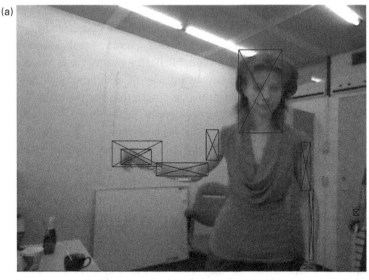

(b)

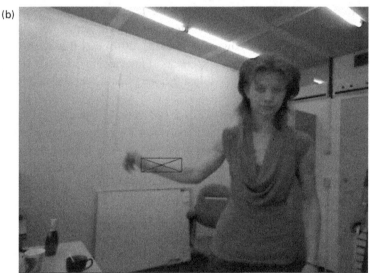

Figure 9.8   Marked regions of interest in images captured by a robot camera. (a) Marked areas denote skin and motion area, respectively. (b) The marked areas denote the average position of the fastest moving skin color objects. Tracking of multiple objects is possible because of the parallel processing framework.

states can be expressed naturally through waving. In fact our goal is not to be confined to the type of movement, but to extract dynamic primitives that are typical for a certain emotion.

Figure 9.9 depicts pairs of four emotional waving patterns recorded in an experimental scenario as shown in Figure 9.8, using color images of 640×480 pixels at a speed of 29 frames per second. The image processing consists of detection of a combination of skin color and motion with the aim of tracking a single body part per person that can be associated with the emotional waving movement. The black rectangular regions capture the center and the boundaries of the skin color areas, green areas capture moving objects, and the blue areas give a combination of a moving skin-colored area.

Recordings of 20 seconds were made where performers were asked to demonstrate happiness, anger, sadness, or politeness. In each plot the acceleration profile was obtained by taking the second derivative of the central point of the tracked object.

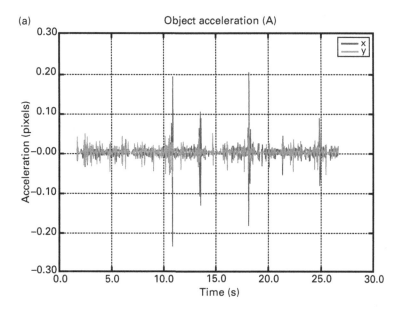

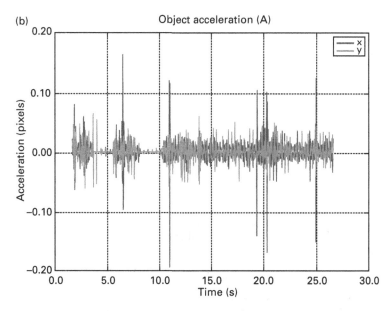

Figure 9.9   Waving patterns showing typical acceleration profile for (a) happiness, (b) anger, (c) sadness, and (d) politeness.

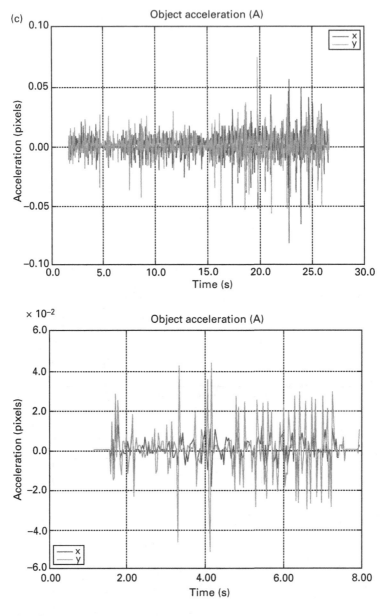

Figure 9.9   (*cont.*)

Examples for all four different emotional states are depicted in Figure 9.9. From this figure the following can be observed.

1. Happy waving provides a regular waving pattern with a relatively high frequency.
2. Anger demonstrates bursts with tremendous acceleration.
3. Sadness demonstrates a profile of low acceleration; its frequency is relatively low and appears to have a lower frequency compared with the other three emotions.

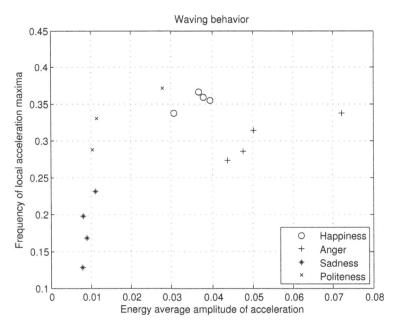

Figure 9.10   Distinct emotion profiles are revealed by average frequency and acceleration.

4. Politeness that demonstrates a "Queen Elizabeth" type of waving profile is a regular pattern with a high frequency that is obtained by using minimal energy.

In an average acceleration-frequency plot of the recorded movements, four distinctive clusters were formed (Figure 9.10). The plots in Figure 9.9 were found by a robot observer to be distinctive, as seen from the clustering shown in Figure 9.10. This implies that the robot is able to classify the emotional states of a human based on the emotional primitives that are extracted by the observable motion.

9.5   Game scenarios for training autistic people

9.5.1   Training gross motor skills, imitation, and turn taking

We created a number of game scenarios that train imitation and turn-taking skills. First, it is well known that children with autism have problems with imitation. Different studies have established that autistic children would imitate either the goal of the imitation, or the particular movement behavior. Combining both, however, has shown to be challenging for the children. Second, facilitating turn taking is particularly important because of the weak social responsiveness of autistic children. We believe that training the children's sensitivity to the contingencies involved in cooperative play may produce turn taking and variability in their play behavior.

Earlier research indicated that if children with autism are asked to make a verbal description of the acted-out target behavior before imitating, it helped them to initiate and sustain cooperative play, which resulted in longer play episodes and more variation in play (Jahr *et al.*, 2000). To address the problem of turn taking through imitation of the goal of an action, we used a task similar to those of Jahr *et al.* (2000) where actors were demonstrating actions to the children. Being requested to undertake social interaction with new people can make it unnecessarily stressful for the child to attend the training. So to minimize the stress levels, we asked the same actor to demonstrate all the scenarios. To further reduce this stress, we created video scenarios instead of using a physically present actor, similar to the study by Charlop-Christy and colleagues (2004).

The i-blocks platform is used in the game. There is one active block, which can change the colors of other blocks, and five passive blocks, which can be subject to a color change. There are sheets of colored paper at the four corners of the table. The task for the children is to match the color of the blocks to the pieces of colored paper positioned in front of the children. For example, a colorless passive receiving block lying on red piece of paper should be colored red. This can be done by turning the active sending block to red and holding it close to the passive receiving block. Turning of the active block changes its color and this is the behavior that the child has to imitate. A child could explore the blocks by himself or herself and later color the blocks together with someone else.

Three scenarios have been performed and tested in the following way. First, the child and the coordinator view the video scenario on a computer or TV. After that the coordinator asks the child to describe what actions were performed by the actor. If the scenario is described correctly the child can start imitating the scenario; if not, the video scenario is replayed until the child explains the actions correctly. The child plays the scenario with the coordinator. Snapshots of the three scenarios are shown in Figure 9.11.

In the first scenario, the blocks are placed in front of the actor, the passive blocks are on the colored pieces of paper, and the active block is in the middle. The actor picks up the active block and starts turning it until the block acquires the color of the paper in front of him. The actor transfers the color to the passive block on the piece of paper. He does so for all the three paper–block combinations. The scenario is finished when all passive blocks are colored according to the underlying piece of paper.

The goal of this scenario is training of gross motor skills; also the aim is that the child becomes familiar with the interaction possibilities of the blocks and the concept of the game. By the second and third scenario, the complexity of the task increases, and imitation and turn-taking behaviors between a child and a caregiver take place. Within the video modeling, the first actor colors a block and then shares the block with the second actor who, on his turn, colors his block. By the third scenario the active block is shared once more by the first actor. Following the video modeling, the coordinator and the child have to complete a longer scenario, where they share the blocks twice.

Two user tests were performed with groups of five autistic children. The first test was meant to optimize the concept and the experimental setting. The second, actual test was done with children of four and five years of age. Two of them were diagnosed with PDD-NOS (P1, P2), one PDD-NOS or classic autism (P3), one classic autism and ADHD (P4) and for the fifth child there were no definite outcomes of diagnosis (P5). All the children managed to finish two or three of the scenarios.

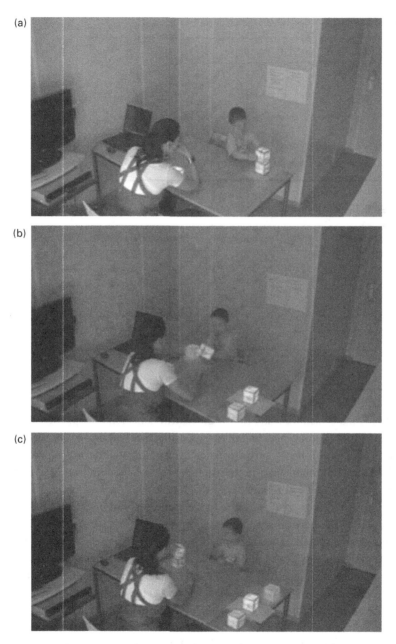

Figure 9.11 Snapshots from scenario 3. (a) Child colors second block, (b) child shares a block (cooperates), (c) coordinator colors second block.

The children were prepared for the test by their development coordinator, who was also the turn-taking partner in the scenarios with the children, and who made a qualitative evaluation of the tests. Four out of five children could perform the imitation and turn-taking properly. With one exception, most of the children could perform the

Table 9.1 Number of distractions during the pre-test

Participant	Total distractions	Distracted by blocks
P1	13	13
P2	2	0
P3	6	3
P4	4	3
P5	12	9
P6	19	13

Table 9.2 Number of distractions during the final test

Participant	Total distractions	Distracted by blocks
P1	7	2
P2	1	0
P3	2	0
P4	21	2
P5	1	0

imitation and turn-taking behaviors. Some individual achievements were as follows. A participant, who normally has trouble sustaining one-on-one play, was able to concentrate on the scenarios and follow the instructions. Another participant, who usually shows minimal group play and play variability (i.e. he plays every day with the same training scenario), had a surprising achievement in that he followed the instructions and let the coordinator join in the game. However, he didn't manage to complete the scenario, because he became heavily distracted.

With such a short-term exposure to the game, it is not possible to judge the effect of the game on the general social behavior of the children: that is, whether the children would be able to generalize the imitation and turn-taking skills to a different real-life situation. Using the blocks did not have a distraction effect on the children during the imitation and turn-taking tasks. In Tables 9.1 and 9.2, the number of distractions of the children during the test with the first and second group is shown. Although the total distraction by the blocks still varies widely per person, the distractions considerably decreased for the second test, which was conducted with a different group of autistic children, due to better preparation of the children by the coordinator.

We have implemented an accelerometer that makes the blocks sensitive to holding with a hand and has possibilities for implementing and testing many behaviors related to grasping, imitation, and other interaction behaviors. In the future, we will test the children's ability of mimicry or "blind" imitation, of goal imitation, or of the overall process of imitation proper. In this study, goal imitation was used to further facilitate turn taking. We showed that when all the actions were well understood by the autistic children, they performed turn-taking behaviors willingly, which is not normally the case.

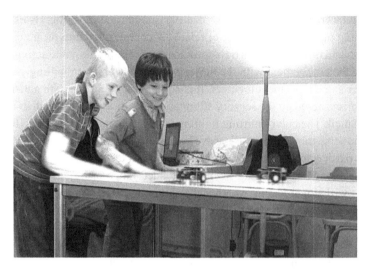

Figure 9.12 When the children perform the same movement, the robots imitate, enhance, or contradict the movement pattern.

In another game scenario (Figure 9.12), aiming to encourage pairs of children to cooperate and imitate each other, mobile robots were used. As already shown in several studies, children with autism understand that they are imitated and find this experience rewarding and pleasurable. We used this finding to stimulate collaboration between pairs of autistic children. The children first observed a set of behaviors that had been performed by mobile robots. If the pair of children chooses to perform one of these behaviors, the robots will start to imitate it. The robots can enhance or contradict the movement and in this way cause the children to negotiate possible actions to further control the robots.

In summary, the children were enthusiastic about playing with the blocks and the mobile robots despite normally not showing variation in play. The proposed method shows a potential in supporting autistic children in learning imitation and turn-taking behaviors at a very early age, as summarized in the following observations.

1. Most of the children managed to imitate the play scenarios with the i-blocks and with the mobile robots. The children took part in turn taking by sharing the active block with the caregiver.
2. The video modeling was shown to be a suitable way to teach the children how to understand and imitate the target behavior.
3. The stress levels of the children stayed lower than in actual social contact with a new person, as observed by the coordinator, and they could get well prepared for the upcoming scenario.

Earlier studies have shown that the basic principles of this method, namely using videomodeling and making the children verbalize the behavior that has to be imitated, can improve the social skills of the children. We changed the setting by introducing a multi-agent system of tangible interaction blocks that were especially designed for autistic children and were tested to be perceived as pleasurable and engaging. By using physical and engaging play objects, training of relatively complex and untypical behaviors such as imitation and turn taking was transformed into a pleasurable game activity. Similarly, because of the engagement with the moving robots, the children willingly collaborated to make the same movement together. It is common for children with autism to choose the play objects based on the sensory stimulation that they provide, such as color, touch, sound, or smell. The color-emitting lighting blocks, which emit pleasing, dimmed light through the semi-transparent walls, have been well accepted by all autistic children that have been participating in different experiments with the blocks so far.

We plan a longitudinal study with an extended range of imitative and turn-taking games that will aim at testing whether the children will be able to transfer the learned cooperative play behaviors to different, preferably real-life situations. In the current research, the play of children and a caregiver in a prepared environment has been observed. We intend to explore the effect of this method in a natural environment and in realistic everyday interactions, such as at school, with autistic and typical children.

9.5.2   Understanding and imitation of emotional behaviors

In this section we aim to go beyond sensory–motor interaction in robotic models of embodied cognition by also including the interactive aspects of autonomy. This means that sensory–motor interaction has to be enriched with intentional, emotional, and reward features. Specifically, we focus on the emotions that are conveyed by movement behaviors. Keltner and Kring (1998) point out a highly dependent link between emotion and social meaning. They argue that emotions serve a set of functions that are critical for coordinating social interactions. These functions are: to provide information to the peers about the surrounding environment (e.g. fear may indicate the presence of a danger); to elicit both complementary and similar emotions in others, depending on the context; and to be an incentive that promotes social relationships. This motivates us to pursue a more general social learning framework with robots that include emotional facial expressions, bodily posture, and actions of others, and that trigger appropriate emotional responses.

Although it is not shown that emotional resonance (response to perceived emotion) and understanding and recognition of emotion are related components of the emotional system (Nadel et al., 2006), any teaching to recognize emotions alone will be beneficial to children with autism (Barakova and Lourens, 2010).

For the purpose of mediation of play between children, a robot that can engage in reciprocal social interaction through movement was used. In particular, we are designing behaviors to support collective games for e-puck and the humanoid robot NAO. The game scenarios that are constructed on the basis of these interactive behaviors were aimed at helping children with autism learn to recognize emotional movements from a robot partner and to produce similar movements.

The Laban movement guidelines as suggested by Camurri et al. (2003) were used to design emotional behaviors on a mobile robot. Note that for this experiment we did not directly use the human emotional movement primitives.

To test solely the perceived emotion from the movement, the experiments were performed with the e-puck robot (www.e-puck.org) that had neither anthropomorphic nor zoomorphic shape. A control user group of 42 typically developing children were asked to observe and categorize the emotional behaviors enacted by the robots. The outcome of the tests showed a good recognition of several basic emotions. The first row (light bars) of the chart in Figure 9.13 shows the recognition rate in percentage of the designed emotional behaviors for each emotion. It is important to mention that the children were not provided with a list of possible emotions.

To analyze the robot behaviors we attached the Wiimote to the robot when it performed the emotional movements. The plots did not show the typical acceleration profile as seen by the emotional movements enacted by a human demonstrator, as shown in Section 9.4. The recording of the acceleration profiles from human motion patterns were a substantial step in redesigning the emotional behavior of the robot. The second row of bars (dark gray) in Figure 9.13 shows the recognition rate in percentages by a group of participants (children from a different school), after we had redesigned the robot behaviors according to the findings from human recordings.

The emotional behaviors of the robots based on human data were included in a game for promoting associative play (Barakova and Lourens, 2010) by children with autism. The emotional behaviors consist of a robotic sequence of movements that were shown to be perceived as expressing a certain emotion (Figure 9.13, the darker bars). To design the game, the following shortcomings of the children were targeted: inability to share and socially interact, inability to understand expression of emotions and link them to context, and preference to learn by examples and logic rather than by trial and error.

To account for these problems, a combined approach was taken to design a game that requires negotiations and working towards a common goal, together with recognition of emotional states. The game uses a storyline that describes various situations involving different emotions. When the children recognize the emotion described in the story they have to command a robot to either perform or contradict this emotion. The robot is commanded by the collective physical behavior of the children. At least

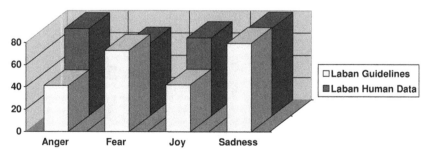

Figure 9.13 The outcomes of the two user tests on perceiving emotional behaviors from robot movement. For the first test (the light bars) the robot behaviors are designed according to Laban theory guidelines. In the second test (the dark bars) we used human data, from which we extracted movement primitives. The emotional content of the movements was evaluated by independent certified movement analysts.

two children have to step on one site of a large disk to make the disk tilt (Figure 9.14). The disk can be tilted in several directions, denoted with arrows lit by colored LED lights. The tilted disk will trigger a movement of a robot that expresses corresponding emotion. The LED arrows have the color that resembles the emotion in a similar way to the traffic light metaphor that was used in schools for autistic children to illustrate children's emotions. To change the robot's emotional behavior, the children had to agree on their next position and move together. When conflicting views occurred, it was an opportunity for the children to learn to negotiate and become aware that they need the help of others.

The two experiments in this section showed that expressing and interpreting emotions by humans and robots are done on the basis of the same signals. LMA was used

(a)

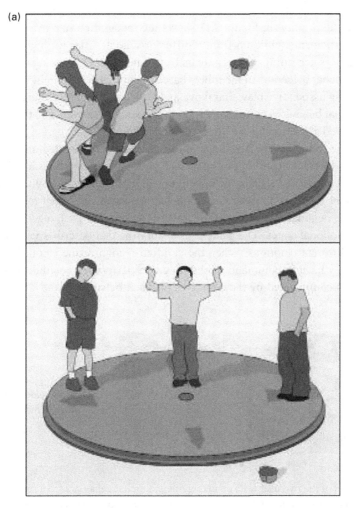

Figure 9.14   Fragments from game scenarios and flowchart of the game platform. (a) The robot is drawn as a small object near the platform. (b) The information flow from the robot to the life-size disk through a notebook.

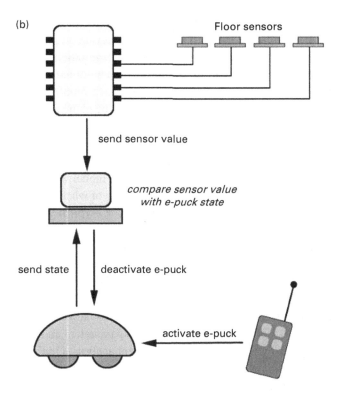

Figure 9.14   (*cont.*)

for a qualitative evaluation of the human as well as the robot movements and the robot movement behaviors were incorporated in a simple game with the e-puck robot. LMA, therefore, incorporates on a functional level the common coding (mirroring) principle. Scenarios that involve recognition and simulation of emotional movements on the humanoid robot NAO are currently being developed.

9.6   Discussion

Using robots for behavioral training of autistic children through games and interactive scenarios is a topic of growing interest. We have shown how using brain-inspired and cognitive models to emulate human-like features on robots can add to this line of research. Our hypothesis that training motor skills at an early age can contribute to the development of social skills in autistic people was confirmed in several cases. Autistic children could play games that targeted imitation of behavior. In addition, they became involved in taking turns, by exchanging tangible objects. Both behaviors, imitation and turn taking, are not typical in the everyday activities of the autistic children. The robots and tangibles especially contributed to accomplishment of these behaviors. The engaging light-emitting i-blocks, which also trigger the curiosity and logical thinking of the children, are a powerful stimulation to help the children accomplish the social interaction scenarios. Controlling mobile robots was another pleasurable activity for the children. Children willingly imitated each other's movement patterns in order to control the robots. A further step was instigating the negotiations that the children had to engage with: firstly, they had to recognize the emotional pattern to be able to change the robot mood (the experiment with the e-puck robot); and secondly, the open-ended play made the children discuss the goal of the game and thus communicate more often.

We simulated human-like behaviors in robots in two ways. First, we showed that neural models of sensory integration could approximate instrumental behaviors by autistic and typical people. Using the dynamic neural field model we created a realistic simulation of autistic and typical behavior. Independently of whether the delay in sensory integration is the actual mechanism that causes the atypical grasping behavior, the behavioral emulations on a robot showed realistic movement patterns that can be used for behavioral training. The difference in the autistic and typical grasping behavior is detected by the tangible devices, for instance by the i-blocks during the imitation scenarios. Further games that stimulate the usage of the visual cue can be created. The grasping behavior can be precisely emulated by a robot.

Second, for enacting and recognition of emotional body language by humans, we used a method that finds correlations between signal parameters and qualitative analysis of emotional signals by certified Laban movement analysts. On the basis of these correlations, we created emotional primitives that can be used for recognition as well as for emulation of emotional behavior by robots. Constructing robot behaviors based on this method showed a much better recognition rate by the children than the behaviors that were built solely on the recommendation of the Laban guidelines. The constructed robot behaviors have been used in games with mobile robots. The scenarios that will use a humanoid robot, NAO, are under development in collaboration with autism clinics.

References

Adolphs, R. (2002) Neural systems for recognizing emotion. *Current Opinion in Neurobiology.* **12**, 169–177.

Alers, S. H. M. and Barakova, E. I. (2009). Multi-agent platform for development of educational games for children with autism. In *IEEE ICE CIG 2009*, pp. 47–53, ISBN: 978–1–4244–4459–5.

Amari, S.-I. (1977). Dynamical study of formation of cortical maps. *Biological Cybernetics*, **27**(2), 77–87.

Barakova, E. I. and Chonnaparamutt, W. (2009). Timing sensory integration for robot simulation of autistic behavior. *IEEE Robotics and Automation Magazine*, **16**(3), 51–58.

Barakova, E. I. and Lourens, T. (2005). Event based self-supervised temporal integration for multimodal sensor data. *Journal of Integrative Neuroscience*, **4**(2), 265–282.

Barakova, E. I. and Lourens, T. (2010). Expressing and interpreting emotional movements in social games with robots. *Personal and Ubiquitous Computing*, **14**, 457–467.

Barakova, E. I., van Wanrooij, G., van Limpt, R., and Menting, M. (2007). Using an emergent system concept in designing interactive games for autistic children. In *Proceedings of the 6th International Conference on Interaction Design and Children (IDC07)*, pp. 73–77. ACM 978–1–59593–747–6.

Barakova, E. I., Gillessen, J., and Feijs, L. (2009). Social training of autistic children with interactive intelligent agents. *Journal of Integrative Neuroscience*, **8**(1), 23–34.

Bauman, M. L. (1992) Motor dysfunction in autism. In Joseph, A. B. and Young, R. R. (eds.), *Movement Disorders in Neurology and Neuropsychiatry*. Boston, MA: Blackwell Scientific, pp. 658–661.

Bekker, T., Sturm, J., and Barakova, E. (2010). Design for social interaction through physical play in diverse contexts of use. *Personal and Ubiquitous Computing*, **14**(5), 381–383, doi: 10.1007/s00779–009–0269–9.

Bolognini, N., Frassinetti, F., Serino, A., and Ladavas, E. (2005). "Acoustical vision" of below threshold stimuli: interactions among spatially converging audiovisual inputs. *Experimental Brain Research*, **160**(3), 273–282.

Brock, J., Brown, C. C., Boucher, J., and Rippon, G. (2002). The temporal binding deficit hypothesis of autism. *Developmental Psychopathology*, **14**(2), 209–224.

Camurri, A., Lagerlöf, I., and Volpe, G. (2003). Recognizing emotions from dance movement: comparison of spector recognition and automated techniques. *International Journal of Human-Computer Studies*, **59**(1/2), 213–225.

Charlop-Christy, M. H., Le, L., and Freeman, K. A. (2004). A comparison of video modeling with in vivo modeling for teaching children with autism. *Journal of Autism and Developmental Disorders*, **30**(6), 537–552.

Craighero, L., Bello, A., Fadiga, L., and Rizzolatti, G. (2002). Hand action preparation influences the responses to hand pictures. *Neuropsychologia*, **40**, 492–502.

Damasio, A. R. and Maurer, R. G. (1978). A neurological model for childhood autism. *Archives of Neurology*, **35**, 777–786.

Decety, J. (2002). Is there such a thing as functional equivalence between imagined, observed, and executed action? In Meltzoff, A. and Prinz, W. (eds.), *The Imitative Mind: Development, Evolution, and Brain Bases*. Cambridge, UK: Cambridge University Press, pp. 291–310.

De Gelder, B. (2006). Towards the neurobiology of emotional body language. *Nature Reviews Neuroscience*, **7**(3), 242–249.

Dinstein, I., Thomas, C., Humphreys, K. *et al.* (2010). Normal movement selectivity in autism. *Neuron*, **66**(3), 461–469.

Dott, L. P. (1995). Aesthetic listening: contributions of dance/movement therapy to the psychic understanding of motor stereotypes and distortions in autism and psychosis in childhood and adolescence. *The Arts in Psychotherapy* (European Consortium for Arts Therapy Education), **22**(3), 241–247.

Emery, N. J. and Amaral, D. G. (2000). The role of the amygdala in primate social cognition. In Lane, R. D. and Nadel, L. (eds.), *Cognitive Neuroscience of Emotion*. New York: Oxford University Press, pp. 156–191.

Erlhagen, W. and Schöner, G. (2002). Dynamic field theory of motor preparation. *Psychological Review*, **109**, 545–572.

Fadiga, L., Fogassi, L., Pavesi, G., and Rizzolatti, G. (1995). Motor facilitation during action observation: a magnetic stimulation study. *Journal of Neurophysiology*, **73**, 2608–2611.

Fagerberg, P., Ståhl, A., and Höök, K. (2003). Designing gestures for affective input: an analysis of shape, effort and valence. In *Proceedings of the 3rd ACM Conference on Mobile and Ubiquitous Multimedia, MUM2003*.

Faubel, C. and Schöner, G. (2006). Fast learning to recognize objects – dynamic fields in label-feature spaces. In *Proceedings of the 5th IEEE International Conference on Development and Learning*.

Foroud, A. and Pellis, S. M. (2003). The development of "roughness" in the play fighting of rats: a Laban movement analysis perspective. *Developmental Psychobiology*, **42**(1), 35–43, doi:10.1002/dev.10088.

Foroud, A. and Whishaw, I. Q. (2006). Changes in the kinematic structure and non-kinematic features of movements during skilled reaching after stroke: a Laban movement analysis in two case studies. *Journal of Neuroscience Methods*, **158**(1), 137–149.

Gallese, V., Fadiga, L., Fogassi, L., and Rizzolatti, G. (1996). Action recognition in the premotor cortex. *Brain*, **119**, 593–609.

Gepner, B., Deruelle, C., and Grynfeltt, S. (2001). Motion and emotion: a novel approach to the study of face processing by young autistic children. *Journal of Autism and Developmental Disorders*, **31**(1), 37–45.

Hecht, H., Vogt, S., and Prinz, W. (2001). Motor learning enhances perceptual judgement: a case for action-perception transfer. *Psychological Research*, **65**, 3–14.

Iacoboni, M. and Dapretto, M. (2006). The mirror neuron system and the consequences of its dysfunction. *Nature Reviews Neuroscience*, **7**(12), 942–951. doi:10.1038/nrn2024. PMID 17115076.

Iarocci, G. and McDonald, J. (2006). Sensory integration and the perceptual experience of persons with autism. *Journal of Autism and Development Disorders*, **36**(1), 77–90.

Iossifidis, I. and A. Steinhage, A. (2001). Controlling an 8 DOF manipulator by means of neural fields. In Halme, A., Chatila, R. and Prassler, E. (eds.), *Proceedings of the IEEE International Conference on Field and Service Robotics (FSR2001)*. Helsinki: Yleisjäljennös–Painopörssi, pp. 269–274.

Jahr, E., Eldevik, S., and Eikeseth, S. (2000). Teaching children with autism to initiate and sustain cooperative play. *Research in Developmental Disabilities*, **21**, 151–169.

Jeannerod, M. (2001). Neural simulation of action: a unifying mechanism for motor cognition. *Neuroimage*, **14**, S103–109.

Keltner, D. and Kring, A. M. (1998). Emotion, social function, and psychopathology. *Review of General Psychology*, **2**, 320–342.

Laban, R. and Lawrence, F. C. (1947). *Effort*. London: Macdonald & Evans.

Leary, M. R. and Hill, D. A. (1996). Moving on: autism and movement disturbance. *Mental Retardation*, **34**(1), pp. 39–53.

Malone, T. W. and Lepper, M. R. (1987). Making learning fun: a taxonomy of intrinsic motivations for learning. In Snow, R. E. and Farr, M. J. (eds.), *Aptitude, Learning and Instruction*. Vol. III: *Cognitive and Affective Process Analysis*. Hillside, NJ: Lawrence Erlbaum Associates, pp. 223–253.

Manjiviona, J. and Prior, M. (1995). Comparison of Asperger syndrome and high-functioning autistic children on a test of motor impairment. *Journal of Autism and Developmental Disorders*, **25**, 23–39.

Marti, P., Giusti, L., Moderini, C., and Pollini, A. (2009). A robotic toy for children with special needs: from requirements to design. In *Proceedings of the 11th IEEE International Conference on Rehabilitation Robotics*, held June 23–26, Kyoto, Japan.

Masterton, B. A. and Biederman, G. B. (1983). Proprioceptive versus visual control in autistic children. *Journal of Autism and Developmental Disorders*, **13**(2), 141–152.

Meltzoff, A. N. and Moore, M. K. (1997). Explaining facial imitation: a theoretical model. *Early Development and Parenting*, **6**, 179–192.

Mottron, L. and Burack, J. (2001). Enhanced perceptual functioning in the development of autism. In Burack, J. A., Charman, T., Yirmiya, N., and Zelazo, P. R. (eds.), *The Development of Autism: Perspectives from Theory and Research*. New York: Oxford University Press, pp. 131–148.

Murata, A., Fadiga, L., Fogassi, L., *et al.* (1997). Object representation in the ventral premotor cortex (area F5) of the monkey. *Journal of Neurophysiology*, **78**, 2226–2230.

Nadel, J. (2004). Early imitation and a sense of agency. In Berthouze, L., Kozima, H., Prince, C. G., *et al.* (eds.), *Proceedings of the 4th International Workshop on Epigenetic Robotics*. Lund University Cognitive Studies 117. Lund, Sweden: Lund University, pp. 15–16.

Nadel, J., Simon, M., Canet, P., *et al.* (2006). Human responses to an expressive robot. In *Proceedings of the 6th International Workshop on Epigenetic Robotics*. Lund University Cognitive Studies 128. Lund, Sweden: Lund University, pp. 79–86.

O'Riordan, M., Plaisted, K., Baron-Cohen, S., and Driver, J. (2001). Superior target detection in autism. *Journal of Experimental Psychology, Human Perception and Performance*, **27**(3), 719–730.

Ozonoff, S., Strayer, D. L., William, M., McMahon, W. M., and Filloux, F. (1994). Executive function abilities in autism and Tourette syndrome: an information processing approach. *Journal of Child Psychology and Psychiatry*, **35**, 1015–1032.

Pierno, A. C., Morena, M., Dean L., and Umberto, C. (2008). Robotic movement elicits visuo-motor priming in children with autism. *Neuropsychologia*, **46**(2), 448–454.

Rauterberg, M. (2004). Positive effects of entertainment technology on human behaviour. In Jacquart, R. (ed.), *Building the Information Society*. IFIP World Computer Congress 2004. Norwell, MA: Kluwer Academic Press, pp. 51–58.

Rizzolatti, G. and Luppino, G. (2001). The cortical motor system. *Neuron*, **31**, 889–901.

Rizzolatti, G., Fogassi, L., and Gallese, V. (2001). Neurophysiological mechanisms underlying the understanding and imitation of action. *Nature Reviews Neuroscience*, **2**, 661–670.

Rizzolatti, G., Fadiga, L., Fogassi, L, and Gallese, V. (2002). From mirror neurons to imitation: facts and speculations. In Meltzoff, M. and Prinz, W. (eds.), *The Imitative Mind: Development, Evolution, and Brain Bases*. Cambridge, UK: Cambridge University Press, pp. 247–266.

Robins, B., Dautenhahn, K., Dickerson, P., and Stribling, P. (2004). Robot mediated joint attention in children with autism. *Interaction Studies*, **5**, 161–198.

Rotshtein, P., Malach, R., Hadar, U., Graif, M., and Hendler, T. (2001). Feeling or features: different sensitivity to emotion in high-order visual cortex and amygdala. *Neuron*, **32**, 747–757.

Russo, N., Flanagan, T., Iarocci, G., *et al.* (2007). Deconstructing executive deficits among persons with autism: implications for cognitive neuroscience. *Brain Cognition*, **65**(1), 77–86.

Sauser, E. L. and Billard, A. G. (2006). Biologically inspired multimodal integration: interferences in a human–robot interaction game. In *Proceedings of 2006 IEEE/RSJ International Conference on Intelligent Robots and Systems*, pp. 5619–5624.

Schauer, C. and Gross, H.-M. (2004). Design and optimization of Amari neural fields for early auditory-visual integration. In *Proceedings of the 2004 IEEE International Joint Conference on Neural Networks*, Vol. 4, pp. 2523–2528.

Schoner, G., Dose, M., and Engels, C. (1995). Dynamics of behavior: theory and applications for autonomous robot architectures. *Robotics and Autonomous Systems*, **16**(4), 213–245.

Smith, M. and Bryson, S. E. (1994). Imitation and action in autism: a critical review. *Psychological Bulletin*, **116**(2), 259–273.

Stein, B. E., London, N., Wilkinson, L. K., and Price, D. D. (1989). Enhancement of perceived visual intensity by auditory stimuli: a psychophysical analysis. *Journal of Cognitive Neuroscience*, **1**(1), 12–24.

Steinhage, A. (2000). The dynamic approach to anthropomorphic robotics. In *Proceedings of the 4th Portuguese Conference on Automatic Control*, Portuguese Association of Automatic Control (APCA), pp. 1175–1181.

Stone, W. L., Ousley, O. Y., and Littleford, C. D. (1997). Motor imitation in young children with autism: What's the object?' *Journal of Abnormal Child Psychology*, **25**(6), 475–485.

Strafella, A. P. and Paus, T. (2000). Modulation of cortical excitability during action observation: a transcranial magnetic stimulation study. *NeuroReport*, **11**, 2289–2292.

Sumby W. H. and Pollack, I. (1954). Visual contribution to speech intelligibility in noise. *Journal of the Acoustical Society of America*, **26**(2), 212–215.

Teitelbaum, P., Teitelbaum, O., Nye, J., Fryman, J., and Maurer, R. G. (1998). Movement analysis in infancy may be useful for early diagnosis of autism. *Proceedings of the National Academy of Sciences of the USA*, **95**, 13 982–13 987.

Thelen, E., Schner, G., Scheier, C., and Smith, L. B. (2001). The dynamics of embodiment: a field theory of infant preservative reaching. *Behavioral and Brain Sciences*, **24**(1), 1–34; discussion 34–86.

Umiltà, M. A., Kohler, E., Gallese, V., *et al.* (2001). I know what you are doing: a neurophysiological study. *Neuron*, **31**, 155–165.

Van Beers, R. J., Sittig, A. C., and van der Gon, J. J. D. (1998). The precision of proprioceptive position sense. *Experimental Brain Research*, **122**(4), 367–377.

Van Berckelaer-Onnes, I. A. (2003). Promoting early play. *Autism*, **7**(4), 415–423.

Vasey, P., Foroud, A., Duckworth, N., and Kovacovsky, S. (2006). Male/female and female/female mounting in Japanese macaques: a comparative study of posture and movement. *Archives of Sexual Behavior*, **35**(2), 116–128.

Vilensky, J. A., Damasio, A. R., and Maurer, R. G. (1981). Gait disturbances in patients with autistic behaviour. *Archives in Neurology*, **38**, 646–649.

Vogt, S. (1995). On relations between perceiving, imagining and performing in the learning of cyclical movement sequences. *British Journal of Psychology*, **86**, 191–216.

Vogt, S. (1996). The concept of event generation in movement imitation neural and behavioral aspects. *Corpus, Psyche et Societas*, **3**, 119–132.

Vygotsky, L. S. (1966). Play and its role in the mental development of the child. *Voprosy Psikhologii*, **12**, 62–67.

Williams, J. H. G. (2008). Self–other relations in social development and autism: multiple roles for mirror neurons and other brain bases. *Autism Research*, **1**(2), 73–90. doi:10.1002/aur.15. PMID 19360654.

Part IV

Philosophical and theoretical considerations

10 From hardware and software to kernels and envelopes: a concept shift for robotics, developmental psychology, and brain sciences

Frédéric Kaplan and Pierre-Yves Oudeyer

10.1 From hardware and software to kernels and envelopes

At the beginning of robotics research, robots were seen as physical platforms on which different behavioral programs could be run, similar to the hardware and software parts of a computer. However, recent advances in developmental robotics have allowed us to consider a reversed paradigm in which a single software, called a kernel,[1] is capable of exploring and controlling many different sensorimotor spaces, called envelopes. In this chapter, we review studies we have previously published about kernels and envelopes to retrace the history of this concept shift and discuss its consequences for robotic designs and also for developmental psychology and brain sciences.

This chapter is based on other studies we have published on various aspects of this subject (Kaplan and Oudeyer, 2007a, 2007b, 2008, 2009). Its aim is to reframe these works into a coherent structure in order to give a more global overview of this concept shift. The first section of this chapter discusses in more detail the epistemological transition from the classical dualism that views a robot as fixed body into which different programs can be plugged to the new dualism based on kernel and envelopes. Each important conceptual step in this evolution is illustrated with concrete examples and experiments. The main point of this first section is to introduce this concept shift and not to define precisely what kind of systems can be considered a kernel and what kind of systems cannot. The kernel is simply defined as what is stable across applications and independent of the particular trajectory of one agent. Typically "metalearning" algorithms are good candidates to be part of a kernel as long as they can be considered task and embodiment independent. In contrast, memory used by the learning systems (weight of neural networks, list of prototypes, data in general) would typically not be part of the kernel. The main goal of this first section is to articulate how the kernel/ envelope dichotomy opens the way to new kinds of experimental studies. In particular,

---

[1] The term *kernel* is currently used with different meanings in computer science. The term is used here in a different way from that in the machine learning community (e.g. kernels of support vector machines).

Neuromorphic and Brain-Based Robots, eds. Jeffrey L. Krichmar and Hiroaki Wagatsuma. Published by Cambridge University Press. © Cambridge University Press 2011.

we discuss the case of generic algorithms capable of learning to control a robotic body without knowing its characteristics beforehand. With such kinds of algorithm, experiments can be performed, which can precisely characterize the importance of the embodiment in the final behavior, simply by changing the embodiment and keeping the kernel stable.

This new kind of experiment opens a different perspective on data obtained by research in developmental science and neuroscience. In the following section, we argue why children's development can indeed be seen as a succession of temporary embodiments corresponding not necessarily to physical changes but to the acquisition of new skills. A child learning how to walk or how to play the piano discovers whole new spaces to explore. As he learns, he experiences a kind of metamorphosis. Likewise, to perform basic tasks, a child's body envelope extends itself to include objects, clothes, tools, or even vehicles. What stays the same in this developmental and behavioral process is the kernel, the origin of the motivation and action of the child. We discuss how this view allows us to reinterpret developmental psychology data from the development of sensorimotor dexterity to the acquisition of language.

Finally, we review different hypotheses about the possible underlying neural substrate for kernels and envelopes. In particular we discuss the putative role of subcortical systems in the process of envelope creation, the possible importance of tonic dopamine as a learning progress signal and the kind of computation that could be performed by microcortical circuits. The chapter ends with the discussion of an evolutionary scenario illustrating how an old brain circuitry optimized for specific extrinsic needs could have evolved into a subcortical kernel, possibly at the origin of the formidable cortical extension that characterizes the human brain.

10.2   A concept shift for robotics

10.2.1   The reunited body

Between the 1950s and the 1980s, the classical gap between the builders of robotic bodies and the researchers trying to model "intelligence" had some direct consequences on the performances of the machines produced. The artificial intelligence (AI) algorithms, designed to manipulate predefined unambiguous symbols, show clearly their inadequacy when it comes to dealing with the complexity and the unpredictability of the real world. Consider for instance the problem of programming the walking behavior of a four-legged robot using a classical AI algorithm. The set of joints of a robotic body are not a set of abstract symbols but rather a complex system, with positions that can easily end up being out of equilibrium, especially if it is made of rigid parts, as most robots are. The type of ground and the degree of friction have a direct influence on the behavior of the machine. With a symbolic AI approach, but also with many approaches in control theory, it is important that the system is not only equipped with the precise model of the robot body, but also with the environment in which the robot is embedded. It many cases this is just impossible. Viewed from this angle, walking on four legs can reveal itself to be a harder problem than demonstrating mathematical theorems.

To resolve this impasse, a new school of thought emerged at the end of the 1980s, with the work of researchers like Rodney Brooks, Luc Steels, and Rolf Pfeifer. The so-called embodied artificial intelligence, or new AI, strongly criticized the disembodied and symbolic approach of the "classical" artificial intelligence, claiming that intelligence could not be considered without reference to the body and the environment (Pfeifer and Scheier, 1999). Rodney Brooks added that bodies and environments are impossible to model and that therefore research should not try to build models of external reality but on the contrary concentrate on direct situated interaction: "the world is its own best model" (Steels, 1994; Brooks, 1999).

This change of perspective introduced a renewal of robotic experiments and in some ways a return to conception and experimentation methods that were characteristics of robotics *before* the advent of the digital computer. Grey Walter's cybernetic "tortoises" built in 1948 are taken as a canonical example of what good conception is, integrating seamlessly the physical design of the machine with the targeted behavior. These analogical robots were capable of complex behavior, without the need for any internal "representation" (Grey Walter, 1953). Their design was taking into account that they were physical machines, on which many kinds of "forces" had an influence, from gravity to friction, and that perception itself was primarily the result of their own movement and behavior (a concept later known as "enaction" (Varela *et al.*, 1991). The nature and positioning of their sensors enabled them to solve complex tasks, such as returning to their charging station, without the need to make any kind of complex "reasoning."

Inspired by von Uexküll's writings (von Uexküll, 1909), researchers of the new AI defined the behavior of their robot, taking into account their "Umwelts": the very nature and structure of their body immersed them in a specific ecological niche where certain stimuli are meaningful and others not. This research was also supported by the reappraisal of a nondualistic philosophical trend which in the tradition of Merleau-Ponty views cognition as being situated and embodied in the world (Merleau-Ponty, 1942, 1945; Varela *et al.*, 1991).

To try to convince the cognitivists to view intelligence only as a form of sophisticated computation, researchers in embodied AI tried to define the kind of *morphological computation* realized by the body itself (Pfeifer and Bongard, 2007). To solve a problem like four-legged walking, it is easier and more efficient to build a body with the right intrinsic physical dynamics instead of building a more complex control system. One can replace the rigid members and powerful motors of the robot by a system of elastic actuators inspired by the muscle–tendon dichotomy that is typical of the anatomy of quadruped animals. With such a body, one just needs a simple control system producing a periodic movement on each leg to obtain an elegant and adapted walking behavior. Once put on a given ground the robot stabilizes itself after a few steps and converges towards its "natural" gait. With such a system, the walking speed can not be arbitrarily defined but corresponds instead to attractors of this dynamical system. Only an important perturbation can enable the robot to leave its natural walking gait and enter another attractor corresponding for instance to "trotting" (Pfeifer and Bongard, 2007).

Thus, in an attempt to suppress the gap inherited from the post-war field division, embodied artificial intelligence emphasized the crucial importance of the body and illustrated its role for the elaboration of complex behavior: body morphological structure and animation processes must be thought of as a coherent whole.

10.2.2   Stable kernels

In the beginning of the 1990s, robotic experiments from the new AI perspective focused essentially on reenacting insect adaptive behavior, examples strategically far from the classical AI programs playing chess. In the following years, some researchers tried to extend this embodied approach to build robots capable of learning in the same way as young children do. The idea was not to address one particular step in a child's development (like learning how to walk or how to talk), but to capture the open-ended, versatile nature of children learning. In just a few months children incrementally learn to control their body, to manipulate objects, and to interact with peers and caregivers. They acquire everyday novel complex skills that open them to new kinds of perception and actions. How could a machine ever do something similar? The objective of child-like general learning capabilities was not new as it was already clearly expressed in one of Turing's classic articles on artificial intelligence (Turing, 1950). However, the sensorimotor perspective developed by the embodied approach gave to this challenge a novel dimension.

In asking how a machine could learn in an open-ended manner, researchers in epigenetic or developmental robotics (Lungarella et al., 2003; Kaplan and Oudeyer, 2006; Asada et al., 2009) partially challenged the basis of the embodied artificial intelligence approach and introduced a methodological shift. The importance of the body was still central as the focus was on developing sensorimotor skills intrinsically linked with a specific morphology and the structure of a given environment. However, while following an holistic approach, it seemed logical to identify, inside a robotic system, a process independent of any particular body, ecological niche, or task. Indeed, by definition, a mechanism that could drive the learning of an open-ended set of skills cannot be specific to a particular behavior, environment, or body. It must be general and disembodied.

Thus, the just reunited body must again be divided. But the division is not the one inherited from the punch-cards and the digital computer; that is, the software/hardware gap. In this new methodological dualism, the objective is to separate (1) a potentially changing body envelope corresponding to a sensorimotor space and (2) a kernel, defined as a set of general and stable processes capable of controlling any specific embodied interface. By differentiating a generic process of *incorporation* and fluid body envelopes, the most recent advances in epigenetic/developmental robotics allow us to consider the body from a new point of view. Unlike the traditional body schemata, grounded in anatomical reality, body envelopes are ephemeral spaces associated with a particular task or skill. Contrary to easily changeable animation programs used in robotics, we now consider a stable kernel, acting as an engine driving developmental processes. It is not the body that stays and the programs that change. It is precisely the opposite: the program stays, the embodiment changes.

Several kinds of kernels can be envisioned. Some of them lead to open developmental trajectories, others don't. Let us imagine a control room equipped with a set of measurement devices, a panel of control buttons, and most importantly, *no labels* on any of these devices. Imagine now an operator trying to guess how the whole system works despite the absence of labels. One possible strategy consists of randomly pushing buttons and observing the kind of signals displayed on the measurement devices. However, blindly finding correlation between these inputs and outputs could be very difficult. For the operator, a better strategy is to identify the contexts in which he or she progresses in understanding the effects of certain buttons and to explore further the corresponding actions.

It is possible to construct an algorithm that drives such smart exploration. Given a set of input and output channels, the algorithm will try to construct a predictive model of the effect of the input on the output, given its history of past interactions with the system. Instead of trying random configuration, the algorithm detects situations in which its predictions progress maximally and chooses the input signal in order to optimize its own progress. Following this principle, the algorithm avoids the subspaces where the outputs are too unpredictable, or on the contrary too predictable, in order to focus on the actions that are most likely to make it progress (Figure 10.1). We call these zones "progress niches".[2] The use of such an algorithm results in an organized exploration of an unknown space, starting with the simplest subspaces to progressively explore zones more difficult to model. The term "kernel" is relevant for several reasons to describe the behavior of this algorithm. It is a *central* process, stable, and unaffected by the peripheral embodied spaces. It is also the *origin* and the starting point of all the observed behavior.

Details of one version of this progress-driven kernel can be found in Oudeyer *et al.* (2007) and also in the Appendix to this chapter (see also earlier versions in Kaplan and Oudeyer, 2003, and Oudeyer *et al.*, 2005). Many variants of such intrinsic motivation systems have been or are currently being explored (see Oudeyer and Kaplan, 2007, for a taxonomy). To our knowledge, the first computational system exploring progress-driven exploration was described by Schmidhuber in 1991 (Schmidhuber, 1991). He suggested giving intrinsic reward to a reinforcement-learning controller in proportion to the predictor's error reductions, in order to motivate the controller to create actions that generate more data to maximize the predictor's future cumulative expected learning progress. In following papers, Schmidhuber described various techniques to obtain a similar behavior of the controller (Storck *et al.*, 1995; Schmidhuber, 2006).[3] More recently, different types of intrinsic motivation systems were explored, mostly in software simulations (Huang and Weng, 2002; Marshall *et al.*, 2004; Steels, 2004). The term "intrinsically motivated reinforcement learning" has been used by Barto in this context (Barto *et al.*, 2004). Interestingly, the mechanisms developed in these papers

---

[2] To discover these progress niches, the algorithm must explore regularly the entire space of possible actions. For such exploration the classical trade-off between exploration and exploitation applies. The algorithm must be programmed to balance the exploitation of the best progress niches and the constant exploration to discover some new ones. Please refer to the Appendix for a detailed implementation.

[3] See Schmidhuber's website for a complete list: www.idsia.ch/~juergen/html.

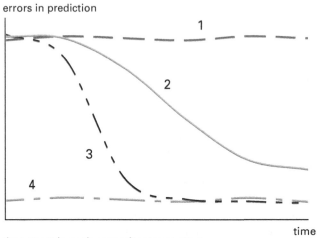

errors in prediction

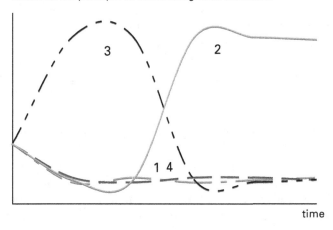

time spent in each sensorimotor context
based on the principle of maximizing error reduction

Figure 10.1   Confronted with four sensorimotor contexts characterized by different learning profiles, the exploration strategy of a progress-driven kernel consists in avoiding situations already predictable (context 4) or too difficult to predict (context 1), in order to focus first on the context with the fastest learning curve (context 3) and eventually, when the latter starts to reach a "plateau" to switch to the second most promising learning situation (context 2).

also show strong similarities with mechanisms developed in the field of statistics, where it is called "optimal experiment design" (Fedorov, 1972).

Coming back to our walking case study, let us now consider an experiment where a progress-driven kernel controls the movement of the different motors. For each motor, it chooses the period, the phase, and the amplitude of a sinusoidal signal. The prediction system tries to predict the effect of the different set of parameters in the way the image captured by a camera placed on the robot's head is modified. This indirectly reflects the movement of its torso. At each iteration the kernel produces the values for the next parameter set in order to maximize the reduction of the prediction error (Figure 10.2).

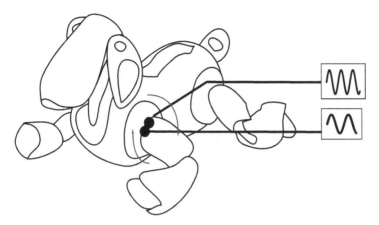

Figure 10.2   A robot can learn to walk just by exploring smartly a sensorimotor space. In the experiment, a progress-driven kernel controls the movement of the different motors of a four-legged robot. For each motor, it chooses the period, the phase, and the amplitude of a sinusoidal signal. The prediction system tries to predict the effect of the different set of parameters in the way the image captured by a camera placed on the robot's head is modified. This indirectly reflects the movement of its torso. At each iteration the kernel produces the values for the next parameter set in order to maximize the reduction of the prediction error.

When one starts an experiment like this one, several sets of parameters are explored for a few minutes. The robot's legs wobble in an apparently disorganized manner. Most of these attempts have very predictable effects: the robot just doesn't move. Errors in prediction stay at a minimal level: these situations are not interesting for the kernel. By chance, after thirty minutes or so, one movement leads the robots to make a slight move – in most cases a step backward. This new situation results first in an increase of the error in prediction but as the robot experiences similar movements again, this error tends to decrease: the kernel has discovered a "progress niche."

Then the robot will start exploring different ways to move backwards. During this exploration, it is likely that it discovers that certain modification of the parameters could lead to some sort of rotation movement, at least from an external observer's point of view. This is a new set of progress niches that the robot will learn to exploit when the skills for walking backwards have essentially been mastered.

In most experiments, it takes typically three hours for the kernel to find several subsets of parameters resulting in moving forward, backwards, sideways and to turn left and right. At no time in the process was the robot given the objective of learning to walk. Guided by the principle of maximizing the reduction of error in prediction, the robot ends up developing versatile locomotion skills. Actually, this versatility is the result of the unspecific nature of the kernel. A robot artificially motivated to go towards a specific object may not have learned to walk backwards or to spin.[4]

---

[4] There exist many different gait patterns for four-legged robots. In the discussed experiment only a "walking" gait was discovered by the robot. We do not know whether other gaits, like trotting, could be discovered using the same approach.

The fact that walking backwards revealed itself to be a parameter subset easier to discover was not easy to foresee. Given the morphological physical structure of the robot and the kind of ground the robot was placed on during the experiments, the walking backwards movement happened to be the first to be discovered. To know whether this progress niche is actually an attractor for most developmental trajectories, it is necessary to set up a bench of experimental trials, changing systematically the initial conditions, including the morphology of the robot itself. With such an experimental approach it becomes possible to study the developmental consequences of a physical modification of the body. A longer leg or a more flexible back can considerably change the structure of the progress niches and therefore the trajectory explored by the kernel. From a methodological point of view, the body becomes an *experimental variable*.

These robotic experiments naturally lead to novel questions addressed at other fields, including neurosciences (Can we identify the neural circuits that act as a kernel? Kaplan and Oudeyer, 2007a), developmental psychology (Can we reinterpret the developmental sequences of young children as progress niches? Kaplan and Oudeyer, 2007c) or in linguistics (Can we reconsider the debate on innateness in language learning by reconsidering the role of the body in this process? Kaplan et al., 2007).

10.2.3   Fluid body envelopes

A simple way to change the body envelope of a robot is to equip it with a tool. Figure 10.3(a) shows how the body of a four-legged robot can be simply extended by a helmet that plays the role of a prosthetic finger. With this simple extension the robot can now push buttons, press on hard surfaces, even switch on or off other devices. This is a new space to explore. Figure 10.3(b) shows the same idea with a pen holder. With this simple extension, the robot can now leave traces and use the environment as an external memory. A drawing is the temporal integration on a paper of a sequence of gestures. This simple pen holder opens a whole new space of exploration where the machine can learn to predict the relationship between a sequence of actions and particular kinds of representations. Such a kind of anticipation is likely to be a fundamental milestone on the road towards higher-level cognition (Steels, 2003).

Figure 10.3(c) shows a small scooter adapted to the morphology of the robot. Learning how to move with this device is not very different from learning how to walk. As in all the other cases, the progress-driven kernel discussed in Section 10.2.2 can be applied (Kaplan et al., 2006). The body changes but the program stays the same.

The progress-driven kernel only gives a partial understanding of the general process of incorporation. We illustrated how it could act on a single space, a single body envelope, such as the parameter space resulting in versatile walking skills, but we have not shown how it could be used to shift between them. Incorporation as we described in our introduction involves complex sequences of body envelope transformations. It involves recursive and hierarchical processes. Typically, once a robot has learned how to control its body to walk, it should be able to use these newly discovered walking primitives as basic elements for performing the exploration of new spaces. A walking robot will certainly discover new objects, a new environment for learning. Let's take for instance the

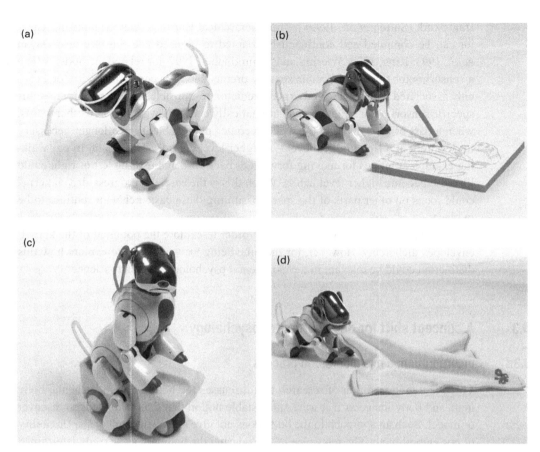

Figure 10.3   (a) A helmet-finger extension. (Design: ECAL (Ecole cantonale d'Art de Lausanne)/Stéphane Barbier-Bouvet.) (b) A pen holder extension. (Design: ECAL/Bénédicte Meynet, Olivier Burgisser, Xavier Rui, Sébastien Wildi and Siméon Reymond.) (c) A scooter. (Design: ECAL/ Clément Benoît and Nicolas Moro.) (d) A blanket with a special handle. (Design: ECAL/ Bénédicte Meynet, Olivier Burgisser, Xavier Rui, Sébastien Wildi and Siméon Reymond.) (Photos: ECAL/Milo Keller.)

case of the graspable blanket of Figure 10.3(d). This blanket is equipped with a special handle adapted to the robot's "mouth." Learning to grasp the blanket is quite similar to learning to grasp the pen holder we have just mentioned. Once the robot had learned how to grasp this object, it could explore the specific space corresponding to walking with a blanket. This compositional process could continue endlessly.

Going from the exploration of a single envelope to a generic kernel capable of easily switching between hierarchical envelopes is a difficult issue. In particular, it involves a mechanism permitting the formation of habits. The possibility of implementing these different features in a single generic kernel remains to be shown. However, several state-of-the-art methods are able to move towards this goal and envision how such a kernel could work. Multilayer recurrent neural network architectures (such as those considered in Schmidhuber, 1992; Tani and Nolfi, 1999; Tani, 2007) or the option framework (Sutton *et al.*, 1999) permit hierarchical learning where chunks of behavior can be compiled and continuously adapted to be used later on (see also Dayan *et al.*, 1993; Ring, 1994; Wiering and Schmidhuber, 1997, for related methods). When a sensorimotor trajectory becomes easily predictable, it becomes implicitly or explicitly associated with a dedicated expert predictor, responsible for both recognizing this specific sensorimotor situation and automatically choosing what to do. In other words, when a part of the sensorimotor space becomes predictable it is no longer necessary to explore it at a fine grained level – a higher-level control is sufficient. In our walking example, routines for moving forward or backward and turning left or right could likewise become higher-level habits. When this is the case, the progress-driven kernel could focus on other parts of the space, assuming these basic behavior routines to be in place.

Many challenges remain to be faced in order to explore the potential of the kernel/ envelopes dichotomy. However, for the time being we would like to explore how this distinction could be relevant in developmental psychology and neuroscience.

10.3   A concept shift for developmental psychology

10.3.1   Incorporation: a misunderstood process

There is a long tradition of research that discusses the notion of body schema, body map, and body image as if it were some stable notion that the child needs to discover or model. Such an approach to the body does not give a good account of the flexibility of our embodiment. The relevance of considering the body not as a fixed, determined entity but as a fluid, perceptually changing space has been argued by several philosophers (Merleau-Ponty, 1945), psychologists (Schilder, 1935), ethnographers (Warnier, 1999), and neuroscientists (Head and Holmes, 1911, or for instance Iriki *et al.*, 1996, for more recent studies). However, we are still far from having a precise model of this process and its relationship with attention, memory, and learning.

In many respects, our skin is not the limit of our body. When we interact with tools and technical devices, our body extends its boundaries, changes shape. The stick, the hammer, the pen, the racket, and the sword extend our hand and become, after some training, integral parts of our body envelope. Without thinking about it, we bend a bit more when we wear a hat and change the way we walk when we wear special shoes. This is also true for more complex devices. We are the car that we are driving. It took us many painful hours of training to handle our car the right way. At the beginning it was an external body element, reacting in unpredictable ways. But once we got used to the dynamics of the machine, the car became like our second skin. We are used to the space it occupies, and the time necessary to slow down. Driving becomes as natural as walking, an unconscious experience.

Compared with a fixed body, the concept of envelopes that would be extensibles, stretchables, constantly changing, seems more relevant. If we want to fix a nail on wall, we will first pick up a hammer. At this stage, the tool is *abstracted* from the environment. A few seconds later, when we hammer the nail, we temporarily extend our body envelope to include the tool in our hand. It disappears from our attention focus as a direct extension of our hand. It is *incorporated*. Once our goal has been reached, we put back the hammer and the tool again becomes an external object, ready to be used, but separated. This is the fundamental and misunderstood process of *incorporation*.

The first time we use a hammer, we fail to control it perfectly. Every time we fail to predict where the hammer will fall, the tool again becomes abstracted, back in our attention focus. It takes time until we can successfully predict the consequences of our action with this "extended" hand, and it is only when prediction errors are very low that the object is fully incorporated (Figure 10.4).

Before picking up a hammer, we must first choose it among the other tools abstracted from our toolbox. Once chosen, new objects – nails – become relevant for the pursuit of our goal. We don't think any more of our extended hand; instead we focus on these new abstracted objects. In general, incorporation is a recursive process. At a given state of incorporation, certain objects are abstracted from the environment and become

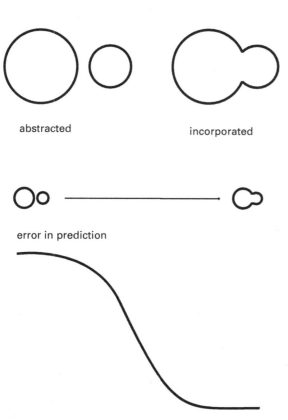

abstracted   incorporated

error in prediction

Figure 10.4 Illustration of the incorporation process. Objects can either be abstracted from the environment or incorporated as an extension of our body. The process of incorporation takes time. Surprise or failure causes an incorporated object to be abstracted again. When one learns to use an object, error in prediction corresponds to disincorporation of the object. The fewer the errors the more the object is incorporated.

Figure 10.5   Incorporation is a recursive process. At a given state of incorporation, certain objects are abstracted from the environment and become affordants. When one of these objects starts to be controlled and therefore incorporated, new objects become abstracted.

affordants. When one of these objects starts to be controlled and therefore incorporated, our attentional space changes and new objects become abstracted (Figure 10.5).

These processes can be understood in a rather simple way if we consider the kernel/ envelopes distinction. In the rest of this section we will discuss the existence of a kernel, in which it plays the role of an intrinsic motivation system, capable of driving the developmental and learning dynamics occurring for particular body envelopes. First, we will see that although the term "kernel" was not used in this context, such a construct has been discussed in various forms in psychology literature. Then we will illustrate how some child developmental milestones can be interpreted in this framework.

10.3.2   A kernel for active exploration: history of a construct

In psychology, an activity is characterized as intrinsically motivated when there is no apparent reward except the activity itself (Ryan and Deci, 2000). People seek and engage in such activities for their own sake and not because they lead to extrinsic reward. In such cases, the person seems to derive enjoyment directly from the practice of the activity. Following this definition, most children's playful or explorative activities can be characterized as being intrinsically motivated. Also, many kinds of adult behavior seem to belong to this category: free problem-solving (solving puzzles, crosswords), creative activities (painting, singing, writing during leisure time), gardening, hiking, etc. Such situations are characterized by a feeling of effortless control, concentration, enjoyment, and a contraction of the sense of time (Csikszenthmihalyi, 1991).

The first bloom of investigations concerning intrinsic motivation occurred in the 1950s. Researchers started by trying to give an account of exploratory activities on the basis of the theory of drives (Hull, 1943), which are non-nervous-system tissue deficits like hunger or pain, which the organisms try to reduce. For example, Montgomery (1954) proposed a drive for exploration and Harlow (1950) a drive to manipulate. This drive naming approach had many shortcomings which were criticized in detail by White (1959): intrinsically motivated exploratory activities have a fundamentally different dynamics. Indeed, they are not homeostatic: the general tendency to explore is never satiated and is not a consummatory response to a stressful perturbation of the organism's body. Moreover, exploration does not seem to be related to any non-nervous-system tissue deficit.

Some researchers then proposed another conceptualization. Festinger's theory of cognitive dissonance (Festinger, 1957) asserted that organisms are motivated to reduce dissonance; that is, the incompatibility between internal cognitive structures and the situations currently perceived. Fifteen years later a related view was articulated by Kagan, stating that a primary motivation for humans is the reduction of uncertainty in the sense of the "incompatibility between (two or more) cognitive structures, between cognitive structure and experience, or between structures and behavior" (Kagan, 1972). However, these theories were criticized on the basis that much human behavior is also intended to *increase* uncertainty, and not only to reduce it. Humans seem to look for some forms of optimality between completely uncertain and completely certain situations.

In 1965, Hunt developed the idea that children and adults look for optimal incongruity (Hunt, 1965). He regarded children as information-processing systems and stated that interesting stimuli were those where there was a discrepancy between the perceived and standard levels of the stimuli. For Dember and Earl, the incongruity or discrepancy in intrinsically motivated behaviors was between a person's expectations and the properties of the stimulus (Dember and Earl, 1957). Berlyne developed similar notions as he observed that the most rewarding situations were those with an intermediate level of novelty, between already familiar and completely new situations (Berlyne, 1960). Whereas most of these researchers focused on the notion of optimal incongruity at the level of psychological processes, a parallel trend investigated the notion of optimal arousal at the physiological level (Hebb, 1955). As overstimulation and understimulation situations induce fear (e.g. dark rooms, noisy rooms), people seem to be motivated to maintain an optimal level of arousal. A complete understanding of intrinsic motivation should certainly include both psychological and physiological levels.

Eventually, a later group of researchers preferred the concept of challenge to the notion of optimal incongruity. These researchers stated that what was driving human behavior was a motivation for effectance (White, 1959), personal causation (De Charms, 1968), and competence and self-determination (Deci and Ryan, 1985).

In more recent years, the concept of intrinsic motivation has been less present in mainstream psychology but has flourished in social psychology and the study of practices in applied settings, in particular in professional and educational contexts. Building on studies suggesting that extrinsic rewards (money, high grades, prizes) actually destroy intrinsic motivation (an idea articulated by Bruner in the 1960s; Bruner, 1962), some employers and teachers have started to design effective incentive systems based on intrinsic motivation. However, this view is currently at the heart of many controversies (Cameron and Pierce, 2002).

In summary, most psychological approaches of intrinsic motivation postulate that "stimuli worth investigating" are characterized by a particular relationship (incompatibility, discrepancy, uncertainty, or on the contrary predictability) between an internal predictive model and the actual structure of the stimulus. This invites us to consider intrinsically motivating activities not only at the descriptive behavioral level (no apparent reward except the activity itself) but primarily in respect to particular internal models built by an agent during its own personal history of interaction and to postulate the existence of an intrinsic motivation system, namely a kernel.

10.3.3   Reinterpretation of developmental patterns

How can we reinterpret particular developmental processes as being the result of a kernel playing the role of an intrinsic motivation system driving the infant into situations expected to result in maximal learning progress? Following on from preliminary experimental results, we discussed in Kaplan and Oudeyer (2007b) a scenario presenting the putative role of the progress drive for the development of early imitation. We argue in particular that the kernel/envelope distinction could help in understanding why children focus on specific imitative activities at a certain age and how they progressively organize preferential interactions with particular entities present in their environment.

The kernel pushes the agent to discover and focus on situations which lead to maximal learning progress. As already mentioned, we call these situations, neither too predictable nor too difficult to predict, "progress niches." Once discovered, progress niches gradually disappear as they become more predictable. The notion of progress niches is related to Vygotsky's *zone of proximal development*, where the adult deliberately challenges the child's level of understanding. Adults push children to engage in activities beyond their current mastery level, but not too far beyond so that they remain comprehensible (Vygotsky, 1978). We could interpret the zone of proximal development as a set of potential progress niches organized by the adult in order to help the child learn. But it should be clear that independently of the adults' efforts, what is and what is not a progress niche is ultimately defined from the child's point of view. Progress niches share also similarities with Csikszenthmihalyi's *flow experiences* (Csikszenthmihalyi, 1991). Csikszenthmihalyi argues that some activities are *autotelic* when challenges are appropriately balanced with the skills required to cope with them (see also Steels, 2004). We prefer to use the term "progress niche," by analogy with ecological niches, as we refer to a transient state in the evolution of a complex "ecological" system involving the embodied agent and its environment.

The experiments we described with robots illustrated how an agent can (1) separate its sensorimotor space into zones of different predictability levels and (2) choose to focus on the one which leads to maximal learning progress, called a "progress niche." With this kind of operant model, it could be speculated that meaningful sensorimotor distinctions (self, others, and objects in the environment) may be the result of discriminations constructed during a progress-driven process, where different envelopes are constructed and actively explored.

More specifically, we can offer an interpretation of several fundamental stages characterizing infants' development during their first year.

It has been argued that simple forms of imitative behavior are present just after birth. They could constitute a process of early identification. Some totally or partially nativist explanations could account for this early "like-me" stance (Meltzoff and Gopnick, 1993; Moore and Corkum, 1994). This would suggest the possibility of an early distinction between persons and things. If an intermodal mapping facilitating the match between what is seen and what is felt exists, the hypothesis of a kernel for active exploration would suggest that infants will indeed create a discrimination between such easily predictable couplings (interaction with peers) and unpredictable situations (all the other cases) and that they will focus on the first zone of their sensorimotor space that constitutes a "progress niche." Neonatal imitation (when it occurs) would be the result of the exploitation of the most predictable coupling present just after birth.[5]

During the first two months of their life, infants perform repeated body motions. They kick their legs repeatedly; they wave their arms. This process is sometimes referred as "body babbling." However, nothing indicates that this exploratory behavior is randomly organized. Rochat argues that children are in fact performing self-imitation, trying to imitate themselves (Rochat, 2002). This would mean that children are structuring their own behavior in order to make it more predictable and form "circular reactions" (Baldwin, 1925; Piaget, 1952). Such self-imitative behaviors can be well explained by the progress drive hypothesis. Sensorimotor trajectories directed towards the child's own body can be easily discriminated from trajectories directed towards other people by comparing their relative predictability. In many respects, making progress in understanding primary circular reactions is easier than in the cases involving other agents: Self-centered types of behavior are "progress niches." In such a scenario the "self" emerges as a meaningful discrimination for achieving better predictability. Once this distinction is made, progress for predicting the effects of self-centered actions can rapidly be made.

After two months, infants become more attentive to the external world and particularly to people. Parental scaffolding plays a critical role in making the interaction with the child more predictable (Schaffer, 1977). Parents adapt their own responses so that interactions with the child follow the normal social rules that characterize communicative exchanges (e.g. turn taking). Moreover, if an adult imitates an infant's own actions, it can trigger continued activity in the infant. This early imitative behavior is referred as "pseudo-imitation" by Piaget (1962). Pseudo-imitation and focus on scaffolded adult behavior could be seen as predictable effects of the progress drive. As the self-centered trajectories start to be well mastered (and no longer constitute "progress niches"), the child's focus shifts to another branch of the discrimination tree, the "self–other" zone.

After five months, attention shifts again from people to objects. Children gain increased control over the manipulation of some objects on which they discover "affordances" (Gibson, 1986). Parents recognize this shift and initiate interactions about those affordant objects. However, children do not easily alternate their attention between the object and their caregiver. A progress-driven process can account for this discrimination between affordant objects and unmastered aspects of the environment. Although this stage is typically not seen as imitative, it could be argued that the exploratory process involved in the discovery of the object affordances shares several common features with the one involved for self-centered activities: the child structures its world looking for "progress niches."

---

[5] This particular interpretation of neotanal imitation shows an example of how the kernel/envelope approach may lead to rethinking the innate/learned distinction. In such a case, the "innateness" of the behavior is not "coded" in the genes, but is a direct result of the coupling between a socially structured environment and an innate bias towards behaviors leading to learning progress.

The concepts of kernel and envelope lead to robotic experiments that can be used as a "tool for thoughts" in developmental psychology. In that sense, it may help in formulating new concepts useful for the interpretation of the developmental dynamics underlying children's development. For example, the existence of a kernel could explain why certain types of imitative behavior are produced by children at a certain age and stop being produced later on. It could also explain how discrimination between actions oriented towards the self, towards others, and towards the environment may occur. However, we do not argue that a drive for maximizing learning progress could be the only motivational principle driving children's development. The complete picture is likely to include a complex set of drives.[6] Developmental dynamics are certainly the result of the interplay between intrinsic and extrinsic forms of motivations, particular learning biases, as well as embodiment and environmental constraints. We believe that computational and robotic approaches can help to specify the contribution of these different components in the overall observed patterns and shed new light on the particular role played by intrinsic motivation in these complex processes.

10.4   A concept shift for neuroscience

10.4.1   Can we identify neural circuits corresponding to a kernel in the human brain?

Can we identify neural circuits that could play the role of a kernel? Or is it just a conceptual tool to understand how the brain learns? In neuroscience, dominant views in behavioral neuropsychology have long impeded discussions about putative intrinsic causes of behavior. Learning dynamics in brain systems are still commonly studied in the context of external reward seeking (food, sex, etc.) and very rarely as resulting from endogenous and spontaneous processes. Actually, the term "reward" has been misleading, as it has different meanings in neuropsychology and in machine learning (White, 1989; Wise, 1989; Oudeyer and Kaplan, 2007). In behavioral neuropsychology, rewards are primarily thought of as objects or events that increase the probability and intensity of behavioral actions leading to such objects: "rewards make you come back for more" (Thorndike, 1911). This means the function of rewards is based primarily on behavioral effects interpreted in a specific theoretical paradigm. As Schultz puts it "the exploration of neural reward mechanisms should not be based primarily on the physics and the chemistry of reward objects but on specific behavioral theories that define reward function" (Schultz, 2006, p. 91).

In computational reinforcement learning, a reward is only a numerical quantity used to drive an action-selection algorithm so that the expected cumulated value of this quantity is maximal in the future. In such context, rewards can be considered primarily as internal measures rather than external objects (as clearly argued by Sutton and Barto, 1998). This may explain why it is much easier from a machine learning perspective to

---

[6] The model we discuss in this chapter and present in more detail in the Appendix can be easily extended to account for this situation, just by transforming the intrinsic reward function into a linear combination of several reward sources.

consider the intrinsic motivation construct as a natural extension of the reinforcement learning paradigm, whereas dominant behavioral theories and experimental methodology in neuroscience do not permit consideration of such a construct. This is certainly one reason why complex behaviors that do not involve any consummatory reward are rarely discussed.

In the absence of experimental studies concerning intrinsically motivated behaviors, we can consider what resembles them the most: that is, exploratory behaviors. The extended lateral hypothalamic corridor, running from the ventral tegmental area to the nucleus accumbens, has been recognized as a critical piece of a system responsible for exploration. Pankseep calls it the SEEKING system (Panksepp, 1998) (different terms are also used as, for instance, behavioral activation system: Gray, 1990; or behavioral facilitation system: Depue and Iacono, 1989). "This harmoniously operating neuroemotional system drives and energizes many mental complexities that humans experience as persistent feelings of interest, curiosity, sensation seeking and, in the presence of a sufficiently complex cortex, the search for higher meaning" (Panksepp, 1998, p. 145). This system, a tiny part compared with the total brain mass, is where one of the major dopamine pathways originates (for a discussion of anatomical issues one can refer, for instance, to Stellar, 1985; Rolls, 1999).

The roles and functions of dopamine are known to be multiple and complex. Dopamine is thought to influence behavior and learning through two, somewhat decoupled, forms of signal: phasic (bursting and pausing) responses and tonic levels (Grace, 1991). A set of experimental evidence shows that dopamine activity can result from a large number of arousing events including novel stimuli and unexpected rewards (Hooks and Kalivas, 1994; Schultz, 1998; Fiorillo, 2004). In contrast, dopamine activity is suppressed by events that are associated with reduced arousal or decreased anticipatory excitement, including the actual consumption of food reward and the omission of expected reward (Schultz, 1998). More generally, dopamine circuits appear to have a major effect on our feeling of engagement, excitement, creativity, and our willingness to explore the world and to make sense of contingencies (Panksepp, 1998). More precisely, growing evidence currently supports the view of dopamine as a crucial element of incentive salience ("wanting processes") different from hedonic activation processes ("liking processes") (Berridge, 2007). Injections of GABA in the ventral tegmental area and of a dopamine receptor antagonist in the nucleus accumbens cause rats to stop searching for a sucrose solution, but still drink the liquid when moved close to the bottle (Ikemoto and Panksepp, 1999). Parkinsonian patients who suffer from degeneration of dopaminergic neurons experience not only psychomotor problems (inability to start voluntary movement) but more generally an absence of desire to engage in exploratory behavior and a lack of interest for pursuing cognitive tasks (Bernheimer et al., 1973). When the dopamine system is artificially activated via electrical or chemical means, humans and animals engage in eager exploration of their environment and display signs of interest and curiosity (Panksepp, 1998). Likewise, the addictive effects of cocaine, amphetamine, opioids, ethanol, nicotine, and canabinoid are directly related to the way they activate dopamine systems (Carboni et al., 1989; Pettit and Justice, 1989; Yoshimoto et al., 1991). Finally, too much dopamine activity is thought to be at the origins of uncontrolled speech and movement (Tourette's syndrome), obsessive-compulsive disorder, euphoria, over-excitement, mania, and psychosis in the context of schizophrenic behavior (Bell, 1973; Weinberger, 1987; Grace, 1991; Weiner and Joel, 2002).

Things get even more complex and controversial when one tries to link these observations with precise computational models. Hypotheses concerning phasic dopamine's potential role in learning have flourished in the last ten years. Schultz and colleagues have conducted a series of recordings of midbrain dopamine neurons firing patterns in awake monkeys under various behavioral conditions which suggested that dopamine neurons fire in response to unpredicted reward (see Schultz, 1998, for a review). Building on these observations, they develop the hypothesis that phasic dopamine responses drive learning by signaling an error that labels some events as "better than expected." This type of signaling has been interpreted in the framework of computational reinforcement learning as analogous to the prediction error signal of the temporal difference (TD) learning algorithm (Sutton, 1988). In this scheme, a phasic dopamine signal interpreted as TD-error plays a double role (Barto, 1995; Houk et al., 1995; Montague et al., 1996; Schultz et al., 1997; Suri and Schultz, 2001; Baldassarre, 2002; Doya, 2002; Khamassi et al., 2005). First, this error is used as a classical training signal to improve future prediction. Second, it is used for finding the actions that maximize reward. This so-called actor–critic reinforcement learning architecture has been presented as a relevant model to account for both functional and anatomical subdivisions in the midbrain dopamine system. However, most of the simple mappings that were first suggested, in particular the association of the actor to matrisome and the critic to the striosome part of the striatum, are now claimed to be inconsistent with the known anatomy of these nuclei (Joel et al., 2002).

Computational models of phasic dopamine activity based on the error signal hypothesis have also raised controversy for other reasons. One of them, central to our discussion, is that several stimuli that are *not* associated with reward prediction are known to activate the dopamine system in various ways. This is particularly the case for novel, unexpected "never-rewarded" stimuli (Hooks and Kalivas, 1994; Ikemoto and Panksepp, 1999; Horvitz, 2000, 2002; Fiorillo, 2004). The classic TD-error model does account for novelty responses. As a consequence, Kakade and Dayan suggested extending the framework to include, for instance, "novelty bonuses" (Kakade and Dayan, 2002) that distort the structure of the reward to include novelty effects (in a similar way that "exploration bonuses" permit continued exploration in theoretical machine learning models; Dayan and Sejnowski, 1996). More recently, Smith and colleagues presented another TD-error model in which phasic dopamine activation is modeled by the combination of "Surprise" and "Significance" measures (Smith et al., 2006). These attempts to reintegrate novelty and surprise components into a model elaborated in a framework based on extrinsic reward seeking may successfully account for a larger number of experimental observations. However, this is done at the expense of the complexification of a model that was not meant to deal with such types of behavior.

Some authors developed an alternative hypothesis to the reward prediction error interpretation, namely that dopamine promotes behavioral switching (Oades, 1985; Redgrave et al., 1999). In this interpretation, dopaminergic-neuron firing would be an essential component for directing attentional processes to unexpected, behaviorally important stimuli (related or unrelated to rewards). This hypothesis is supported by substantial evidence but stays at a general level of explanation. Actually, Kakade and Dayan argued that this interpretation is not incompatible with the reward error-signaling hypothesis provided that the model is modified to account for novelty effect (Kakade and Dayan, 2002).

The incentive salience hypotheses, despite their psychological foundations, are not yet supported by many computational models. But they do suggest some progress in this direction. In 2003, McClure and colleagues argued that incentive salience interpretation is not incompatible with the error signal hypothesis and presented a model where incentive salience is assimilated to expected future reward (McClure *et al.*, 2003). Another recent interesting investigation can be found in Niv *et al.* (2006) concerning an interpretation of tonic responses. In this model, tonic levels of dopamine are modeled as encoding "average rate of reward" and used to drive response vigor (slower or faster responding) into a reinforcement learning framework. With this dual model, the authors claim that their theory "dovetails neatly with both computational theories which suggest that the phasic activity of dopamine neurons reports appetitive prediction errors and psychological theories about dopamine's role in energizing responses" (Niv *et al.*, 2006).

In summary, despite many controversies, converging evidence seems to suggest that (1) dopamine plays a crucial role in exploratory and investigation behavior, and (2) the mesoaccumbens dopamine system is an important brain component to rapidly orient attentional resources to novel events. Moreover, current hypotheses may favor a dual interpretation of dopamine's functions where phasic dopamine is linked with prediction error and tonic dopamine is involved in processes of energizing responses.

10.4.2 Tonic dopamine as a signal of expected prediction of error decrease

We have reviewed above several elements of the current complex debate on the role and function of dopamine in action selection and learning. Building on the investigation we conducted using the kernel/envelope dichotomy, we would like to introduce yet another interpretation of the potential role of dopamine by formulating the hypothesis that tonic dopamine acts as a signal of "progress niches"; that is, states where prediction error of some internal model is expected to decrease. As experimental research in neuroscience has not really studied intrinsically motivated activities per se, it is not possible at this stage to decide whether this hypothesis is compatible or incompatible with the other interpretation of dopamine we have reviewed. Nevertheless, we can discuss how this interpretation fits with existing hypotheses and observations of dopamine's functions. We have just discussed the interpretation of tonic dopamine as a "wanting" motivational signal (incentive salience hypothesis). In the context of intrinsically motivated behavior, we believe this view is compatible with the hypothesis of dopamine as a signal of "progress niches." Dopamine acts as an invitation to investigate these "promising" states. This interpretation is also consistent with investigations that were conducted concerning human affective experience during stimulation of the dopamine circuits. When the lateral hypothalamus dopamine system is stimulated (part of the SEEKING system previously discussed), people report a feeling that "something very interesting and exciting is going on" (Panksepp, 1998, p.149, based on experiments reported in Heath, 1963; Quaade *et al.*, 1974). This corresponds to subjective affective states linked with intrinsically motivating activities (Csikszenthmihalyi, 1991).

In addition, Berridge articulates the proposition that "dopamine neurons code an informational consequence of learning signals, reflecting learning and prediction that are generated elsewhere in the brain but do not cause any new learning themselves" (Berridge, 2007, p. 405). In this view, dopamine signals are a consequence and not a cause of learning phenomena happening elsewhere in the brain. This is consistent with the fact that dopamine neurons originating in the midbrain are recognized to have only sparse direct access to the signal information that needs to be integrated by an associative learning mechanism. All the signals that they receive are likely to be "highly processed already by forebrain structures before dopamine cells get much learning-relevant information" (Berridge, 2007, p. 406; see also Dommett *et al.*, 2005).

In the model of a kernel presented in the Appendix to this chapter, this progress signal is used as a reinforcement to drive action-selection and behavioral switching. This aspect of our architecture could lead to a similar interpretation of the role of dopamine in several previous (and now often criticized) actor–critic models of action selection occurring in the basal ganglia (Barto, 1995; Houk *et al.*, 1995; Montague *et al.*, 1996; Schultz *et al.*, 1997; Suri and Schultz, 2001; Baldassarre, 2002; Doya, 2002; Khamassi *et al.*, 2005). Let us recall that the dorsal striatum receives glutamate inputs from almost all regions of the cerebral cortex. Striatal neurons fire in relation to movement of a particular body part but also to preparation of movement, desired outcome of a movement, to visual and auditory stimuli, and to visual saccades toward a particular direction. In most actor–critic computational models of the basal ganglia, dopamine responses originating in the substantia nigra are interpreted as increasing the synaptic strength, between currently active striatal input and output elements (thus shaping the policy of the actor in an actor–critic interpretation). With this mechanism, if the striatal outputs corresponds to motor responses and the dopamine cells become active in the presence of an unexpected reward, the same pattern of inputs should elicit the same pattern of motor outputs in the future. One criticism of this interpretation is that "if dopamine neurons respond to surprise/arousing events, regardless of appetitive or aversive values, one would postulate that dopamine activation does not serve to increase the likelihood that a given behavioral response is repeated under similar input conditions" (Horvitz, 2002, p. 70). Progress niches can be extrinsically rewarding (e.g. progress in playing poker sometimes results in gaining some money) or aversive (e.g. risk-taking behavior in extreme sports). Therefore, we believe our hypothesis is compatible with interpretations of the basal-ganglia-based action-selection circuits that control the choice of actions during cortico-striato-thalamo-cortical loops.

However, the precise interpretation of this reinforcement learning architecture is at this stage very open. A seductive hypothesis would be that the much studied reinforcement learning architectures based on short-prediction error phasic signals could be just reused with an internal self-generated reward, namely expected progress. This should lead to a complementary interpretation of the role of phasic and tonic dopamine in intrinsically motivated behavior in reinforcement. An alternative hypothesis is that tonic dopamine is directly used as a reinforcement signal. As previously discussed, Niv and colleagues assimilated the role of tonic dopamine in an average reward signal into a recent computational model (Niv *et al.*, 2006), a view which seems to contradict the hypothesis articulated a few years ago that the tonic dopamine signal reports a long-run average punishment rate (Daw *et al.*, 2002). Our hypothesis is based on the difference of two long-run average prediction error rates (Equation 10.3 of the model presented in the Appendix). We will now discuss how and where this progress signal could be measured.

10.4.3 Cortical microcircuits as both prediction and metaprediction systems

Following our hypothesis that tonic dopamine acts as signal of prediction progress, we must now guess where learning progress could be computed. For this part, our hypothesis will be that cortical microcircuits act as both prediction and metaprediction systems and therefore have the possibilty of directly computing regional learning progress, through an unsupervised regional assignment, as this is done in the computational model we have presented.

However, before considering this hypothesis let us briefly explore some alternative ones. The simpler one would be that progress is evaluated in some way or another in the limbic system itself. If indeed, as many authors suggest, phasic responses of dopamine neurons report prediction errors in certain contexts, their integration over time could be easily performed just through the slow accumulation of dopamine in certain parts of the neural circuitry (hypothesis discussed in Niv *et al.*, 2006). By comparing two running averages of the phasic signals, one could get an approximation of Equation (10.1) of the model presented in the Appendix. However, to be appropriately measured, progress must be evaluated in a regional manner, by local "expert" circuits. Although it is not impossible to imagine an architecture that would maintain such types of regional specialized circuitry in the basal ganglia (see for instance the multiple expert actor–critic architectures described in Khamassi *et al.*, 2005), we believe this is not the most likely hypothesis.

As we argued, scalability considerations in real-world structured inhomogeneous spaces favor architectures in which neural resources can be easily recruited or built for different kinds of initially unknown activities. This still leaves many possibilities. Kawato argues that, from a computational point of view, "it is conceivable that internal models are located in all brain regions having synaptic plasticity, provided that they receive and send out relevant information for their input and output" (Kawato, 1999). Doya suggested a broad computational distinction between the cortex, the basal ganglia, and the cerebellum, each of these associated with a particular type of learning problem: unsupervised learning, reinforcement learning, and supervised learning, respectively (Doya, 1999). Another potential candidate location, the hippocampus, has often been described as a comparator of predicted and actual events (Gray, 1982) and fMRI studies revealed that its activity was correlated with the occurrence of unexpected events

(Ploghaus *et al.*, 2000). Among all these possibilities, we believe the most promising direction of exploration is the cortical one, essentially because the cortex offers the type of open-ended, unsupervised "expert circuits" recruitment that we believe is crucial for the computation of learning progress.

A single neural microcircuit forms an immensely complicated network with multiple recurrent loops and highly heterogeneous components (Mountcastle, 1978; Shepherd, 1988; Douglas and Martin, 1998). Finding what type of computation could be performed with such a high dimensional dynamical system is a major challenge for computational neuroscience. To explore our hypothesis, we must investigate whether the computational power and evolutionary advantage of columns can be unveiled if these complex networks are considered not only as predictors but also as performers of both prediction and metaprediction functions (by anticipating not only future sensorimotor events but also their own errors in prediction and learning progress).

In recent years, several computational models explored how cortical circuits could be used as prediction devices. Maas and colleagues suggested viewing a column as a liquid state machine (LSM) (Maas *et al.*, 2002) (which is somewhat similar to Echo State Networks described by Jaeger: Jaeger, 2001; Jaeger and Haas, 2004). Like the Turing machine, the model of a LSM is based on a rigorous mathematical framework that guarantees, under idealized conditions, universal computing power for time series problems. More recently, Deneve *et al.* (2007) presented a model of a Kalman filter based on recurrent basis function networks, a kind of model that can be easily mapped onto cortical circuits. Kalman filters share some similarity with the kind of metaprediction machinery we have discussed in this chapter, as they also deal with modeling errors made by prediction of internal models. However, we must admit that there is currently no definitive experimental evidence or computational model that supports precisely the idea that cortical circuits actually compute their own learning progress.

If indeed we could show that cortical microcircuits can signal this information to other parts of the brain, the mapping with our model based on a stable kernel for the active exploration of many different envelopes would be rather straighforward. Lateral inhibition mechanisms, specialization dynamics, and other self-organizing processes that are typical of cortical plasticity should allow us to perform without problems the type of regionalization of the sensorimotor space that an architecture like the one presented in the Appendix features. Moreover, hierarchical organization that has been identified in neocortical dynamics would naturally extend one of the main weaknesses of the present computational architecture: its difficulty in dealing with hierarchical forms of learning. As previously argued, action selection could then be realized by some form of subcortical actor–critic architecture, similar to the one involved in the optimization of extrinsic forms of rewards.

We believe this hypothesis is consistent from an evolutionary perspective, or at least that an "evolutionary story" can be articulated around it. The relatively "recent" invention of the cortical column circuits correlates roughly with the fact that only mammals seem to display intrinsically motivated behavior. Once discovered by evolution, cortical columns multiplied, leading to the highly expanded human cortex. (Humans have the largest number of cortical neurons, 10^{10}, among all animals, closely followed by large cetaceans and elephants (Roth and Dicke, 2005), giving over a thousandfold expansion from mouse to man to provide 80% of the human brain. What can make them so advantageous from an evolutionary point of view? It is reasonable to suppose that the kernel responsible for intrinsically motivated exploration appeared after (or on top of) an existing machinery dedicated to the optimization of extrinsic motivation. For an extrinsically motivated animal, value is linked with specific stimuli, particular visual patterns, movement, loud sounds, or any bodily sensations that signal basic homeostatic physiological needs like food or physical integrity are (or are not) being fulfilled. These animals can develop behavioral strategies to experience the corresponding situations as often as possible. However, when an efficient strategy is found, nothing pushes them further towards new activities. Their development stops there.

The appearance of a basic cortical circuit that not only acts as predictor but also as metapredictor capable of evaluating its own learning progress can be seen as a major evolutionary transition. The brain manages now to produce its own reward, a progress signal, internal to the central nervous system with no significant biological effects on non-nervous-system tissues. This is the basis of an adaptive internal value system for which sensorimotor experiences that produce positive value evolve with time. This is what drives the acquisition of novel skills, with increasing structure and complexity. This is a revolution, yet it is essentially based on the old brain circuitry that evolved for the optimization of specific extrinsic needs. If we follow our hypothesis, the unique human cortical expansion has to be understood as a coevolutionary dynamical process linking larger "space" for learning and more things to learn. In some way, it is human culture, as a huge reservoir of progress niches, that has put pressure on having more of these basic processing units.

The attentive reader should have noticed that there is something peculiar about the hypotheses we present here. We hypothesize that the cortical circuits offer the neural substrate for representing a very large number of sensorimotor spaces corresponding to our concept of body envelope. Additionally we suppose that they can perform the local computation necessary for the evaluation of learning progress that is then relayed by subcortical structures. This means that in this view it would be wrong to associate the subcortical structures with the stable kernel and the cortical ones with the fluid envelopes, as some of the crucial computational operations of the kernel are presumed to be performed locally by the cortical areas.

10.5   Concluding remarks

Recent research in robotics sets the stage, both theoretically and experimentally, for a new conception of the embodiment process that views the experience of the body as a fluid, constantly changing space. By extracting, on the one hand, the concept of a generic and stable kernel, origin of movement and action, and, on the other hand, the notion of changing body envelopes, robotics offers a novel framework for considering deep and complex issues linked with development and innateness. Indeed, what is development if not a succession of embodiment: not only a body that changes physically but the discovery of novel embodied spaces. Each newly acquired skill changes the space to explore. Through incorporation, the body extends temporarily to include objects, tools, musical interfaces, or vehicles as novel envelopes to explore, with no fundamental differences from their biological counterpart (Warnier, 1999; Clark, 2004).

By pushing further this notion of fluid body envelopes, couldn't we consider symbolic reasoning and abstract thought as merely special forms of body extension? Lakoff and Nunez suggested very convincingly that there is a direct correspondence between sensorimotor manipulation and very abstract notion in mathematics (Lakoff and Nunez, 2001). Metaphorical transfer, one of the most fundamental processes to bootstrap higher levels of cognition, can be relevantly considered as a process of incorporation (Lakoff and Johnson, 1998). Eventually, couldn't we consider linguistic communication itself as just one particular case of embodied exploration (Oudeyer and Kaplan, 2006)? All these spaces could be explored relevantly by a progress-driven kernel like the one we have discussed in this chapter.

Robots have always played a pivotal role in philosophical debates (Kaplan, 2004, 2005; Asada *et al.*, 2009). They help us think about ourselves by comparison. Studying the development of robots with embodied spaces very different from our own is probably the most promising way to study the role of our body in our own developmental processes. In that sense, robots are not models. They are physical *thought experiments*. That is why they can permit us to consider apparently impossible splits, like the ones separating the body from the animation processes or, more recently, the distinction between a stable kernel and fluid body envelopes.

Appendix: a kernel for progress-driven exploration of sensorimotor envelopes

Building a kernel permitting a continuous search for learning progress implies complicated and deep issues. The idealized problem illustrated in Figure 10.1 allowed us to make more concrete the intuition that focusing on activities where prediction errors decrease most can generate organized developmental sequences. Nevertheless, the reality is in fact not as simple. Indeed, in this idealized problem, four different sensorimotor situations/activities were predefined. Thus it was assumed that when the idealized machine would produce an action and make a prediction about it, it would be automatically associated with one of the predefined kinds of activities. Learning progress would then be simply computed by, for example, comparing the difference between the mean of errors in prediction at time t and at time $t - \theta$. On the contrary, infants do not come to the world with an organized predefined set of possible kinds of activities. It would in fact be contradictory, since they are capable of open-ended development, and most of what they will learn is impossible to know in advance. It is the same for a developmental robot, for which the world is initially a fuzzy blooming flow of unorganized sensorimotor values. In this case, how can we define learning progress? What meaning can we attribute to "maximizing the decrease of prediction errors"?

A first possibility would be just to compute learning progress at time t as the difference between the mean prediction errors at time t and at time $t - \theta$. But implementing this on a robot quickly shows that it is in fact nonsense. For example, the behavior of a robot motivated to maximize such a progress would be typically an alternation between jumping randomly against walls and periods of complete immobility. Indeed, passing from the first behavior (highly unpredictable) to the second (highly predictable) corresponds to a large decrease in prediction errors, and so to a large internal reward. So we see that there is a need to compute learning progress by comparing prediction errors in sensorimotor contexts that are similar, which leads us to a second possible approach.

In order to describe this second possibility, we need to introduce a few formal notations and precisions about the computational architecture that will embed intrinsic motivation. Let us denote a sensorimotor situation with the state vector $x(t)$ (e.g. a given action performed in a given context), and its outcome with $y(t)$ (e.g. the perceptual consequence of this action). Let's call M a prediction system trying to model this function, producing for any $x(t)$ a prediction $y'(t)$. Once the actual evolution $y(t)$ is known, the error $e_x(t) = |y(t) - y'(t)|$ in prediction can be computed and used as a feedback to improve the performances of M. At this stage, no assumption is made regarding the kind of prediction system used in M. It could be for instance a linear predictor, a neural network, or any other prediction method currently used in machine learning. Within this framework, it is possible to imagine a first way of computing a meaningful measure of learning progress. Indeed, one could compute a measure of learning progress $p_x(t)$ for every single sensorimotor situation x through the monitoring of its associated prediction errors in the past; for example, with the formula:

$$p_x(t) = <e_x(t-\theta)> - <e_x(t)>, \tag{10.1}$$

where $< e_x(t) >$ is the mean of e_x values in the last τ predictions. Thus, we here compare prediction errors in exactly the same situation x, and so we compare only identical sensorimotor contexts. The problem is that, whereas this is an imaginable solution in small symbolic sensorimotor spaces, this is inapplicable to the real world for two reasons. The first reason is that, because the world is very large, continuous, and noisy, an organism never experiences exactly the same sensorimotor state twice. There are always slight differences. A possible solution to this limit would be to introduce a distance function $d(x_m, x_n)$ and to define learning progress locally in a point x as the decrease in prediction errors concerning sensorimotor contexts that are close under this distance function:

$$p_x(t) = <e_x^\delta(t-\theta)> - <e_x^\delta(t)>, \tag{10.2}$$

where $<e_x^\delta$ denotes the mean of all $\{e_{x1}|d(x,x_1)<\delta\}$ values in the last τ predictions, and where δ is a small fixed threshold. Using this measure would typically allow the machine to manage to repeatedly try roughly the same action in roughly the same context and identify all the resulting prediction errors as characterizing the same sensorimotor situation (and thus overcoming the noise). Now, there is a second problem which this solution does not solve. Many learning mechanisms, and in particular the one used by infants, are fast and characterized by "one-shot learning." In practice, this means that typically, an infant who observes the consequence of a given action in a given context will readily be able to predict what happens if exactly the same action occurs in the same context again. Learning machines such as memory-based algorithms also show this feature. As a consequence, if learning progress is defined locally as explained above, a given sensorimotor situation will be typically interesting only for a very brief amount of time, and will hardly direct further exploration. For example, using this approach, a robot playing with a plastic toy might try to squash it on the ground to see the noise it produces, experiencing learning progress in the first few times it tries, but would quickly stop playing with it and typically would not try to squash it for example on the sofa or on a wall to hear the result. This is because its measure of potential learning progress is still too local.

Thus, we conclude that there really is a need to build broad categories of activities (e.g. squashing plastic toys on surfaces or kicking small objects) as those pre-given in the initial idealized problem. The computation of learning progress will only become both meaningful and efficient if an automatic mechanism allows for the mental construction of these categories of activities, typically corresponding to not-so-small regions in the sensorimotor space. We have presented a possible solution, based on the iterative splitting of the sensorimotor space into regions R_n. Initially, the sensorimotor space is considered as one big region, and progressively regions are split into subregions containing more homogeneous kinds of actions and sensorimotor contexts (the mechanisms of splitting are detailed in Oudeyer *et al.*, 2007). In each region R_n, the history of prediction errors $\{e\}$ is memorized and used to compute a measure of learning progress that characterizes this region:

$$PR_n(t) = \; < eR_x(t-\theta)> - < eR_n(t)>, \qquad (10.3)$$

where $<eR_n(t)>$ is the mean of $\{e_x | x \in R_n\}$ values in the last τ predictions.

Given this iterative region-based operationalization of learning progress, there are two general ways of building a neural architecture that uses it to implement intrinsic motivation. A first kind of architecture, called monolithic, includes two loosely coupled main modules. The first module would be the neural circuitry implementing the prediction machine M presented earlier, and learning to predict the $x \rightarrow y$ mapping. The second module would be a neural circuitry *metaM* organizing the space into different regions R_n and modeling the learning progress of M in each of these regions, based on the inputs $(x(t), e_x(t))$ provided by M. This architecture makes no assumption at all on the mechanisms and representations used by the learning machine M. In particular, the splitting of the space into regions is not informed by the internal structure of M. This makes this version of the architecture general, but makes the scalability problematic in real-world structured inhomogeneous spaces where typically specific neural ressources will be recruited/built for different kinds of activities.

This is why we have developed a second architecture, in which the machines M and *metaM* are tightly coupled. In this version, each region R_n is associated with a circuit M_{R_n} called an expert, as well as with a regional meta machine *meta M_{R_n}*. A given expert M_{R_n} is responsible for the prediction of y given x when x is a situation which is covered by R_n. Also, each expert M_{R_n} is only trained on inputs (x, y) where x belongs to its associated region R_n. This leads to a structure in which a single expert circuit is assigned for each nonoverlapping partition of the space. The metamachine *meta M_{R_n}* associated

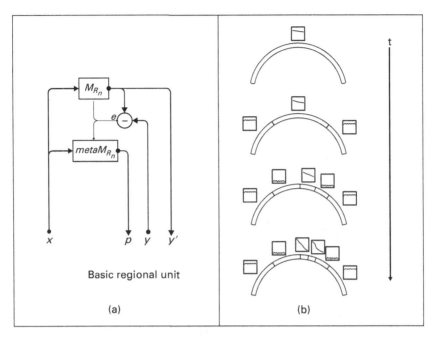

Figure 10.6 (a) An intrinsic motivation system is based on a population of regional units, each comprising an expert predictor M_{R_n} that learns to anticipate the consequence y of a given sensorimotor context x belonging to its associated region of expertise R_n, and a metapredictor *meta* M_{R_n} modeling the learning progress of M_{R_n} in the close past. The learning progress defines the saliency of situations belonging to a given context, and actions are chosen in order to reach maximally interesting situations. Once the actual consequence is known, M_{R_n} and *meta* M_{R_n} get updated; *meta* M_{R_n} reevaluates the error curve linked with this context and computes an updated measure of the learning progress (local derivative of curve). (b) Illustration of the splitting/assignment process based on a self-organized classification system capable of structuring an infinite continuous space of particular situations into higher-level categories (or kinds) of situations. An expert predictor/metapredictor circuit is assigned to each region.

with each expert circuit can then compute the local learning progress of this region of the sensorimotor space (see Figure 10.6b for a symbolic illustration of this splitting/assignment process). The idea of using multiple experts has been already explored in several works (e.g. Jordan and Jacobs, 1994; Kawato, 1999; Tani and Nolfi, 1999; Baldassarre, 2002; Doya *et al.*, 2002; Khamassi *et al.*, 2005).

The basic circuits we just described allow us to compute an internal reward $r(t) = PR_n(t)$ each time an action is performed in a given sensorimotor context, depending on how much learning progress has been achieved in a particular region R_n. An intrinsic motivation to progress corresponds to the maximization of the amount of this internal reward. Mathematically, this can be formulated as the maximization of future expected rewards (i.e. maximization of the return), that is

$$E\{r(t+1)\} = E\{\sum_{t \geq t_n} \gamma^{t-t_n} r(t)\},$$

where $\gamma(0 \le \gamma \le 1)$ is the discount factor, which assigns less weight to the reward expected in the far future. We can note that, at this stage, it is theoretically easy to combine this intrinsic reward for learning progress with the sum of other extrinsic rewards $r_e(t)$ coming from other sources, for instance in a linear manner with the formula $r(t) = \alpha.PR_n(t)+(1-\alpha)r_e(t)$ (the parameter α measuring the relative weight between intrinsic and extrinsic rewards).

This formulation corresponds to a reinforcement learning problem (Sutton and Barto, 1998) and thus the techniques developed in this field can be used to implement an action-selection mechanism which will allow the system to maximize future expected rewards efficiently (e.g. Q-learning: Walkins and Dayan, 1992; TD-learning: Sutton, 1988, etc.). However, forecasting prediction error reduction is, by definition, a highly nonstationary problem (progress niches appear and disappear in time). As a consequence, traditional "slow" reinforcement learning techniques are not well adapted in this context. In Oudeyer *et al.* (2007), we describe a very simple action-selection circuit that avoids problems related to delayed rewards and makes it possible to use a simple prediction system which can predict $r(t + 1)$, and so evaluate $E\{r(t + 1)\}$. Let us consider the problem of evaluating $E\{r(t + 1)\}$ given a sensory context $\mathbf{S(t)}$ and a candidate action $\mathbf{M(t)}$, constituting a candidate sensorimotor context $\mathbf{SM(t)} = x(t)$ covered by region R_n. In our architecture, we approximate $E\{r(t + 1)\}$ with the learning progress that was achieved in R_n with the acquisition of its recent exemplars: that is, $E\{r(t+1)\} \approx PR_n\,(t-\theta_{Rn})$ where $t-\theta_{Rn}$ is the time corresponding to the last time region R_n when the associated expert circuit processed a new exemplar. The action-selection loop goes as follows:

- In a given sensory $\mathbf{S(t)}$ context, the robot makes a list of the possible values of its motor channels $\mathbf{M(t)}$ which it can set; if this list is infinite, which is often the case since we work in continuous sensorimotor spaces, a sample of candidate values is generated.
- Each of these candidate motor vectors $\mathbf{M(t)}$ associated with the sensory context $\mathbf{S(t)}$ makes a candidate $\mathbf{SM(t)}$ vector for which the robot finds out the corresponding region R_n; then the formula we just described is used to evaluate the expected learning progress $E\{r(t + 1)\}$ that might be the result of executing the candidate action $\mathbf{M(t)}$ in the current context.
- The action for which the system expects the maximal learning progress is chosen with a probability $1 - \epsilon$ and executed, but sometimes a random action is selected (with a probability ϵ, typically 0.35 in the following experiments).
- After the action has been executed and the consequences measured, the system is updated.

More sophisticated action-selection circuits could certainly be envisioned (see, for example, Sutton and Barto, 1998). However, this one was revealed to be surprisingly efficient in the real-world experiments we conducted.

References

Asada, M., Hosoda, K., Kuniyoshi, Y., *et al.* (2009). Cognitive developmental robotics: a survey. *IEEE Transactions on Autonomous Mental Development*, **1**(1), 12–34.

Baldassarre, G. (2002). A modular neural-network model of the basal ganglia's role in learning and selection motor behaviors. *Journal of Cognitive Systems Research*, **3**(1), 5–13.

Baldwin, J. M. (1925). *Mental Development in the Child and the Race.* New York: Macmillan.

Barto, A. G. (1995). Adaptive critics and the basal ganglia. In Houk, J. C., Davis, J. L., and Beiser, D. G. (eds.), *Models of Information Processing in the Basal Ganglia.* Cambridge, MA: MIT Press, pp. 215–232.

Barto, A. G., Singh, S., and Chentanez, N. (2004). Intrinsically motivated learning of hierarchical collections of skills. In *Proceedings of the 3rd IEEE International Conference on Development and Learning (ICDL 2004).*

Bell, D. S. (1973). The experimental reproduction of amphetamine psychosis. *Archives in General Psychiatry,* **29,** 35–40.

Berlyne, D. E. (1960). *Conflict, Arousal and Curiosity.* New York: McGraw-Hill.

Bernheimer, H., Birkmayer, W., Hornykiewicz, O., Jellinger, K., and Seitelberger, F. (1973). Brain dopamine and the syndromes of Parkinson and Huntington: clinical, morphological and neurochemical correlations. *Journal of the Neurological Sciences,* **20,** 415–455.

Berridge, K. C. (2007). The debate over dopamine's role in reward: the case of incentive salience. *Psychopharmacology,* **191,** 391–431.

Brooks, R. (1999). *Cambrian Intelligence: The Early History of the New AI.* Cambridge, MA: MIT Press.

Bruner, J. (1962). *On Knowing: Essays for the Left Hand.* Cambridge, MA: Harvard University Press.

Cameron, J. and Pierce, W.D. (2002). *Rewards and Intrinsic Motivation: Resolving the Controversy.* South Hadley, MA: Bergin and Garvey Press.

Carboni, E., Imperato, A., Perezzani, L., and Di Chiara, G. (1989). Amphetamine, cocaine, phencyclidine and nomifensine increases extra cellullar dopamine concentrations preferentially in the nucleus accumbens of freely moving rats. *Neuroscience,* **28,** 653–661.

Clark, A. (2004). *Natural-born Cyborgs: Minds, Technologies and the Future of Human Intelligence.* Oxford, UK: Oxford University Press.

Csikszenthmihalyi, M. (1991). *Flow: The Psychology of Optimal Experience.* New York: Harper Perennial.

Daw, N., Kakade, S., and Dayan, P. (2002). Opponent interactions between serotonin and dopamine. *Neural Networks,* **15,** 603–616.

Dayan, P. and Sejnowski, T. J. (1996). Exploration bonuses and dual control. *Machine Learning,* **25,** 5–22.

Dayan, P., Hinton, G., Giles, C., Hanson, S., and Cowan, J. (1993). Feudal reinforcement learning. In *Advances in Neural Information Processing Systems,* Vol. 5. San Mateo, CA: Morgan Kaufmann, pp. 271–278.

De Charms, R. (1968). *Personal Causation: The Internal Affective Determinants of Behavior.* New York: Academic Press.

Deci, E. L. and Ryan, R. M. (1985). *Intrinsic Motivation and Self-Determination in Human Behavior.* New York: Plenum Press.

Dember, W. N. and Earl, R. W. (1957). Analysis of exploratory, manipulatory and curiosity behaviors. *Psychological Review,* **64,** 91–96.

Deneve, S., Duhamel, J.-R., and Pouget, A. (2007). Optimal sensorimotor integration in recurrent cortical networks: a neural implementation of Kalman filters. *Journal of Neuroscience,* **27**(21), 5744–5756.

Depue, R. A. and Iacono, W. G. (1989). Neurobehavioral aspects of affective disorders. *Annual Review of Psychology,* **40,** 457–492.

Dommett, E., Coizet, V., Blatha, C. D., *et al.* (2005). How visual stimuli activate dopaminergic neurons at short latency. *Science,* **307,** 1476–1479.

Douglas, R. and Martin, K. (1998). Neocortex. In Shepherd, G. M. (ed.), *The Synaptic Organization of the Brain.* Oxford, UK: Oxford University Press, pp. 459–509.

Doya, K. (1999). What are the computations of cerebellum, basal ganglia, and the cerebral cortex? *Neural Networks*, **12**, 961–974.

Doya, K. (2002). Metalearning and neuromodulation. *Neural Networks*, **15**(4–5), 495–506.

Doya, K., Samejima, K., Katagiri, K., and Kawato, M. (2002). Multiple model-based reinforcement learning. *Neural Computation*, **14**, 1347–1369.

Fedorov, V. V. (1972). *Theory of Optimal Experiment.* New York: Academic Press.

Festinger, L. (1957). *A Theory of Cognitive Dissonance.* Evanston, IL: Row, Peterson.

Fiorillo, C. D. (2004). The uncertain nature of dopamine. *Molecular Psychiatry*, **9**, 122–123.

Gibson, J. (1986). *The Ecological Approach to Visual Perception.* Hillsdale, NJ: Lawrence Erlbaum Associates.

Grace, A. A. (1991). Phasic versus tonic dopamine release and the modulation of dopamine system responsivity: a hypothesis for the etiology of schizophrenia. *Neuroscience*, **41**, 1–24.

Gray, J. A. (1982). *The Neuropsychology of Anxiety: An Enquiry into the Functions of the Septo-hippocampal System.* Oxford, UK: Clarendon Press.

Gray, J. A. (1990). Brain systems that mediate both emotion and cognition. *Cognition and Emotion*, **4**, 269–288.

Grey Walter, W. (1953). *The Living Brain.* 2nd edn., 1967, London: Penguin.

Harlow, H. F. (1950). Learning and satiation of response in intrinsically motivated complex puzzle performances by monkeys. *Journal of Comparative and Physiological Psychology*, **43**, 289–294.

Head, H. and Holmes, G. (1911). Sensory disturbances from cerebral lesions. *Brain*, **34**, 102–254.

Heath, R. G. (1963). Electrical self-stimulation of the brain in Man. *American Journal of Psychiatry*, **120**, 571–577.

Hebb, D. O. (1955). Drives and the C.N.S (conceptual nervous system). *Psychological Review*, **62**, 243–254.

Hooks, M. S. and Kalivas, P. W. (1994). Involvement of dopamine and excitatory amino acid transmission in novelty-induced motor activity. *Journal of Pharmacology and Experimental Therapeutics*, **269**, 976–988.

Horvitz, J.-C. (2000). Mesolimbocortical and nigrostriatal dopamine responses to salient non-reward events. *Neuroscience*, **96**(4), 651–656.

Horvitz, J.-C. (2002). Dopamine gating of glutamatergic sensorimotor and incentive motivational input signals to the striatum. *Behavioral and Brain Research*, **137**, 65–74.

Houk, J. C., Adams, J. L., and Barto, A. G. (1995). A model of how the basal ganglia generate and use neural signals that predict reinforcement. In Houk, J. C., Davis, J. L., and Beiser, D. G. (eds.), *Models of Information Processing in the Basal Ganglia.* Cambridge, MA: MIT Press, pp. 249–270.

Huang, X. and Weng, J. (2002). Novelty and reinforcement learning in the value system of developmental robots. In Prince, C., Demiris, Y., Marom, Y., Kozima, H., and Balkenius, C. (eds.), *Proceedings of the 2nd International Workshop on Epigenetic Robotics: Modeling Cognitive Development in Robotic Systems.* Lund University Cognitive Studies 94. Lund, Sweden: Lund University, pp. 47–55.

Hull, C. L. (1943). *Principles of Behavior: An Introduction to Behavior Theory.* New York: Appleton-Century-Croft.

Hunt, J. McV. (1965). Intrinsic motivation and its role in psychological development. In Levine, D. (ed.), *Nebraska Symposium on Motivation*, Vol. 13. Lincoln, NE: University of Nebraska Press, pp. 189–282.

Ikemoto, S. and Panksepp, J. (1999). The role of nucleus accumbens dopamine in motivated behavior: a unifying interpretation with special reference to reward-seeking. *Brain Research Reviews*, **31**, 6–41.

Iriki, A., Tanaka, A., and Iwamura, Y. (1996). Coding of modified schema during tool use by macaque postcentral neurones. *Cognitive Neuroscience and Neuropsychology*, **7**(14), 2325–2330.

Jaeger, H. (2001). *The Echo State Approach to Analyzing and Training Recurrent Neural Networks*. Technical Report, GMD Report 148. Bonn, Germany: German National Research Institute for Computer Science (GMD).

Jaeger, H. and Haas, H. (2004). Harnessing nonlinearity: predicting chaotic systems and saving energy in wireless communication. *Science*, **304**(5667), 78–80.

Joel, D., Niv, Y., and Ruppin, E. (2002). Actor-critic models of the basal ganglia: new anatomical and computational perspectives. *Neural Networks*, **15**, 535–547.

Jordan, M. and Jacobs, R. (1994). Hierarchical mixtures of experts and the EM algorithm. *Neural Computation*, **6**(2), 181–214.

Kagan, J. (1972). Motives and development. *Journal of Personality and Social Psychology*, **22**, 51–66.

Kakade, S. and Dayan, P. (2002). Dopamine: generalization and bonuses. *Neural Networks*, **15**, 549–559.

Kaplan, F. (2004). Who is afraid of the humanoid? Investigating cultural differences in the acceptance of robots. *International Journal of Humanoid Robotics*, **1**(3), 465–480.

Kaplan, F. (2005). *Les machines apprivoisees: comprendre les robots de loisir*. Paris: Vuibert, Collections Automates Intelligents.

Kaplan, F. and Oudeyer, P.-Y. (2003). Motivational principles for visual know-how development. In Prince, C. G., Berthouze, L., Kozima, H., *et al.* (eds.), *Proceedings of the 3rd International Workshop on Epigenetic Robotics: Modeling Cognitive Development in Robotic Systems*. Lund University Cognitive Studies 101. Lund, Sweden: Lund University, pp. 73–80.

Kaplan, F. and Oudeyer, P.-Y. (2006). Trends in epigenetic robotics: Atlas 2006. In Kaplan, F., Oudeyer, P.-Y., Revel, A., *et al.* (eds.), *Proceedings of the Sixth International Workshop on Epigenetic Robotics: Modeling Cognitive Development in Robotic Systems*. Lund University Cognitive Studies 128. Lund, Sweden: Lund University.

Kaplan, F. and Oudeyer, P.-Y. (2007a). In search of the neural circuits of intrinsic motivation. *Frontiers in Neuroscience*, **1**(1), 225–236.

Kaplan, F. and Oudeyer, P.-Y. (2007b). The progress-drive hypothesis: an interpretation of early imitation. In Nehaniv, C. and Dautenhahn, K. (eds.), *Models and Mechanisms of Imitation and Social Learning: Behavioural, Social and Communication Dimensions*. Cambridge, UK: Cambridge University Press, pp. 361–377.

Kaplan, F. and Oudeyer, P.-Y. (2007c). Un robot motivé pour apprendre: le rôle des motivations intrinsèques dans le développement sensorimoteur. *Enfance*, **59**(1), 46–58.

Kaplan, F. and Oudeyer, P.-Y. (2008). Le corps comme variable expérimentale. *La Revue Philosophique*, **2008**(3), 287–298.

Kaplan, F. and Oudeyer, P.-Y. (2009). Stable kernels and fluid body envelopes. *SICE Journal of Control, Measurement, and System Integration*, **48**(1).

Kaplan, F., d'Esposito, M., and Oudeyer, P.-Y. (2006) (October). *AIBO's Playroom*. Online: http://aibo.playroom.fr.

Kaplan, F., Oudeyer, P.-Y., and Bergen, B. (2007). Computational models in the debate over language learnability. *Infant and Child Development*, **17**(1), 55–80.

Kawato, M. (1999). Internal models for motor control and trajectory planning. *Current Opinion in Neurobiology*, **9**, 718–727.

Khamassi, M., Lachèze, L., Girard, B., Berthoz, A., and Guillot, A. (2005). Actor-critic models of reinforcement learning in the basal ganglia. *Adaptive Behavior*, **13**(2), 131–148.

Lakoff, G. and Johnson, M. (1998). *Philosophy in the Flesh: The Embodied Mind and its Challenge to Western Thought.* New York: Basic Books.

Lakoff, G., and Nunez, R. (2001). *Where Mathematics Comes From: How the Embodied Mind Brings Mathematics Into Being.* New York: Basic Books.

Lungarella, M., Metta, G., Pfeifer, R., and Sandini, G. (2003). Developmental robotics: a survey. *Connection Science*, **15**(4), 151–190.

Maas, W., Natschlager, T., and Markram, H. (2002). Real-time computing without stable states: a new framework for neural computation based on perturbations. *Neural Computation*, **14**(11), 2531–2560.

Marshall, J., Blank, D., and Meeden, L. (2004). An emergent framework for self-motivation in developmental robotics. In *Proceedings of the 3rd International Conference on Development and Learning (ICDL 2004).*

McClure, S., Daw, N. D., and Montague, P. R. (2003). A computational substate for incentive salience. *Trends in Neurosciences*, **26**(8), 423–428.

Meltzoff, A. and Gopnik, A. (1993). The role of imitation in understanding persons and developing a theory of mind. In Baron-Cohen, S., Tager-Flusberg, H., and Cohen, D. (eds.), *Understanding Other Minds.* Oxford, UK: Oxford University Press, pp. 335–366.

Merleau-Ponty, M. (1942). *La structure du comportement.* Paris: Presses Universitaires de France.

Merleau-Ponty, M. (1945). *Phénoménologie de la Perception.* Paris: Gallimard.

Montague, P. R., Dayan, P., and Sejnowski, T. J. (1996). A framework for mesencephalic dopamine systems based on predictive Hebbian learning. *Journal of Neuroscience*, **16**, 1936–1947.

Montgomery, K. C. (1954). The role of exploratory drive in learning. *Journal of Comparative and Physiological Psychology*, **47**, 60–64.

Moore, C. and Corkum, V. (1994). Social understanding at the end of the first year of life. *Developmental Review*, **14**, 349–372.

Mountcastle, V. (1978). An organizing principle for cerebral function: the unit model and the distributed system. In Edelman, G. and Mountcastle, V. (eds.), *The Mindful Brain.* Cambridge, MA: MIT Press, pp. 17–49.

Niv, Y., Daw, N. D., Joel, D., and Dayan, P. (2006). Tonic dopamine: opportunity costs and the control of response vigor. *Psychopharmacology*, 507–520.

Oades, R. D. (1985). The role of noradrenaline in tuning and dopamine in switching between signals in the CNS. *Neuroscience Biobehavorial Review*, **9**, 261–282.

Oudeyer, P.-Y. and Kaplan, F. (2006). Discovering communication. *Connection Science*, **18**(2), 189–206.

Oudeyer, P.-Y. and Kaplan, F. (2007). What is intrinsic motivation? A typology of computational approaches. *Frontiers in Neurorobotics*, **1**(1), doi:10.3389/neuro.12.006.2007.

Oudeyer, P.-Y., Kaplan, F., Hafner, V. V., and Whyte, A. (2005). The playground experiment: task-independent development of a curious robot. In Bank, D. and Meeden, L. (eds.), *Proceedings of the AAAI Spring Symposium on Developmental Robotics, 2005*, pp. 42–47.

Oudeyer, P.-Y., Kaplan, F., and Hafner, V. (2007). Intrinsic motivation systems for autonomous mental development. *IEEE Transactions on Evolutionary Computation*, **11**(1), 265–286.

Panksepp, J. (1998). *Affective Neuroscience: The Foundations of Human and Animal Emotions.* New York: Oxford University Press.

Pettit, H. O. and Justice, J. B., Jr. (1989). Dopamine in the nucleus accumbens during cocaine self-administration as studied by in vivo microdialysis. *Pharmacology Biochemistry and Behavior*, **34**, 899–904.

Pfeifer, R. and Bongard, J. (2007). *How the Body Shapes the Way We Think: A New View of Intelligence.* Cambridge, MA: MIT Press.

Pfeifer, R. and Scheier, C. (1999). *Understanding Intelligence.* Boston, MA: MIT Press.

Piaget, J. (1952). *The Origins of Intelligence in Children.* New York: Norton Press.

Piaget, J. (1962). *Play, Dreams and Imitation in Childhood.* New York: Norton Press.

Ploghaus, A., Tracey, I., Clare, S., *et al.* (2000). Learning about pain: the neural substrate of the prediction error of aversive events. *PNAS,* **97**, 9281–9286.

Quaade, F., Vaernet, K., and Larsson, S. (1974). Stereotaxic stimulation and electrocoagulation of the lateral hypothalamus in obese humans. *Acta Neurochirurgica,* **30**, 111–117.

Redgrave, P., Prescott, T., and Gurney, K. (1999). Is the short latency dopamine response too short to signal reward error? *Trends in Neurosciences,* **22**, 146–151.

Ring, M. (1994). Continual learning in reinforcement environments. Ph.D. Thesis, University of Texas at Austin.

Rochat, P. (2002). Ego function of early imitation. In Melzoff, A. and Prinz, W. (eds.), *The Imitative Mind: Development, Evolution and Brain Bases.* Cambridge, UK: Cambridge University Press.

Rolls, E. T. (1999). *The Brain and Emotion.* Oxford, UK: Oxford University Press.

Roth, G. and Dicke, U. (2005). Evolution of the brain and intelligence. *Trends in Cognitive Sciences,* **9**(5), 250–257.

Ryan, R. and Deci, E.L. (2000). Intrinsic and extrinsic motivations: classic definitions and new directions. *Contemporary Educational Psychology,* **25**, 54–67.

Schaffer, H. (1977). Early interactive development in studies of mother-infant interaction. In *Proceedings of Loch Lomonds Symposium.* New York: Academic Press, pp. 3–18.

Schilder, P. (1935). *L'image du corps.* 1968 edn., Paris: Gallimard.

Schmidhuber, J. (1991). Curious model-building control systems. In *Proceedings of the IEEE International Joint Conference on Neural Networks,* Vol. 2, pp. 1458–1463.

Schmidhuber, J. (1992). Learning complex, extended sequences using the principle of history compression. *Neural Computation,* **4**(2), 234–242.

Schmidhuber, J. (2006). Optimal artificial curiosity, developmental robotics, creativity, music, and the fine arts. *Connection Science,* **18**(2), 173–187.

Schultz, W. (1998). Predictive reward signal of dopamine neurons. *Journal of Neurophysiology,* **80**, 1–27.

Schultz, W. (2006). Behavioral theories and the neurophysiology of reward. *Annual Review of Psychology,* **57**, 87–115.

Schultz, W., Dayan, P., and Montague, P. R. (1997). A neural substrate of prediction and reward. *Science,* **275**, 1593–1599.

Shepherd, G. M. (1988). A basic circuit for cortical organization. In Gazzaniga, M. (ed.), *Perspectives in Memory Research.* Cambridge, MA: MIT Press, pp. 93–134.

Smith, A., Li, M., Becker, S., and Kapur, S. (2006). Dopamine, prediction error and associative learning: a model-based account. *Network: Computation in Neural Systems,* **17**, 61–84.

Steels, L. (1994). The artificial life roots of artificial intelligence. *Artificial Life Journal,* **1**(1), 89–125.

Steels, L. (2003). Intelligence with representation. *Philosophical Transactions of the Royal Society A,* **361**(1811), 2381–2395.

Steels, L. (2004). The autotelic principle. In Fumiya, I., Pfeifer, R., Steels, L., and Kunyoshi, K. (eds.), *Embodied Artificial Intelligence.* Lecture Notes in AI 3139. Berlin: Springer Verlag, pp. 231–242.

Stellar, J. R. (1985). *The Neurobiology of Motivation and Reward.* New York: Springer Verlag.

Storck, J., Hochreiter, S., and Schmidhuber, J. (1995). Reinforcement driven information acquisition in non-deterministic environments. In *Proceedings of ICANN 1995: International
Conference on Artificial Neural Networks*, Vol. 2. Paris: EC2, pp. 159–164.

Suri, R. E. and Schultz, W. (2001). Temporal difference model reproduces anticipatory neural
activity. *Neural Computation*, **13**, 841–862.

Sutton, R. S. (1988). Learning to predict by the methods of temporal differences. *Machine
Learning*, **3**(1), 9–44.

Sutton, R. S. and Barto, A. G. (1998). *Reinforcement Learning: An Introduction*. Cambridge,
MA: MIT Press.

Sutton, R. S., Precup, D., and Singh, S. (1999). Between MDPSs and semi-MDPs: a framework
for temporal abstraction in reinforcement learning. *Artificial Intelligence*, **112**, 181–211.

Tani, J. (2007). On the interactions between top-down anticipation and bottom-up regression.
Frontiers in Neurorobotics, **1**.

Tani, J. and Nolfi, S. (1999). Learning to perceive the world as articulated: an approach for hierarchical learning in sensory-motor systems. *Neural Network*, **12**, 1131–1141.

Thorndike, E. L. (1911). *Animal Intelligence: Experimental Studies.* New York: Macmillan.

Turing, A. (1950). Computing machinery and intelligence. *Mind*, **59**, 433–460.

Varela, F. J., Thompson, E., and Rosch, E. (1991). *The Embodied Mind: Cognitive Science And
Human Experience.* Cambridge, MA: MIT Press.

von Uexküll, J. (1909). *Umwelt und Innenwelt der Tiere.* Berlin: Springer.

Vygotsky, L. (1978). *Mind in Society: The Development of Higher Psychological Processes.*
Cambridge, MA: Harvard University Press.

Walkins, C. J. C. H. and Dayan, P. (1992). Q-learning. *Machine Learning*, **8**, 279–292.

Warnier, J-P. (1999). *Construire la culture materielle: l'homme qui pensait avec les doigts.*
Paris: Presses Universitaires de France.

Weinberger, D. R. (1987). Implications of normal brain development for the pathogenesis of
schizophrenia. *Archives in General Psychiatry*, **44**, 660–669.

Weiner, I. and Joel, D. (2002). Dopamine in schizophrenia: dysfunctional information processing
in basal ganglia–thalamocortical split circuits. In Chiara, G. D. (ed.), *Handbook of Experimental
Pharmacology.* Vol 154/II: *Dopamine in the CNS II.* Berlin: Springer, pp. 417–472.

White, N. M. (1989). Reward or reinforcement: what's the difference? *Neuroscience
Biobehavorial Review*, **13**, 181–186.

White, R. N. (1959). Motivation reconsidered: the concept of competence. *Psychological Review*,
66, 297–333.

Wiering, M. and Schmidhuber, J. (1997). HQ-learning. *Adaptive Behavior*, **6**(2), 219–246.

Wise, R. A. (1989). The brain and reward. In Liebman, J. M. and Cooper, S. J. (eds.), *The
Neuropharmacological Basis of Reward.* Oxford, UK: Clarendon Press, pp. 377–424.

Yoshimoto, K., McBride, W.J., Lumeng, L., and Li, T.-K. (1991). Alcohol stimulates the release
of dopamine and serotonin in the nucleus accumbens. *Alcohol*, **9**, 17–22.

11 Can cognitive developmental robotics cause a paradigm shift?

Minoru Asada

11.1 Introduction

This chapter discusses how cognitive developmental robotics (CDR) can make a paradigm shift in science and technology. A synthetic approach is revisited as a candidate for the paradigm shift, and CDR is reviewed from this viewpoint. A transdisciplinary approach appears to be a necessary condition and how to represent and design "subjectivity" seems to be an essential issue.

It is no wonder that new scientific findings are dependent on the most advanced technologies. A typical example is brain-imaging technologies such as fMRI, PET, EEG, NIRS, and so on that have been developed to expand the observations of neural activities from static local images to ones that can show dynamic and global behavior, and have therefore been revealing new mysteries of brain functionality. Such advanced technologies are presumed to be mere supporting tools for biological analysis, but is there any possibility that it could be a means for new science invention?

If robots, as one kind of artifact, could be such a thing, it means that robotics can make a paradigm shift in both science *and* technology. Understanding natural phenomena by constructive or synthetic approaches has been done but has not, as yet, caused any kind of paradigm shift. Is it possible for the consequences of artifact production to go beyond being simply useful tools in our daily life to become a means of impacting existing scientific disciplines? One possibility could be a constructivist approach; that is, a methodology which creates reality by constructing situations. Hashimoto *et al.* (2008) argued that it attempts to verify hypotheses or to find necessary conditions to realize biological behavior through (1) synthesizing the system based on knowledge or a hypothesis of biology, (2) experimenting with the system in real situations, and (3) comparing the consequences of the system with real phenomena, and/or exploring new findings.

Further, the most important issue faced through these processes is how to design a mechanism to be embedded in systems which can contribute to the emergence of a sort of subjectivity or autonomy that the existing disciplines are not good at coping with. This is exactly the target to be attacked by robotics research that aims at shifting paradigms.

In this chapter, we review the meaning and value of CDR, a survey of which is given by Asada *et al.* (2009), and its studies so far. We discuss the methodology and

Neuromorphic and Brain-Based Robots, eds. Jeffrey L. Krichmar and Hiroaki Wagatsuma. Published by Cambridge University Press. © Cambridge University Press 2011.

the consequences of these studies and, in particular, any possibility of causing a paradigm shift.

11.2   The meaning of constructivist approaches

The main purpose of the constructivist approach is to generate a completely new understanding through cycles of hypothesis and verification, targeting the issues that are very hard or almost impossible to solve under existing scientific paradigms. A typical example is evolutionary computation that virtually recreates a past we cannot observe, and shows the evolutionary process (e.g. Hashimoto *et al.*, 2008). If we reduce the timescale, the ontogenetic process (i.e. the individual development process) can be the next target for constructivist approaches. Development of neuromechanisms in the brain and cognitive functions in infants are at considerably different levels. The former has its own history as developmental biology and the researchers' approach to the issue under this discipline. The latter deals with cognitive development in developmental psychology, cognitive science, and so on. Depending on the age, given (already acquired) functions and faculties to be acquired through interactions with the environment, including other agents, should be clearly discriminated.

The subjectivity argued by Hashimoto *et al.* (2008) is only meaningful if we focus on human individuals. That is, the process of self-establishment by infants provides various kinds of research issues in developmental psychology, cognitive science, and sociology, including the issue of communication. Therefore, approaches to the issues that are difficult to solve under a single existing discipline might be found by the constructivist ones. Especially for the infant's cognitive development, developmental psychology largely depends on observations from outside (macroscopic), neuroscience tends to be microscopic, and brain imaging is more difficult to apply to infants than adults. Thus, a single paradigm seems difficult to approach, and it is not easy to verify hypothesized models. Therefore, it is time for the constructivist approaches to begin to play an active role.

11.3   Cognitive developmental robotics as a constructivist approach

A representative constructivist approach is cognitive developmental robotics (a survey is given by Asada *et al.*, 2009). Sandini *et al.* (2004) and Weng *et al.* (2001) take similar approaches, but CDR puts more emphasis on the human/humanoid cognitive development. A slightly different approach is taken by Atkeson *et al.* (2000) who aim to program humanoid behavior through the observation and understanding of human behavior and, by doing so, give a clearer insight into the nature of human behavior. Though partially sharing the purpose of human understanding, they do not exactly deal with the developmental aspect.

Figure 11.1 summarizes the various aspects of the development according to the survey by Lungarella *et al.* (2003) from the viewpoints of external observation, internal

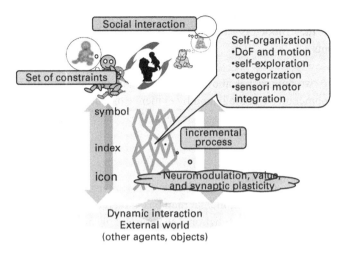

Figure 11.1   Various aspects of the development from viewpoints of external observation, internal structure, its infrastructure, and social structure (based on Lungarella *et al.*, 2003).

structure, its infrastructure, and social structure, focusing especially on the underlying mechanisms in different forms.

Roughly speaking, the developmental process consists of two phases: individual development at an early stage and social development through interaction between individuals at a later stage. The former relates mainly to neuroscience (internal mechanism) and the latter to cognitive science and developmental psychology (behavior observation). Intrinsically, both should be seamless, but there is a big difference between them at the representation level for the research target to be understood. CDR aims not at simply filling the gap between them but, more challengingly, at building a new paradigm that provides new understanding of ourselves while at the same time adding a new design theory of humanoids that is symbiotic with us. So far, CDR has been mainly focusing on computational models of cognitive development, but in order to more deeply understand how humans develop, robots can be used as reliable reproduction tools in certain situations such as psychological experiments. The following is a summary.

A. Construction of computational model of cognitive development:
  1. hypothesis generation: proposal of a computational model or hypothesis based on knowledge from existing disciplines
  2. computer simulation: simulation of the process difficult to implement with real robots, such as physical body growth
  3. hypothesis verification with real agents (humans, animals, and robots), then go to (1).
B. Offer new means or data to better understand human developmental process → mutual feedback with (A):
  1. measurement of brain activity by imaging methods

2. verification using human subjects or animals
3. providing the robot as a reliable reproduction tool in (psychological) experiments.

According to the two approaches above, there are many studies inspired by the observations of developmental psychology and by evidence or findings in neuroscience. The survey by Asada *et al.* (2009) introduces these studies based on the constructive model of development they hypothesize.

11.3.1   A cognitive developmental map

Let us consider a cognitive developmental map based on the various aspects mentioned in the previous section. The major functional structure of the human brain–spine system is a hierarchical one reflecting the evolutionary process, and consists of spine, brainstem, diencephalon, cerebellum, limbic system, basal ganglia, and neocortex. Here, we regard this hierarchy as the first analogy toward the cognitive developmental map, and the flow of functional development is indicated at the center of Figure 11.2: that is, reflex, sensorimotor mapping, perception, voluntary motion, and higher-order cognition.

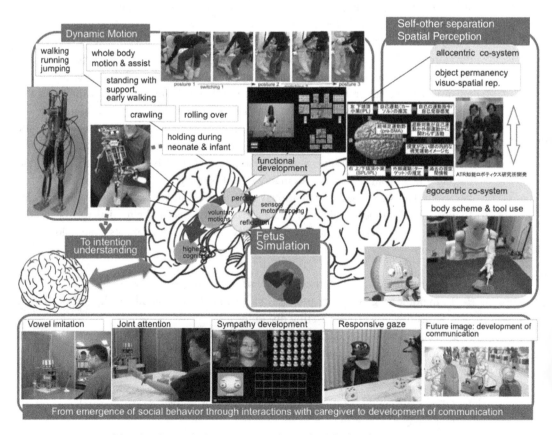

Figure 11.2   A cognitive developmental map (adapted from Fig. 3 in Asada *et al.*, 2009) (© 2009 IEEE).

In Figure 11.2, we show, as much as possible, the correspondence between the developmental processes for individuals and the relationship between objects and individuals to the brain regions in terms of functions. Among these regions, the medial frontal cortex (MFC) is proposed to be closely related to mind development and social cognition by Amodio and Frith (2006). However, it seems that a more global network of the brain works together for such development and cognition, and more importantly, interaction triggered by caregivers (scaffolding) is one of the environmental factors that plays an essential role in various developmental processes, such as vocal imitation (Yoshikawa *et al.*, 2003; Hisashi *et al.*, 2008), joint attention (Sumioka *et al.*, 2008a, 2008b), and empathy development (Watanabe *et al.*, 2007). Making clear the principle of development between individuals in these processes that is seamlessly connected with individual development may increase the possibility of a paradigm shift by CDR.

11.4   Is a paradigm shift possible?

Many studies introduced in the survey by Asada *et al.* (2009) have shown different aspects of CDR, but none of them is sufficient to cause a paradigm shift by themselves. Most of them have only shown the possibilities of realization of cognitive functions with a computational model of learning/development in each aspect. But, as yet, no fully encompassing principle of cognitive development has emerged. One point by Hashimoto *et al.* (2008) is "Conventional scientific methodology is not good at dealing with subjectivity, since scientific research becomes possible by finding an objective entity in which subjective feature is stripped off. But treating subjectivity scientifically is unavoidable."

This is especially true in the case of robotics since robots are supposed to be introduced into our society as independent agents. In such a case, subjectivity is not only a technical issue but more seriously a kind of controversial one: that is, should robots have subjectivity (autonomy) or not? Before making the immediate conclusion for the issue, we should carefully consider the issue from a scientific viewpoint. However, as mentioned above, existing disciplines are not good at dealing with the subjectivity in a scientific manner. This may require us to understand human beings as social agents, which involves psychology, cognitive science, and sociology. Here is a necessary condition to cause a paradigm shift since it seems hard or insufficient under a single scientific paradigm. An interdisciplinary approach seems essential.

What is a sufficient condition? Is it possible just by integrating the existing scientific disciplines? Is CDR completely independent from them? Of course not! By involving them, CDR should raise its meaning by prospecting the limits of the existing scientific disciplines. In this context, the issue to be attacked is "interaction" between neurons or brain regions or individual persons. Communication, a kind of interaction between subjective agents, may involve language development at the level of individual persons, which remains something of a mystery.

What it comes down to is: CDR should

1. integrate the knowledge, evidence, and findings (utilize the existing paradigms and synthesize them),
2. build a model or hypothesis that has no contradiction with the evidence or findings in existing disciplines or resolve the contradiction or controversial issues in these existing disciplines such as brain science and developmental psychology, and
3. find a new fact or provide a solution to the issue through the verification process of the model or the hypothesis by simulations or real experiments.

Item (1) does not imply denying the existing disciplines but rather seeks to involve them. Therefore, CDR researchers should have a minimum amount of knowledge in these disciplines to discuss the issues with researchers in these areas such as developmental psychology and brain science. Item (2) is a key point for CDR researchers to hit on an idea that reflects the integrated knowledge in (1) maximally based on the design principle. If CDR can provoke the emergence of new ideas and theories that could not be predicted or imagined in a single discipline, the role of CDR may change from serving as a bridge between different existing disciplines to being the principal one of the paradigm shift. Item (3) asks us if the consequence of (2) can impact the related areas in (1). One of the most serious issues is whether or not the performance of CDR can be regarded as being superior to that of the existing discipline from a viewpoint of the existing paradigm. To overcome this, CDR should create a new paradigm. This is the final condition of the paradigm shift. What is it?

Regarding the relationship between an infant and its caregiver as a developing process of interaction between individual agents, key issues are neonatal imitation (e.g. Meltzoff and Moore, 1977; Sawa *et al.*, 2007, as a synthetic approach), joint attention (Baron-Cohen, 1995; Moore and Dunham, 1995; Nagai *et al.*, 2003), vocal imitation (Yoshikawa *et al.*, 2003; Jones 2007; Ishihara *et al.*, 2008), peekaboo (Rochat *et al.*, 1999; Ogino *et al.*, 2007), pointing (Tomasello, 1995), delayed imitation (game of make-believe), linkage between lexicon and action, and so on. The common issues are body representation, rhythm and timing, multimodal input/output (vision, auditory, touch, somatosensory, motion, vocalization, etc.), self–other separation, sociality acquisition, and so on. If CDR can provide the constructive and unified form of the representation that can explain and simultaneously design the cognitive development of these issues, instead of representing them separately, this may lead to the paradigm shift. To enable this, the studies of developmental disorders in addition to the studies of normal children may help construction of the unified model of cognitive development.

11.5   Mirror neuron system connects physical embodiment and social entrainment

11.5.1   Rethinking physical embodiment

"Physical embodiment" is a key idea whose meaning has been frequently defined and argued (e.g. Brooks, 1991; Agre, 1995; Asada *et al.*, 1999, 2001; Pfeifer and Scheier,

1999; Sandini *et al.*, 2004; Pfeifer and Bongard, 2006; Vernon *et al.*, 2007). Kuniyoshi *et al.* (2007) described it as follows:

The agent's physical body specifies the constraints on the interaction between the agent and its environment that generate the rich contents of its process or consequences. It also gives the meaningful structure to the interaction with environment, and is the physical infrastructure to form the cognition and action.

The key concept of the above "physical embodiment" is shaped in the context of development as follows. At an early stage of human development (embryo, fetus, neonate, infant, and so on), interactions with various physical environments play a major role in determining the information structuring inside the individual such as body representation, motor image, and object permanency. In contrast, at a later stage, social behaviors such as early communication, joint attention, imitation of various actions including vocalization, empathy, and verbal communication gradually emerge owing to interactions with other agents. Regardless of the premature or mature state of the individual, the common aspect of these developmental processes is a sort of "scaffolding" by the environment including other agents that trigger the sensorimotor mapping and promote the infants' autonomy, adaptability, and sociality, directly or indirectly, and explicitly or implicitly.

Cranial nerve system

The bodies which synthetic approaches have been dealing with so far are limited parts of the nerves–sensor organs–musculoskeleton–body surface system, and have not explicitly dealt with the digestive system, circulatory system, or respiratory system apart from a few studies.[1] For the cranial nerve system, Kuniyoshi and Sangawa (2006) dealt with only parts of the primary motor and primary somatosensory areas. Some brain regions might be mentioned in the architectures of the synthetic approaches, but it seems difficult to have evident correspondence to real ones. The issue becomes more difficult when introducing a viewpoint of development. The following points are suggested.

1. We cannot derive the infants' brain structure and functions from the adults' ones, nor should we do it (Elman *et al.*, 1996; Karmiloff-Smith, 1998; Paterson *et al.*, 1999).
2. Brain regions for function development and function maintenance are not the same. During early language development, damage of the region in the right hemisphere is much more serious than that of the left (Bates, 1997).
3. The attention mechanism develops from the bottom up, such as from the visual saliency map, to the top down needed to accomplish the specified task, and the related brain regions shift from posterior to anterior ones (Posner and Petersen, 1990).

CDR should start from a bottom-up approach (e.g. Mori and Kuniyoshi, 2007) with a minimal implementation, and gradually add more structures and therefore functions that link to modeling interaction with caregivers, of which a design principle should be embedded in the mirror neuron system (MNS).

---

[1] Batteries, electric power lines, and sensor harness may correspond to these organs and systems.

Musculoskeletal system

The fundamental body structure that generates the motions of animals, including humans, is a musculoskeletal system that traditionally corresponds to a link structure in robotics. The big difference between them is the type of actuators used in the system. The former uses the muscle structure while the latter uses electromagnetic motors. This type of motor is the most popular since it is easy to control and therefore easily applied to many products. Separating the target and the method of control, the electromagnetic motors can generate various kinds of motions, such as low speed starting with high torque and continuous driving with low torque, by choosing the method and tuning its control parameters. However, the traditional robot architecture has great difficulty in generating dynamic motion with touch, whereas the musculoskeletal system can realize instantaneous motions such as jumping, landing, punching, kicking, and throwing based on the efficient use of the musculoskeletal body.

In the musculoskeletal structure, multiple muscles can be attached to a single joint and vice versa; that is, one muscle can be expanded across multiple joints, and these structures form the complex system (Neumann, 2002). Therefore, independent control of each joint is difficult, and the whole body movement is generated through the interaction with the environment. At a glance, it seems inconvenient, but this can be a solution to the problem of degrees of freedom (DOF) freezing for robots with many DOF. This was pointed out by Bernstein in 1967 as a fundamental issue of motor development (Sporns and Edelman, 1993).

McKibben pneumatic actuators have been receiving increased attention as such biomimetic artificial muscles. Niiyama and Kuniyoshi (2008), Hosoda *et al.* (2008), and Takuma *et al.* (2008) developed bouncing robots to realize vivid, dynamic motions with very low computational cost. They showed experimentally that the bi-articular muscles strongly governed the coordinated movement of its body, and therefore a simple controller could realize stable bouncing. These robots indicate that control and body structure are strongly connected; that is, we can interpret that the body itself has a role in calculating body control (Pfeifer *et al.*, 2006). One extreme and well-known example is passive dynamic walkers by McGeer (1990) that realize walking on the slope without any explicit control method or actuators. This is important from a viewpoint of energy consumption (resource bounded or fatigue).

CDR focusing on the physical embodiment seeks a seamless development from motor learning to higher cognitive function learning. From this viewpoint, artificial muscles such as McKibben pneumatic actuators that can generate dynamic motions are preferred to conventional electric motors. However, it is still not clear how such a mechanism may affect higher cognitive development; that is, how musculoskeletal systems utilized in motor learning by nonhuman primates or other animals enable the acquisition of human-level cognitive development if CDR aims at acquiring it.

A slight change is suggested. One hypothesis is that the interaction with a social environment, such as a caregiver might provide, may help derive human-specific faculties. A typical one is language. The corresponding language areas in other species, such as nonhuman primates, adapt to other faculties. Children isolated from a social environment for a long time, for example due to child abuse by their parents, suffer from not only disorder of motor development but also impediment of higher cognitive functions (Blakeslee and Blakeslee, 2007). An opposite case where a nonhuman primate was exposed to a social environment is "Kanzi" (Savage-Rumbaugh and Lewin, 1994), who indirectly learned a simple language for communication while his mother failed to do so. This may suggest that even such a primate can develop a sort of language faculty. However, it is still an open question how a musculoskeletal system is necessary for cognitive development.

Body surface (cutaneous sensation)

Due to the limit of current technology, not as many applications of cutaneous sensation for humanoids have been realized, even though it has been recognized as an important and necessary sensation (see Table III in Asada *et al.*, 2009). Recently, CB2 was designed as a research platform for cognitive development in the JST ERATO Asada synergistic intelligence system project and has 200 PVDF sensor elements under the soft silicon skin. Ohmura *et al.* (2006) designed a flexible tactile sensor that can be easily cut and pasted, and attached 2000 of these elements inside a humanoid body surface. Though it is not a whole body attachment, Takamuku *et al.* (2008) developed a bionic hand which consists of a plastic skeleton structure covered by a rubber glove inside which PVDF elements and strain gauges are randomly distributed, and applied it to object classification based on tactile sensation of toes and palm with grasping movements. They applied no sensor calibration, aiming instead at pure self-organization. Though the number of sensors is much fewer than in a human hand, the kinds of mechanoreceptors and layer structure are similar to a human hand, and therefore an extension to learning and development in the study of the grasping skills of humans is expected.

Cutaneous sensation on the body surface is closely connected to the somatosensory system, and a very important and essential sensation to acquire body representations such as body scheme or body image (Blakeslee and Blakeslee, 2007). Considering that the higher cognitive functions are developed based on such fundamental perception, cutaneous sensation is expected to be implemented on humanoids from the viewpoint of CDR. In addition to structuring the information from cutaneous mechanoreceptors, pain is indispensable for animals to survive. Further, its social function is related to empathy, which humanoids symbiotic with us in future are expected to have. Therefore, the implementation of pain sensation should not only be the response to physical impact but also involve the emotional expression of empathy with others' pain that enable deeper communication with us. This is closely related to the MNS which we will mention in the following sections.

11.5.2   Mirror neuron system and infrastructure for social cognitive development

After Gallese *et al.* (1996) found mirror neurons in the ventral premotor cortex of the macaque monkey brain, further evidence has been found from different studies (e.g. Rizzolatti *et al.*, 2008; Ishida *et al.*, 2010):

1. A mirror neuron fires both when an animal acts and when the animal observes the same action performed by another.
2. As long as the goal is shown, a mirror neuron activates even though the intermediate trajectory is invisible. It activates only when the action is a transitive one with an object as a target of the action.
3. A mirror neuron reacts to the sound caused by the action, and also when the monkey does the same action. It is believed that it responds to others' action understanding.
4. Some mirror neurons respond when the monkey observes tool use by another. If the goal is the same, its realization may differ.
5. Other mirror neurons respond to oral communication between monkeys.
6. Mirror neurons exist not only in the ventral premotor cortex but also in the PFG area[2] (neuron activities to somatosensory and visual stimulus) at the inferior parietal lobule which is anatomically connected to the former.
7. Responses of mirror neurons in the PFG area differ depending on action executors.
8. At the peripheral area of the superior temporal sulcus (STS) of the temporal lobule, the visual neurons that respond to others' actions are known. However, they are not called mirror neurons since they do not have any responses related to motions. The response differs depending on gaze; therefore the relation with joint attention is suggested.
9. The ventral premotor cortex F5, the PFG area at the inferior parietal lobule, and the peripheral area of STS are anatomically connected and constitute a system called a "mirror neuron system."
10. Mirror neurons related to reaching are recorded at the dorsal premotor cortex.

Since the ventral premotor cortex of the macaque monkey brain may correspond to the human brain regions close to the Broca area related to language faculty, Rizzolatti and Arbib (1998) suggested the relationship between MNS and language acquisition. There has since been further speculation on the process whereby humans acquire cognitive functions such as imitation, action understanding, and further language faculty. Some can be found in the book edited by Arbib (2006).

One unsolved issue is how another person's action is realized in one's own brain; that is, the capability to simulate the other's internal state in oneself (Gallese and Goldman, 1998). This relates to self–other discrimination, action understanding, joint attention, imitation, theory of mind, empathy, and so on. Ishida *et al.* (2010) and Murata and Ishida (2007) suggested the following based on the above, and related, findings.

- Coding another's body parts occurs in the same area that encodes one's own body parts, and the map of one's own body parts is referred to in perception of others' bodies.
- As a step to self body cognition, the coincidence of efference copy and sensory feedback forms the sense of self-motion. In fact, Murata's group found the neurons in the parietal area related to integration of information from the efference copy and the sensory feedback (Murata and Ishida, 2007).

---

[2] The PFG area is between PF and PG areas, and PF, PG and PFG are vernacular terms for monkey brain regions. Actually, PF and PG correspond to gyrus supramarginalis (Brodmann areas 7b) and gyrus angularis (7a), respectively.

- Originally, mirror neurons had visually coded motions and worked as sensory feedback during motion execution regardless of self or other's motions. Through the evolutionary and developmental processes, the current MNS has been constructed after integration with motion information.
- Mirror neurons concern the cognition of self and others' bodies in addition to others' motion recognition.
- It is unclear whether the parietal area detects the coincidence between efference copy and sensory feedback (consciousness of "self") or their difference (consciousness of "other") (it is suggested that the human parietal area detects the difference).

Similar to the position by Ishida *et al.* (2010) and Murata and Ishida (2007), Shimada (2009) also proposed the following model for the activity of mirror neurons with two terms: the externalized body representation (mainly based on vision) and the internalized body representation (proprioception and efference copy). In the visual area, the externalized body is represented and its consistency with the internalized body representation is checked. During this process, the difference caused by self–other discrimination is not available, but the internalized body representation is adjusted so that this difference can be canceled, and as a result the motor and sensory areas are activated. The processing flow from the externalized body representation to the internalized one seems sufficiently possible considering that the movement is always adjusted based on the visual feedback. He points out that the integration process of different senses (vision, tactile, auditory, somatosensory, and motor commands) related to the externalized and internalized body representation is shared by the self–other discrimination and the MNS.

Such a process of sharing and discriminating the internal states of both self and other does not only seem limited to motor experiences, but other modalities too. Examples are the sensation of being touched when observing others touched by someone (somatosensory and parietal association areas are activated), another one of pleasure or displeasure when observing another person smelling (an emotional circuit responds), and also a feeling of pain by observing others' pain directly. These are the supposed origins of empathy. The fact that the self experience and that of the other are represented in the common area in the brain can be interpreted as a mechanism that processes the other's experience like the self's, and such a "mirror-like" property is supposed to be a neural infrastructure for the capability of sharing and understanding the other's internal state, including emotion (Fukushima and Hiraki, 2009).

Thus, the MNS contributes to learning and development of social behavior through becoming aware of self and other based on commonality and difference between self and other. However, it does not seem clear to what extent the MNS is innate and how much is learned through experience. Mirror neurons in monkeys only respond to goal oriented (actions of transitive verbs) with a visible target, while in the case of humans they also respond to actions of intransitive verbs without any target (Rizzolatti *et al.*, 2008). How can we interpret this difference?

One plausible interpretation is as follows. In the case of monkeys, due to higher pressure to survive, goal-oriented behavior needs to be established and used early. Whereas, in the case of humans, owing much to caregivers, such pressure is reduced and therefore the MNS works not only for goal-oriented behavior but also behavior without goals. Consequently, much room for learning and structuring for generalization is left, and this leads to more social behavior acquisition and extension to higher cognitive capabilities. As Shimada (2009) mentioned, "the difference caused by self–other discrimination is not available, but the internalized body representation is adjusted so that this difference can be canceled, and as a result the motor and sensory areas are activated." If so, repeating such behavior is supposed to be a link to imitation and communication. In the case of monkeys, the motivation to cancel this difference seems low due to high pressure to survive, and therefore not a link to imitation. Actually, monkeys are not known to have the ability to imitate.

11.6   Sociality developmental model by CDR

Explanation and design of the developmental process from fetus to child by a synthetic approach is given from a viewpoint of sociality development. The basic policy is as follows:

1. Since we argue on the level of not phylogeny but ontogeny, we minimize the embedded structure and maximize the explanation and design of the learning process. Body structure, especially brain regions and sensory organs, configuration of the muscle–skeleton system, and their connections are embedded structures. Other developmental changes (e.g. connectivity and synaptic efficacy) are considered at each stage of sociality development.
2. According to the level of self–other cognition, the axis of sociality is formed. Changes from implicit others (including the environment), who can be perceived as non-self, to the explicit others, similar to the self, comprises the fundamental axis of development.
3. During this process, the role of the MNS should be made clear, and we discuss some possibilities of its construction and use.
4. As learning methods, we use Hebbian learning and self-organizing maps (SOM). In fact, most synthetic approaches so far have used them.

Figure 11.3 shows the process of establishing the concept of self and other(s). Starting from the undifferentiated state of self and other, an agent is supposed to gradually discriminate self/non-self, and then self/objects/others, according to Neisser (1993). There are no clear boundaries between the states, but the state transition is continuous, and the changes in the development process are not homogeneous depending on the modality and the cognitive capability. Rather, it is an interesting issue how this nonhomogeneity affects the interactions among them. It would be more accurate to say that the structure which allows the emergence of the states corresponding to the discrimination of self/objects/others during dynamic interactions is desired rather than a structure that constructs an exact representation.

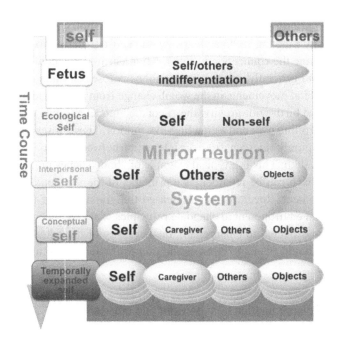

Figure 11.3 Early development of sociality.

11.6.1 Self/others undifferentiated state

Recent progress of visualization technology such as 4D sonar enables us to reveal various fetal behaviors and capabilities in the womb (e.g. Myowa-Yamakoshi and Takeshita, 2006). During this period, the state is supposed to be an undifferentiated one of self/other, and the light and sound as stimuli from inside and outside the mother's womb interact with the fetus as implicit others.

The onset of the first sensation, tactile, is supposed to start from 10 weeks after conception, and vision from 18 to 22 weeks. It is easy to hypothesize that the self body representation can be acquired to some extent from motor and somatosensory learning before perceiving others' bodies visually, supposing that the body representation can be obtained based on a cross-modal one.

While the visual and auditory systems begin to work during this period, their connection to vocalization and limb movements does not seem strong, and therefore each of them is in an undifferentiated and immature state. However, coordinated motions between the lips and hands such as thumb sucking, seem innate or already learned due to the body posture constraint in the womb (e.g. the hand moves towards the fetus' lips when its mouth is opened; Myowa-Yamakoshi and Takeshita, 2006). As with the infrastructure of the MNS, the individual motor library starts to be acquired in this period.

Kuniyoshi and Sangawa (2006) constructed a simulated model of a fetus and showed that various meaningful motor patterns emerge after the birth without "innate" motor primitives. The model consists of a musculoskeletal body floating in a uterus environment (elastic wall and liquid), and a minimal nervous system consisting of a spine, medulla, and primary sensory/motor cortical areas. Connection weights between brain regions are initially random. Hebbian learning and self-organizing mapping methods are used to determine the connection weights. After learning, the configuration of the muscle units – more generally, the cortex map for somatosensory and motor areas – is acquired, and the fetal movements in the womb change from random to ordered. In the simulation after the birth with gravity, the "neonate" model exhibits emergent motor behaviors such as rolling over and a crawling-like motion. These observed whole-body motor patterns are purely emergent from the interaction between the body, environment, and the nervous system. This is a typical example of "body shapes brain" (Kuniyoshi, 2008). Their approach can be regarded as a principle of the synthetic approaches for individual development. Recently, they increased the granularity of their simulation for brain, body, and environment to elucidate principles of social behavior. A structure such as a MNS is expected to emerge, and the necessity of the external structure of the environment should be made clear in addition to the infrastructure of the innate internal structure.

11.6.2   The beginning of discrimination between self and non-self

Neonatal imitation found by Meltzoff and Moore (1977), in particular, has been a hot topic causing a controversial argument between what is "innate" and what is "learned." As mentioned from 4D ultrasound imaging of the fetus movements, the fetuses start touch motions with their body parts such as face and arm at least 14 or 15 weeks after gestation. Hand movements toward its lips are often observed, and these body parts have a high density distribution of tactile sensor organs. Could these provide clues as to the "innate" or "learned" nature of neonatal imitation?

From the viewpoint of CDR, we propose two main causes. One is a physical constraint on body structure (posture constraint): a fetus assumes the pose of folded arms much more than extending them inside the tight space of the womb; thus there is a high probability of the hands being positioned close to the face, especially its mouth. In this case, little freedom of its hand–arm movements is given to the fetus owing not simply to joint structure but also to muscle attachment layout. Another one is the information maximization tendency; that is, touching its lip with its hand may acquire more information than touching other body parts due to high density distribution of tactile sensory organs of the hands and lips. Further, the oral cavity differs from the body surface and is an interesting target for its exploratory behavior.

In fetal and neonatal periods, self sensorimotor mapping and, especially, hand movements close to the mouth and the lip are acquired. This may be a period in which the concept of others has not been matured but the ecological self and non-self concepts begin to discriminate. The fundamental issue is self body cognition. On the basis of the contingency principle of self body cognition, Miyazaki and Hiraki (2006) argued its cognitive sensitivity of infants in terms of the delay of visual sensation. As a computational model of self/other discrimination, Asada *et al.* (1999) proposed a method based on state and its order estimation. The method can extract a static environment, self body, or objects which move in synchronization with the self body, that is, tools, based on a fact that

Table 11.1. Infant development and learning targets

Months	Behaviors	Learning targets
5	Hand regard	Forward and inverse models of the hand
6	Finger the other's face	Integration of visuo-tactile sensation of the face
6	Observe objects from different viewpoints	3D object recognition
7	Drop objects and observe the result	Causality and permanency of objects
8	Hit objects	Dynamics model of objects
9	Drum or bring a cup to mouth	Tool use
10	Imitate movements	Imitation of invisible movements
11	Fine grasp and carry objects to others	Action recognition and generation, cooperation
12	Pretend	Mental simulation

(body) observation is directly related to self-induced motion. In this case, the state order is one. The state order greater than one includes others or the objects manipulated by the others. However, there is no exact representation of others similar to the self.

11.6.3 The existence of explicit others

After birth, infants gradually develop body representations, categories for graspable objects, mental simulation capabilities, and so on, through their learning processes. For example, hand regard at the fifth month means learning of the forward and inverse models of the hand. Table 11.1 shows the typical behavior of infants and the corresponding targets to learn them. Through these processes, the infant establishes the ecological self and non-self; and furthermore the comprehension of interpersonal self, explicit others, and a trinomial relationship (self, other, and an object) is acquired.

Cognition that self and others are similar seems to be a precondition to estimate the internal state of others in sociology. In accordance with preceding studies, Sanefuji and Ohgami (2008) argued that infants can discover the similarity of themselves in someone else's body or behavior based on their given understanding of self/others' similarities. Also, they can relate to changes in another's mind caused by the behavior. That is, the understanding of self/others' similarity is thought to be the infrastructure which supports one aspect of the following social cognitive development such as understanding of the other's demands, intention, and emotion (Meltzoff, 2007).

From the viewpoint of CDR, the basic requirements for understanding of similarity are the localization of self's facial parts, facial pattern detection in visual observation of others, and the correspondence of facial parts between self and the other. Sawa *et al.* (2007) proposed a possible learning model that enables a robot to acquire a body image for parts of its body that are invisible to itself (that is, in their case, "face"). The model associates spatial perception based on motor experience and motor image with perception based on the activations of touch sensors and tactile image, both of which are supported by visual information. Further, they proposed a method to detect facial parts such as eyes, nose, and mouth, each of which has a unique tactile pattern observed by hand touching and scanning on its face. Information on these detected facial parts can be used to construct a correspondence of face between the self and the other.

The understanding of face similarity between oneself and another leads to the understanding of the similarity between one's body and another's, and further, that of the other's behavior. Before going on to the next issue of understanding the other's behavior, we need to solve the coordinate transformation problem between oneself and another. That is, to absorb the apparent difference of the same motion but performed by different agents (self or other). Ogawa and Inui (2007) suggest that the parietal area executes the coordinate transformation between the egocentric and allocentric bases. From the viewpoint of CDR, we would like to search for any possibility of learning such a transformation after birth, rather than supposing that it is innate. How is it possible?

One possibility is based on the scheme of reinforcement learning where a value is assigned to each state according to the distance to the goal regardless of difference between apparent motions. Therefore, if we know the goal and can measure the distance to the goal from the current state, the different views (states) due to the observation from the different coordinate systems can be regarded as identical if their values are the same.[3]

In such a set of states with the same value, the states can be regarded as the same from a viewpoint of goal achievement, and apparent differences among them are assumed to be caused by the differences of the coordinate systems. Since the purpose of the coordinate transformation is to equalize the states beyond the apparent difference, it can be seen that the coordinate transformation is realized if an agent knows the values of all states (views) including the observation of another's behavior in addition to its own.

11.6.4   Interaction between the self and a caregiver as the other

The concept of others, especially a caregiver who has an exact role, is going to be established during the period of infancy, and at the same time, the conceptual self should be established. Typical issues are joint attention, imitation, and the development of empathy.

Approaches to joint attention so far have mainly dealt with gaze control (e.g. Nagai *et al.*, 2003, 2006), and it seems difficult to agree with Emery *et al.*'s (1997) statement that "joint attention has a necessary condition that an agent gaze at a object which is found after following the other's gaze aiming at attending that target object." Any scheme for self/other discrimination and other's behavior recognition is supposed to enable an agent to develop from gaze control as a fundamental behavior of joint attention to joint visual attention as purposeful behavior to follow the other's gaze by inferring the target that the other attends (Butterworth and Jarrett, 1991). During these processes, the person's attention is represented inside the self, and then it is shared such

---

[3] Takahashi *et al.* proposed a more relaxed method by which the tendency (goal approaching or not) is utilized to discriminate other's intention of motion.

that both the self and the other person's attention is the same (Shimada, 2009). This can be regarded as exactly what the MNS is doing. Through these processes, the agent is expected to acquire social behaviors such as social referencing, which is gaze behavior designed to awaken the other's attention.

Regardless of its explicit or implicit representation, the coordinate transformation between the self and the other would significantly aid imitation. The corresponding issue in vocal imitation is the transformation of, especially, each vowel between the self and the other, often an infant and its caregiver, in the formant space. The consequence of this correspondence means sharing each symbol (vowel) such as //a//, //e//, //i//, //o//, or //u// between them. A synthetic approach assuming a strong bias that a caregiver provides the goal-oriented information regardless of its explicit or implicit representation has been carried out by Yoshikawa *et al.* (2003) who have shown that mutual imitation accelerates the learning. They assume that an infant's preference for imitation itself, is a precondition for learning. Again, the adjusting structure suggested by Shimada (2009) may link to this preference.

In the previous section, the importance of "face" was pointed out as a part of the starting point for understanding of similarity between the self and others. The technical issues entail improving face recognition and understanding facial expressions. Behavior generation based on recognition of the other's facial expression, including detection of his/her gaze, is extremely important in communication. Therefore, CDR should overcome the difficulty in designing and building artificial faces.

Watanabe *et al.* (2007) built a face robot that empathizes with its caregiver based on an assumption of intuitive parenting (Papousek and Papousek, 1987). A typical example is when a caregiver mimics or exaggerates a child's emotional expressions. This is considered a good opportunity for teaching children how to feel in real time, and most adults possess this skill. Children are thus able to understand the meaning of facial expressions and develop empathy toward others as the process is reinforced through emphasis on the facial expressions of their caregivers. This is because children empirically learn the connection between their internal state and the facial expressions of others. Since this study focused on this aspect, there was no self/other discrimination in the child's emotional space. Towards developing a conceptual self, cognition of others who are similar, but not completely the same, causes the continuous process of filling the gap between oneself and another, and this process links to imitation and communication.

11.6.5 Social development of self concept and MNS

We have viewed the relationship between social development of self concept and the MNS from the viewpoint of synthetic approaches and shown the issues of CDR. As mentioned above, instead of representing the self independently depending on the cognitive functions during that period of development, a consistent representation of the self (and others) built synthetically that explains and designs cognitive development is needed to link the emergence of a new paradigm. That is, the development of the self concept as shown in Figure 11.3 is not a sequence of isolated representations of different selves but expected as a consequence of emergence or development of a consistent structure. Since it is so difficult, we cannot expect an immediate and unique solution to the issue yet. Therefore, we need to cut the whole issue into several parts, allowing overlaps, and attack each of them separately. Attention should be paid to the separation between already acquired cognitive functions and those expected after learning and development. Also, the relationship among them should be focused upon. For example, dynamic changes associated with independent development, mutual acceleration, and interference are important relationships to study. Through the accumulation of these studies, we may shed light on self-development, which links the creation of a new paradigm.

Solving the issues of language and theory of mind is a symbolic goal for CDR. During the developing processes of self and other concepts, development of vocal communication from an action-based one is also expected (Arbib, 2006). To cope with these issues, development of other research platforms is important and necessary. Other essential developments include the issue of time and memory. To have the concept of time, a robot needs to realize the decay of its physical body, and an emotional state such as sadness is originally based on the self body. A body design considering these issues is needed.

11.7   Discussion

We have reviewed the synthetic approaches in CDR seeking any possibility of designing subjectivity, and argued how MNS can help the issue. However, MNS itself is somewhat controversial (Hickok, 2009); therefore we should be careful of too much speculation. Instead, we should focus on an essential mechanism or principle that plays the same role that MNS is expected to play. Instead of designing the function of MNS directly, a more general and fundamental structure might be needed. Among several candidates, one is synchronization of oscillations, which is widely observed in neural assemblies in the brain.

Yamaguchi (2008) investigated theta rhythms in rat hippocampus and in human scalp electroencephalograms in order to clarify the computational principle in these systems with essential nonlinearity. She claimed that synchronization can crucially contribute to computation through unification among heterogeneous developing systems in real time. Further, Homae et al. (2007), Watanabe et al. (2008), and Nakano et al. (2009) found, based on the measurement of brain activities by near-infrared spectroscopy, that there was synchronization of brain activities, especially correlation between the frontal regions at two or three months and between the frontal and occipital regions at six months. One idea would be to introduce a concept of "synchronization" to explain and design the emergence of subjectivity, more correctly, as a phenomenon such that an agent can be regarded as having its subjectivity. The following is a story about the development of "self" representation.

At an early stage, synchronization with objects (more generally, environment) through rhythmic motions such as beating, hitting, knocking, and so on, or reaching behavior is observed. Tuning and predicting synchronization are the main activities of the agent.

If completely synchronized, the phase is locked (phase difference is zero), and both the agent and the object are mutually entrained into the synchronized state. In this phase, we may say the agent has its own representation: so-called "ecological self."

Next, a caregiver works as one who can synchronize with the agent. The caregiver helps the agent consciously and sometimes unconsciously in various manners such as motherese (Kuhl *et al.*, 1997) or motionese (Nagai and Rohlfing, 2009). Such synchronization may be achieved through turn taking, which includes catching and throwing a ball, giving and taking an object between the caregiver and agent, or calling each other. In this phase, an explicit representation of others occurs in the agent whereas no explicit representation of others has occurred in the first phase even though the caregiver is interacting with the agent. The phase difference in turn taking is assumed to be 180 degrees. Due to the explicit representation of others, the agent may have its own self-representation: so-called "interpersonal self." At the later stage of this phase, the agent is expected to learn when it should inhibit its behavior by detecting the phase difference so that turn taking between the caregiver and itself can occur.

This learning is extended in two ways. One is recognition, assignment, and switching of roles such as throwing and catching, giving and taking, and calling and hearing. The other is learning to desynchronize from the synchronized state with one person and to start synchronization with another person for some reason, such as sudden leaving of the first person (passive mode) or any attention to the second person (active mode). In particular, the latter needs active control of the synchronization (switching), and this active control facilitates the agent to take a virtual role in make-believe play. At this stage, the target to synchronize is not limited to the person but also to objects. However, it is not the same as in the first phase when real objects are used, but virtualized ones such as a virtualized mobile phone, virtualized food in make-believe play of eating or giving, and so on, are used. If such behavior is observed, we can say that the agent has the representation of "conceptual self."

The above story seems too ideal and optimistic, but the development process of subjectivity can be explained and at the same time designed to some extent based on the principle of synchronization. I hope this can trigger future discussions that may lead to the paradigm shift.

Acknowledgment

The author would like to thank group leaders and researchers of my projects (JST ERATO Asada Synergistic Project: www. jeap.org), especially Dale Thomas, a researcher at JST ERATO Asada Synergistic Intelligence Project, for his helpful comments on the draft of this chapter.

References

Agre, P. E. (1995). Computational research on interaction and agency. *Artificial Intelligence*, **72**, 1–52.

Amodio, D. M. and Frith, C. D. (2006). Meeting of minds: the medial frontal cortex and social cognition. *Nature Reviews Neuroscience*, **7**, 268–277.

Arbib, M. A. (2006). The mirror system hypothesis on the linkage of action and languages. In Arbib, M. A. (ed.), *Action to Language Via the Mirror Neuron System*. New York: Cambridge University Press, pp. 3–47.

Asada, M., Uchibe, E., and Hosoda, K. (1999). Cooperative behavior acquisition for mobile robots in dynamically changing real worlds via vision-based reinforcement learning and development. *Artificial Intelligence*, **110**, 275–292.

Asada, M., MacDorman, K. F., Ishiguro, H., and Kuniyoshi, Y. (2001). Cognitive developmental robotics as a new paradigm for the design of humanoid robots. *Robotics and Autonomous Systems*, **37**, 185–193.

Asada, M., Hosoda, K., Kuniyoshi, Y., *et al.* (2009). Cognitive developmental robotics: a survey. *IEEE Transactions on Autonomous Mental Development*, **1**(1), 12–34.

Atkeson, C. G., Hale, J. G., Pollick, F., *et al.* (2000). Using humanoid robots to study human behavior. *IEEE Intelligent Systems*, **15**(4), 46–56.

Baron-Cohen, S. (1995). *Mindblindness*. Cambridge, MA: MIT Press.

Bates, E. (1997). Plasticity, localization and language development. In Broman, S. H. and Fletcher, J. M. (eds.), *The Changing Nervous System: Neurobehavioral Consequences of Early Brain Disorders*. New York: Oxford University Press, pp. 214–253.

Blakeslee, S. and Blakeslee, M. (2007). *The Body Has a Mind of Its Own: How Body Maps in Your Brain Help You Do (Almost) Everything Better*. New York: Random House.

Brooks, R. (1991). Intelligence without representation. *Artificial Intelligence*, **47**, 139–159.

Butterworth, G. E. and Jarrett, N. L. M. (1991). What minds have in common is space: spatial mechanisms serving joint visual attention in infancy. *British Journal of Developmental Psychology*, **9**, 55–72.

Elman, J., Bates, E. A., Johnson, M., *et al.* (1996). *Rethinking Innateness: A Connectionist Perspective on Development*. Cambridge, MA: MIT Press.

Emery, N. J., Lorincz, E. N., Perrett, D. I., and Oram, M. W. (1997). Gaze following and joint attention in rhesus monkeys (*Macaca mulatta*). *Journal of Comparative Psychology*, **111**, 286–293.

Fukushima, H. and Hiraki, K. (2009). Whose loss is it? Human electrophysiological correlates of non-self reward processing. *Social Neuroscience*, **4**(3), 261–275.

Gallese, V. and Goldman, A. (1998). Mirror neurons and the simulation theory of mind-reading. *Trends in Cognitive Science*, 493–501.

Gallese, V., Fadiga, L., Fogassi, L., and Rizzolatti, G. (1996). Action recognition in the premotor cortex. *Brain*, **119**(2), 593–609.

Hashimoto, T., Sato, T., Nakatsuka, M., and Fujimoto, M. (2008). Evolutionary constructive approach for studying dynamic complex systems. In Petrone, G. and Cammarata, G. (eds.), *Recent Advances in Modelling and Simulation*. I-Tech Education and Publishing, ch. 7. Available from: www.intechopen.com/

Hickok, G. (2009). Eight problems for the mirror neuron theory of action understanding in monkeys and humans. *Journal of Cognitive Neuroscience*, **21**, 1229–1243.

Hisashi, I., Yoshikawa, Y., Miura, K., and Asada, M. (2008). Caregiver's sensorimotor magnets guide infant's vowels through auto mirroring. In *Proceedings of the 7th IEEE International Conference on Development and Learning (ICDL'08)*.

Homae, F., Watanabe, H., Nakano, T., and Taga, G. (2007). Prosodic processing in the developing brain. *Neuroscience Research*, **59**, 29–39.

Hosoda, K., Takayama, H., and Takuma, T. (2008). Bouncing monopod with bio-mimetic muscular-skeleton system. In *Proceedings of IEEE/RSJ International Conference on Intelligent Robots and Systems 2008 (IROS '08)*.

Ishida, H., Nakajima, K., Inase, M., and Murata, A. (2010). Shared mapping of own and others' bodies in visuotactile bi-modal area of monkey parietal cortex. *Journal of Cognitive Neuroscience*, **22**(1), 83–96.

Ishihara, H., Yoshikawa, Y., Miura, K., and Asada, M. (2008). Caregiver's sensorimotor magnets lead infant's vowel acquisition through auto mirroring. In: *Proceedings of the 7th IEEE International Conference on Development and Learning.*

Jones, S. S. (2007). Imitation in infancy: the development of mimicry. *Psychological Science*, **18**(7), 593–599.

Karmiloff-Smith, A. (1998). Development itself is the key to understanding developmental disorders. *Trends in Cognitive Science*, 389–398.

Kuhl, P., Andruski, J., Chistovich, I., *et al.* (1997). Cross-language analysis of phonetic units in language addressed to infants. *Science*, **277**, 684–686.

Kuniyoshi, Y. (2008). Body shapes brain: emergence and development of behavior and mind from embodied interaction dynamics. In Asada, M., Hallam, J. C. T., Meyer, J.-A., and Tani, J. (eds.), *From Animals to Animats 10: Proceedings of the 10th International Conference on the Simulation of Adaptive Behavior (SAB08)*, held in Osaka, Japan, July 2008. Lecture Notes in Computer Science 5040. Berlin: Springer.

Kuniyoshi, Y. and Sangawa, S. (2006). Early motor development from partially ordered neural-body dynamics: experiments with a cortico-spinal-musculo-skeletal model. *Biological Cybernetics*, **95**, 589–605.

Kuniyoshi, Y., Yorozu, Y., Suzuki, S., *et al.* (2007). Emergence and development of embodied cognition: a constructivist approach using robots. *Progress in Brain Research*, **164**, 425–445.

Lungarella, M., Metta, G., Pfeifer, R., and Sandini, G. (2003). Developmental robotics: a survey. *Connection Science*, **15**(4), 151–190.

McGeer, T. (1990). Passive walking with knees. In *Proceedings of the 1990 IEEE International Conference on Robotics and Automation.*

Meltzoff, A. N. (2007). The "like me" framework for recognizing and becoming an intentional agent. *Acta Psychologica*, 26–43.

Meltzoff, A. N., and Moore, M. K. (1977). Imitation of facial and manual gestures by human neonates. *Science*, 74–78.

Miyazaki, M. and Hiraki, K. (2006). Video self-recognition in 2-year-olds. In *Proceedings of the XVth Biennial International Conference on Infant Studies*. International Society on Infant Studies.

Moore, C. and Dunham, P. (eds.) (1995). *Joint Attention: Its Origins and Role in Development*. Hillsdale, NJ: Lawrence Erlbaum Associates.

Mori, H. and Kuniyoshi, Y. (2007). A cognitive developmental scenario of transitional motor primitives acquisition. In Berthouze, L., Prince, C. G., Littman, M., Kozima, H., and Balkenius, C. (eds.), *Proceedings of the 7th International Conference on Epigenetic Robotics*. Lund University Cognitive Studies, 135. Lund, Sweden: Lund University.

Murata, A. and Ishida, H. (2007). Representation of bodily self in the multimodal parieto-premotor network. In Funahashi, S. (ed.), *Representation and Brain*. Tokyo: Springer.

Myowa-Yamakoshi, M. and Takeshita, H. (2006). Do human fetuses anticipate self-directed actions? A study by four-dimensional (4D) ultrasonography. *Infancy*, **10**(3), 289–301.

Nagai, Y. and Rohlfing, K. J. (2009). Computational analysis of motionese toward scaffolding robot action learning. *IEEE Transactions on Autonomous Mental Development*, **1**(1), 44–54.

Nagai, Y., Hosoda, K., Morita, A., and Asada, M. (2003). A constructive model for the development of joint attention. *Connection Science*, **15**, 211–229.

Nagai, Y., Asada, M. and Hosoda, K. (2006). Learning for joint attention helped by functional development. *Advanced Robotics*, **20**(10), 1165–1181.

Nakano, T., Watanabe, H., Homae, F., and Taga, G. (2009). Prefrontal cortical involvement in young infants' analysis of novelty. *Cerebral Cortex*, **19**, 455–463.

Neisser, U. (ed.) (1993). *The Perceived Self: Ecological and Interpersonal Sources of Self Knowledge*. New York: Cambridge University Press.

Neumann, D. A. (2002). *Kinesiology of the Musculoskeletal System*. St Louis, MO: Mosby Inc.

Niiyama, R. and Kuniyoshi, Y. (2008). A pneumatic biped with an artificial musculoskeletal system. In *Proceedings of the 4th International Symposium on Adaptive Motion of Animals and Machines (AMAM 2008)*.

Ogawa, K. and Inui, T. (2007). Lateralization of the posterior parietal cortex for internal monitoring of self versus externally generated movements. *Journal of Cognitive Neuroscience*, **19**, 1827–1835.

Ogino, M., Ooide, T., Watanabe, A., and Asada, M. (2007). Acquiring peekaboo communication: early communication model based on reward prediction. In *Proceedings of the 6th IEEE International Conference on Developoment and Learning*, pp. 116–121.

Ohmura, Y., Kuniyoshi, Y., and Nagakubo, A. (2006). Conformable and scalable tactile sensor skin for curved surfaces. In *Proceedings of the IEEE International Conference on Robotics and Automation*, pp. 1348–1353.

Papousek, H. and Papousek, M. (1987). Intuitive parenting: a dialectic counterpart to the infant's precocity in integrative capacities. *Handbook of Infant Development*, 669–720.

Paterson, S. J., Brown, J. H., Gsodl, M. K., Johnson, M. H., and Karmiloff-Smith, A. (1999). Cognitive modularity and genetic disorders. *Science*, **286**, 2355–2358.

Pfeifer, R. and Bongard, J. C. (2006). *How the Body Shapes the Way We Think: A New View of Intelligence*. Cambridge, MA: MIT Press.

Pfeifer, R. and Scheier, C. (1999). *Understanding Intelligence*. Cambridge, MA: MIT Press.

Pfeifer, R., Iida, F., and Gömez, G. (2006). Morphological computation for adaptive behavior and cognition. *International Congress Series*, **1291**, 22–29.

Posner, M. I. and Petersen, S. E. (1990). The attention system of the human brain. *Annual Review of Neuroscience*, 25–42.

Rizzolatti, G. and Arbib, M. A. (1998). Language within our grasp. *Trends in Neuroscience*, **21**, 188–194.

Rizzolatti, G., Sinigaglia, C., and (trans.) Anderson, F. (2008). *Mirrors in the Brain: How Our Minds Share Actions and Emotions*. New York: Oxford University Press.

Rochat, P., Querido, J. G., and Striano, T. (1999). Emerging sensitivity to the timing and structure of protoconversation in early infancy. *Developmental Psychology*, **35**(4), 950–957.

Sandini, G., Metta, G., and Vernon, D. (2004). RobotCub: an open framework for research in embodied cognition. In *Proceedings of the 4th IEEE/RAS International Conference on Humanoid Robots*.

Sanefuji, W. and Ohgami, H. (2008) Responses to "like-me" characteristics in toddlers with/without autism: self, like-self, and others. In *Abstract Volume of XVIth International Conference on Infant Studies*, held in Vancouver. International Society on Infant Studies.

Savage-Rumbaugh, S. and Lewin, R. (1994). *Kanzi: The Ape at the Brink of the Human Mind*. New York: Wiley.

Sawa, F., Ogino, M., and Asada, M. (2007). Body image constructed from motor and tactle images with visual informaiton. *International Journal of Humanoid Robotics*, **4**, 347–364.

Shimada, S. (2009). Brain mechanism that discriminates self and others [in Japanese]. In Hiraki, K. and Hasegawa, T. (eds.), *Social Brains: Recognition of the Self and Other.* Tokyo: University of Tokyo Press.

Sporns, O. and Edelman, G. M. (1993). Solving Bernstein's problem: a proposal for the development of coordinated movement by selection. *Child Development*, 960–981.

Sumioka, Hu., Yoshikawa, Y., and Asada, M. (2008a). Causality detected by transfer entropy leads acquisition of joint attention. *Journal of Robotics and Mechatronics*, **20**(3), 378–385.

Sumioka, H., Yoshikawa, Y., and Asada, M. (2008b). Development of joint attention related actions based on reproducing interaction causality. In *Proceedings of the 7th IEEE International Conference on Development and Learning (ICDL '08).*

Takamuku, S., Fukuda, A., and Hosoda, K. (2008). Repetitive grasping with anthropomorphic skin-covered hand enables robust haptic recognition. In *Proceedings of the IEEE/RSJ International Conference on Intelligent Robots and Systems 2008 (IROS '08).*

Takuma, T., Hayashi, S., and Hosoda, K. (2008). 3D bipedal robot with tunable leg compliance mechanism for multi-modal locomotion. In *Proceedings of the IEEE/RSJ International Conference on Intelligent Robots and Systems 2008 (IROS '08).*

Tomasello, M. (1995). Joint attention as social cognition. *Joint Attention: Its Origins and Role in Development.* Hillsdale, NJ: Lawrence Erlbaum Associates, pp. 103–130.

Vernon, D., Metta, G., and Sandini, G. (2007). A survey of artificial cognitive systems: implications for the autonomous development of mental capabilities in computational agents. *IEEE Transactions on Evolutionary Computation*, **11**(2), 151–180.

Watanabe, A., Ogino, M., and Asada, M. (2007). Mapping facial expression to internal states based on intuitive parenting. *Journal of Robotics and Mechatronics*, **19**(3), 315–323.

Watanabe, H. Homae, F., Nakano, T., and Taga, G. (2008). Functional activation in diverse regions of the developing brain of human infants. *NeuroImage*, **43**, 346–357.

Weng, J., McClelland, J., Pentland, A., *et al.* (2001). Autonomous mental development by robots and animals. *Science*, **291**, 599–600.

Yamaguchi, Y. (2008). The brain computation based on synchronization of nonlinear oscillations: on theta rhythms in rat hippocampus and human scalp EEG. In Marinaro, M., Scarpetta, S., and Yamaguchi, Y. (eds.), *Dynamic Brain: From Neural Spikes to Behaviors.* LNCS 5286. Berlin: Springer-Verlag.

Yoshikawa, Y., Asada, M., Hosoda, K., and Koga, J. (2003). A constructivist approach to infants' vowel acquisition through mother-infant interaction. *Connection Science*, **15**(4), 245–258.

12 A look at the hidden side of situated cognition: a robotic study of brain-oscillation-based dynamics of instantaneous, episodic, and conscious memories

Hiroaki Wagatsuma

12.1 Introduction

One of the most amazing aspects of brain function is that free will and consciousness emerges from the simple elemental functions of neurons. How do a hundred billion neurons produce global functions, such as intention, mind, and consciousness? As gathering a billion people is not equal to making a civilized society, the brain is not merely a combination of neurons. There would be rules of relation and principles of action. I have been interested for many years in the neurodynamics of situated cognition and contextual decision making, particularly focusing on synchronization mechanisms in the brain. Neural synchronization is well known in spinal motor coordination (e.g. central pattern generators, CPG), circadian rhythms and EEG recordings of human brain activities during mental tasks. Synchronized population activity plays functional roles in memory formation and context-dependent utilization of personal experiences in animal models. However, those experiments and models have dealt with a specific brain circuit in a fixed condition, or at least less attention has been given to an embodied view, where the brain, body, and environment comprise a closed whole loop. The embodied view is the natural setting for a brain functioning in the real world. I have recently become interested in building an online and on-demand experimental platform to link the robotic body with its neurodynamics. This platform is implemented in a remote computer and gives us the advantage of studying brain functions in a dynamic environment, and to offer qualitative analyses of behavioral time, in contradistinction to neuronal time, or mental time. This chapter relates past work to present work in an informal way that might be uncommon in journal papers. By taking advantage of this opportunity, I will use informal speech and explanations, as well as personal anecdotes to guide the reader to understand important trends and perspectives in this topic. Section 12.1 gives an introduction to artificial systems that makes a commitment to biology, and argues a point of

Neuromorphic and Brain-Based Robots, eds. Jeffrey L. Krichmar and Hiroaki Wagatsuma. Published by Cambridge University Press. © Cambridge University Press 2011.

biologically inspired robotics in the viewpoint of being *life*. Section 12.2 overviews the multiple memory systems of the brain in terms of conscious awareness. Section 12.3 describes robotic methodologies by using neural dynamics of oscillatory components to enable the system to provide online decision making in cooperation with involuntary motor controls, and discusses necessities for future work. Section 12.4 summarizes key concepts and future perspectives.

12.1.1 Machine vs. life

Biological organisms survive in dynamic environments and display flexibility, adaptability, and survival capabilities that seem to exceed artificial systems. Over the past decade, robotic technologies have been developed in factory automations that aid in mass and precise production. The precise control of robotic arm movements placed in the automated production line enables the construction of various machines, ranging from tiny electronics to rugged cars. Nowadays, most factories need those machines. Recent expectations show a trend towards the availability of robotic technologies for household and elderly care. Our daily lives, however, are overflowing with unexpected changes which prevent automated machines from being used to help us outside factories; that is, robotic researchers and engineers have encountered difficulties in making an ideal robot that is capable of guessing what we want. A temporary way to avoid these difficulties is to define inputs to the machine from the environment as precisely as possible and to train the machine to recognize a set of input–output relationships through learning from experience. Stable repeatability of the input–output response is necessary for the system to be reliable like a computer, but the drawback here is less flexibility. In other words, the artificial system requires a framework of consistent input–output relationships by the external designer. But, in human social activities, the purpose and meaning of actions can change over time, and then the frame of how one solves the current problem needs to be continuously updated. This implies that biological systems have a critical internal mechanism to solve the frame problem, so that the system sets the purpose and meaning internally and reformulates the frame in accordance with the current situation. In terms of cognitive science, those internal components are called motivation, desire, intention, planning, and so on, and are considered to be coming from brain functions. The brain, or the central nervous system, is the core of the controller of the body and plays principal roles in generating emotions and intentions. It is not only in the case of human brains, but also in animals, because vertebrates, such as fishes, amphibians, reptiles, mammals, and birds, have similar brain structures. Consider the simple behavior of fishes in capturing a target. An Amazonian fish, the arowana, jumps a meter above the water's surface to capture an insect on a tree in a submerged forest in the rainy season (Figure 12.1a). Once an insect is targeted, the fish estimates the power and direction of the behavior before jumping. This requires precise and accurate body control. Without giving much thought to the motion planning, the fish predicts the body movement and balance, and then generates a smooth trajectory of the body to successfully reach the precise target. It may be described in the form of the control theory, or by forward and inverse models

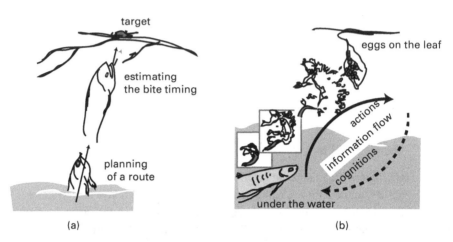

Figure 12.1   Illustrations of complex behaviors of two types of fishes. (a) Arowana jumps a meter above the water surface to capture an insect on a tree of a submerged forest in the rainy season. (b) *Copella arnordi*, a tiny fish swimming and jumping with its partner synchronously outside the water onto a leaf and spawning on the leaf. After spawning, the fish will throw water onto the eggs by shaking its tail toward the leaf until the eggs hatch in a couple of days.

with feedback error corrections. Another amazing behavior we must consider, even in fish, is emotion and cognition (Brown *et al.*, 2006). In the same Amazonian forest, a tiny fish, *Copella arnoldi*, has an interesting behavior. Before spawning, the fish synchronously swims and jumps with a partner to a leaf outside the water, and the couple attaches on the leaf for spawning. After spawning, noticing the target leaf contains their eggs, the fish will throw water on the leaf by shaking its tail to prevent the eggs from drying out in the high temperatures of the Amazonian forest, until eggs hatch in a couple of days (Figure 12.1b).

Even if we disregard the biggest problem of how the fish acquired this kind of complex behavior, possibly referring to the Darwinism controversy, we must consider how fish recognize the situation and what neural basis triggers an intended action from feelings, or a sense of crisis. Llinás and Roy (2009) suggested that the central nervous system's function is to centralize predictions that are internally generated by rapidly comparing properties of the external world with an internal sensorimotor representation of those properties. They hypothesize that the imperative in prediction is the basis for self-awareness. It is a concentration of cognitive or planned actions in time, which differs from prepared reflex/sensorimotor loops. Considering the parallel processing that is ongoing in multiple brain regions and the decision making that occurs in a small time period, there are still other unanswered questions, such as how the centralization is possible, how different timescales are coordinated, and whether the self-awareness appears as a consequence. For this to be a scientific problem, the question should be testable in an experimental framework, and therefore the experimental platform is necessary even if the brain is highly complex and difficult to test in dynamic environments. I shall propose a solution based on an experimental framework that bridges the gap between robotics and neuroscience.

12.1.2   Are we intentional, or perceived?

Autonomous control is an active area of research in robotics. Robotic autonomy can be defined as the ability to act on its own and make decisions independent of any external controller. But, in turn, what the *decision* is has to be clarified beforehand. The implication is that defining autonomy is an endless question, and a profound philosophical problem. An answer is to be found in biological autonomy, and it helps to explain how it exists. Biological autonomy is classified into different types and levels. First, self-maintenance, which implies self-reproduction in a broad sense at the species level, is fundamentally observed as homeostasis in various levels of biological organisms. This appears in the range from the process of membrane formation at the cellular level to the blood pressure and body temperature sustained by the autonomic nervous system in the body. The principle is understandable as sustaining of a certain physical condition in the form of an energy flow or a feedback loop with the environment. Robotic researchers mostly deal with it as self-calibration, self-repairing, and self-refueling of automated machines. Second, self-organization indicates an act to form global structures and patterns as a consequence of cooperation among local elements. This phenomenon is observed in chemical reactions and cell development. Principles of self-organization are studied in mathematics and computer science too by using cellular automata, random graphs, and group theory. Studies of multiagent systems and swarm robotics realize the self-organization phenomenon, as do modular robots, which form a single and constructive body from many elemental robots. Third, self-reference and self- (self–other) awareness are considered as higher order autonomy, referring to cognitive functions in the higher animal, or hierarchical biological systems. For example, human language is noted to have a self-referential nature, which enables us to link words infinitely, and the awareness of *who I am* requires viewing the self out of the frame.

Neuromorphological and brain-based robots would position the emergence of self-referential properties as the ultimate goal, and attempt to build an artificial brain as a container of *self*. Considering the brief overview of biological autonomy, we can take a realistic approach to investigating the self-maintenance and self-organization in scientific research. But, self-reference and self-awareness seem to be still far from scientific approaches. It is possible to draw at least two different perspectives. One is that three listed types of biological autonomy can be explained in a consecutive manner, suggesting the emergence of self-reference is an extension to realizations of self-maintenance and self-organization. A second interpretation is that self-maintenance and self-organization are explained in a physical sense, while self-reference and self-awareness are particularly different and difficult to reproduce in the same manner. Thus, there is a large gap between biological autonomy at the physical levels and cognitive levels.

There are some studies to attempt to bridge this gap between physical and cognitive. In the study of artificial life, a concept of homeodynamics is proposed to form the *self*, which spontaneously discriminates *in* from *out* of the cell membrane, and the source of biological autonomy at the cell level would reach to higher level autonomies (Ikegami and Suzuki, 2008). More realistically, the brain autonomy is discussed as the link between the autonomic nervous system and higher cognitive functions, and some researchers suggest that neural mechanisms that provide emotional responses mediate between them. LeDoux (1996) highlighted underlying brain mechanisms responsible for our emotions to bring unconscious feelings and responses to conscious emotions and intended acts, and Ziemke (2008) argued that a multitiered affectively/emotionally embodied view is necessary to treat biological autonomy in robotics and suggested an *organismic* embodiment in comparison with conventional embodiment approaches in past biologically inspired robotics. Indeed, those rational arguments offer hope of progress. The question is not so much whether those hypotheses are plausible but how we can test them by building a real experimental setup. To answer this question, we must first realize a multilayered system testable platform, which spans from a simple autonomy to a complex one, in a real-time environment. If neuromorphological and brain-based robots are ideal candidates to be the testable platform, we will be able to obtain qualitative and quantitative answers to the further question of whether or not the human brain is an extension of animal brains, in the sense of self-referential properties. In Section 12.3.1, I refer to the fact that the memory system in the brain is a multi-tiered system representing different scales in time and space. Qualitative differences can arise in the human self-referential property because the human being is capable of being aware of time and space simultaneously.

12.2   Investigating brain mechanisms underlying conscious memory

12.2.1   Conscious and unconscious memories in the brain

When discussing types of the long-term memory in the human brain, neuroscience textbooks classify them into explicit (declarative) memory and implicit (nondeclarative, or typically procedural) memory (Tulving, 1972; Squire, 1987; Kandel *et al.*, 2000). This binary classification causes distress for neuroscientists specifically interested in degrees of consciousness. From the background of psychological tests, explicit memory is defined as the conscious, intentional recollection of previous experiences and information. We can ask human subjects questions about their personal histories, for example a question of what they ate at dinner last night, and they can then answer by remembering their past experience. In such tests, psychologists and neurologists certify that this is the case of what the subject consciously remembers and intentionally answers. The definition fundamentally assumes conscious access to the memory content and the operation of thinking, in distinction from automated reactions. For this reason, explicit memory includes facts and events that one has experienced personally in the past.

By contrast, implicit memory includes priming, skills, habits, conditioning, and reflexes, which encode how to do things and which action might be taken in response to a particular stimulus. The implicit memory type is considered to be retrievable without the need for conscious awareness. Accordingly, brain regions underlying these two memory types are separately organized to perform these functions (Kandel *et al.*, 2000) but some regions closely overlap. In animal studies, it is difficult for us to judge the accompaniment of conscious awareness in memory retrieval by external observation, but a common brain structure gives clues to suggest the functional relevance to similar memory capabilities. In tests of episodic memory retrieval, human subjects can explicitly and intentionally recollect what they did in the past, even ten years or more before. Therefore, the episodic recollection seems to virtually travel in time, and allows us to treat past memories as a flexible time length of an episode. Similarly in animal cases, neuroscientists can observe neural correlates to the memory retrieval of experiences having taken place days ago in a form of the behavioral sequence, which demonstrates patterns of neural activity with a modifiable and fluctuating time length for memory retrieval (Lee and Wilson, 2002).

In comparison, conditioning and reflex responses are immediate in principle, and procedure memories provide protocols or sequential actions to proceed with accurate timing. If the conscious state is somehow functional for the establishment of high-level perception in a self-referential manner (Eccles, 1989; Sloman, 2009), an understanding of how brain operations can give rise to thinking in time and space (such as recalling old memories and an imagination of remote places and impossible futures) is a realm of scientific questions and of interest to people who attempt to rebuild a similar system in engineering fields (see Chapters 10, 11, and 13 and Damasio (1999) for details on levels and grades of consciousness, or forms of the *self*).

The medial temporal lobe, or the limbic system, is crucial for the episodic (declarative) memory function. This brain region includes the hippocampus and the amygdala, and these are functionally connected to the prefrontal cortex, which is essential for receiving contextual details of a past experience at the moment of decision making. Interestingly, the limbic system is a contact point between circuits for explicit and implicit memories. The amygdala also serves a dominant role in unconscious emotional responses which serve as a type of implicit memory. Interestingly, LeDoux (1996) noted that emotional responses are spontaneously activated and sometimes implicitly trigger emotional feelings so that humans are aware of what they felt. He suggested the presence of a route of unconscious information to climb up to the conscious state, by referring to the phrase "consciousness is only the tip of the mental iceberg" as originally posited by the neurologist Sigmund Freud.

Another link between two memory types can be found in the nucleus accumbens (NAc), which is part of the basal ganglia. The striatum and basal ganglia are brain regions for procedural memory to execute step-by-step procedures involved in various cognitive and motor skills, without the need for conscious control or attention.

The hippocampal contextual information goes up to the prefrontal cortex through the NAc. Implications of animal studies regarding this linkage are still controversial (Frank *et al.*, 2000; Wood *et al.*, 2000; Ferbinteanu and Shapiro, 2003; Johnson and Redish, 2007; Johnson *et al.*, 2007). However, neuroscientists have a consensus that the hippocampus and related regions carry out a combination of prospective and retrospective information coding designed for the purpose of thinking of remote places that might be visited in the near future and expecting to receive an object according to the past memory. The neural mechanism of prospective and retrospective coding was

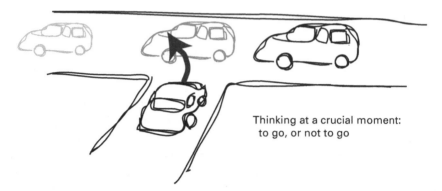

Thinking at a crucial moment:
to go, or not to go

Figure 12.2   A situation regarding driving. A driver is required to decide whether to go or not to go at a single moment. Sensory updates are necessary for timing estimation of oncoming cars and, moreover, a moment of decision making to go depends on individual abilities acquired through past training experiences and personal qualifications for driving. This indicates the importance of the representation of "time" in mental models for contextual decision making and situated cognition.

implemented in the robotic device by Fleischer *et al.* (2007) to investigate the functional coupling between the neural anatomy and internal dynamics.

The question in the present chapter is schematically illustrated in Figure 12.2. In daily life, we rely on implicit memory in the form of the procedural memory; it allows us to remember how to drive a car without needing to think about it consciously. We can simultaneously think of remote places and times; it allows us to imagine the perfect restaurant according to one's appetite and how to get there from here. The conscious awareness does not always disturb ongoing and automated actions such as skills for driving a car, whereas it may interrupt fine-tuned actions in progress at a necessary moment for making a decision. If such processes can conventionally be called top-down processes of the brain, how does the conscious awareness access the subconscious complex, which is supported by a mixture of implicit memory circuits? According to LeDoux (1996), there is a bottom-up process of being aware of unconscious emotions. I consider that top-down and bottom-up brain processes occur, in parallel and occasionally, are for executing contextual decision making and for applying emotionally biased past evidence to the current situation. This hypothesis does not directly imply that the brain consists of conscious and unconscious memory systems in a binary manner, but highlights cooperative working processes between different memory systems to form a consistent intelligence – the personality and perhaps the core of subjective responsibility – which enables us to make a decision immediately even in a novel situation with some degree of confidence. I believe that neuroscientific facts can guide us to build an artificial system to test how these functions work together.

12.2.2   Making a frame at a moment, and the neural basis

Contextual decision making is a central issue in robotics and artificial intelligence research, known as the frame problem (McCarthy and Hayes, 1969). I refer to an anecdote by Dennett (1984) of the robot R2D2, in which the robot is tasked with getting a battery pack in a room where a bomb is located. The robot has to find the battery and leave the room before the explosion of the bomb. But unfortunately the robot was caught in the explosion, because it could not decide which actions should be done first. It thought through everything that could happen and accounted for relevant and irrelevant issues endlessly at rest. The set of "what if" predictions may be countable but conceptually infinite. Although we, human beings, are troubled over what we should do first in complicated situations, the human brain potentially has an ability to escape such situations by finding a solution that is good enough for now. Before thinking of whether or not its temporal solution is intelligent, I focus on the neural basis of making a frame and decision making:

1. to recollect information relevant to the purpose from internal representations and sensory inputs of the external world;
2. to configure a frame, or view, from that information; and
3. to centralize predictions arising in the configured frame and to provide an action that may interrupt ongoing involuntary movements.

Animal experimental studies have been devoted to the elucidation of how these functional roles are realized in the brain.

For explaining the first necessity, Eichenbaum and his colleagues (1999) proposed a memory space hypothesis in which the hippocampus recollects experienced episodes related to the current situation, and provides a temporal memory space to be topological and directional by linking remembered episodes (Eichenbaum, 2001, 2003). They argued that the memory space is not equivalent to a subspace of the environmental geometry representing the physical space in which the animal behaved. They emphasized that the theory is extensible to abilities of transitive inference and class inclusion. As Piaget originally noted (Piaget, 1928), transitive inference is a cognitive assessment to able to organize logical inferences among indirectly related items, and young children acquire this cognitive ability at a certain developmental stage. Dusek and Eichenbaum (1997) tested the hypothesis using a rodent olfactory discriminating task, and concluded that hippocampal information is organized in a form of memory space such that indirectly related items can be remembered by linking together the sequential structure in original episodes. The point of this hypothesis is that links from one item to another one are represented and embedded in a mental metric space, and this property is significant in considering principles to provide "what if" predictions.

On the second necessity, that is, the ability to make a frame, the cognitive map theory is a first step to consider what information structure is formed in the hippocampus, in cases of spatial recognition tasks. The well-known evidence is that, in a rodent exploration task, hippocampal neurons selectively fire when the animal is located in a portion of the environment. The neural activity of these *place cells*, and the corresponding firing field, which is called a *place field*, covers the whole environment of the rat. This experimental evidence was originally discovered by O'Keefe and Dostrovsky (1971) and summarized by O'Keefe and Nadel (1978) as the cognitive map theory. This implies that the hippocampal neuron does not respond to specific sensory stimuli but the population activity represents the current location of the animal in the environment by using a map-like representation. The cognitive map is theoretically explained by the presence of a neural network with neighboring connections of place cells, so that neighboring neurons in the sense of place fields are tightly connected symmetrically (Muller et al., 1991, 1996) to represent a distance without directional information from a place to other places. Thus, the hippocampal recurrent network represents a map in the form of a nondirected graph, or a chart, which consists of nodes and links, and then this network is successfully extended to contain multiple maps that correspond to different environments. This multiplicity and robustness of the spatial representation is clearly demonstrated in experiments (Barnes, 1997; Fyhn et al., 2007), in computational models (Samsonovich and McNaughton, 1997; Káli and Dayan, 2000; Conklin and Eliasmith, 2005), and in the mathematical concept of continuous attractor networks (Amari, 1977; Amit and Tsodyks, 1992; Tsodyks, 1999; Stringer et al, 2004; Wu and Amari, 2005). The issue of how the map representation is utilized as a tool for finding a path to the goal location is discussed in various computational models. Typical models are: a layered neural network with a nondirected map in the first layer and with the following layer representing the allocentric orientation to the goal such as toward the north, south, west, and east (Burgess et al., 1994; 1997), and recurrent neural networks that are capable of encoding both the chart and route by using neighboring connections between neurons with the connection strengths being weakly asymmetric to provide a bias toward the goal orientation (Blum and Abbott, 1996; Redish and Touretzky, 1998; Trullier and Meyer, 2000). The experimental data and models of the neural mechanism have been influential for various applications. In robotic and engineering fields, realistic map-based models have been investigated and developed for giving solutions of simultaneous localization and mapping (SLAM) problems (see also Chapter 5 by Wyeth et al.). By contrast, drawing back to the relevance of the first necessity, the cognitive map theory incorporates an a priori assumption of the map-based representation in the hippocampus, and the question arises of how the map formation is extended to a broad cognitive view to trigger "what if" predictions based on perceptual and behavioral experiences (Eichenbaum, 1999). Some neuroscientists have proposed that the map integrates experienced episodes accompanied with emotional and contextual assessments (Kobayashi et al., 2003; Wagatsuma and Yamaguchi, 2004; Smith and Mizumori, 2006). The question of whether the hippocampus dominantly represents maps or sequences arises with regard to the problem of whether the connectivity is symmetric (distance) or asymmetric (sequence) between two nodes (place cells), as illustrated Figure 12.3. The answer solving this conflict cannot be found only in the structure of connections in the network.

On the third necessity, the centralization of contextual predictions remains an open question. In the neuroscience view, this function is considered to be based on two principal neural mechanisms: the first is a hippocampal function of "guess" or "anticipation" of what will happen next by remembering past experiences, as Eichenbaum (1999) suggested, and the second is a cross-regional hypothesis. The hypothesis focuses on an integration of two resources: the preconfigured frame arising from procedural

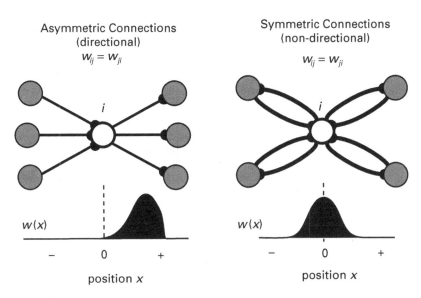

Figure 12.3 Conventional synaptic structures to represent sequence and map. (Left) Typical asymmetric connections provide a chain reaction from left to right. Synaptic weights are distributed with respect to the place field position, and the peak is not located in the original position, the center, but is shifted forward, which provides a propagative activity to retrieve sequential events. (Right) Symmetric connections represent distance so that weight values are increased in inverse proportion to the distance between place cells. This forms a single-peaked activity packet the same as the weight distribution shape, which represents the current location in the environment as a spot on the map.

memory in the striatum, basal ganglia, and other motor-related areas, and the contextual frame as temporal coding of past, present, and possible future, as mentioned above. Grace and his colleagues (Newman and Grace, 1999; Floresco and Grace, 2003; Goto and Grace, 2005) hypothesized that the prefrontal cortex (PFC) is the most likely candidate for the neural basis for the integrative function and experimentally demonstrated a gating action over PFC neural activity, either facilitating or inhibiting firing in the hippocampal–PFC pathway depending on the frequency and relative timing of the arrival of input. The PFC has been implicated in planning complex cognitive behaviors, decision making, and strategy change related to social behavior, known as executive function (Fuster, 2001, 2002). In the human brain, the PFC is thought to integrate thoughts and actions in accordance with internal goals, or purposes. In human society, executive function is important for differentiating among conflicting thoughts, determining good and bad, predicting future consequences of current activities, and predicting the outcomes in social settings, that is, social and contextual decision making. Interestingly, Newman and Grace (1999) explained that the prefrontal gating function is not only coming from the connectivity among relevant brain regions but also arising from a fine tuning of frequency controls of neural oscillations and binding across time, by showing an example of 40-Hz gamma synchronization of sensory cortices and thalamocortical loops. Various types of neural oscillations are observed in the brain depending on conditions and locations. Some researchers suggest functional roles of the gamma rhythm spreading over large cortical regions for visual perception (Rodriguez et al., 1999; Engel et al., 2001) and its link to conscious awareness (Crick and Koch, 2003), although the argument of whether the oscillation is an epiphenomenon or if it has functional roles is still controversial. However, recent findings have fueled a resurgence of interest in the functional roles of neural oscillations.

12.2.3   Functional roles of neural oscillations in the brain

In a series of electrophysiological studies, Buzsaki and his colleagues (2002; 2006; Mizuseki et al., 2009) have investigated neural oscillations in the hippocampus and discussed its possible functional roles. They focused on dynamical and spontaneous changes of hippocampal firing patterns that were strongly modulated by inhibitory oscillations. The experimental data suggest that the hippocampal activity represents not only "memory contents" by its firing rate but also changes its firing timing in a synchronized population, a so-called firing phase, which represents "relations" with other neurons. In recent experimental studies, Diba and Buzsaki (2008) showed that theta rhythm-related activities preserve the time lags between place cell pairs even when the environmental size is changed. This evidence supports the duality of rate- and phase-coding in their theoretical model. Another plausible contribution of neural oscillations to cognitive assessments was hypothesized by Lisman and his colleagues in the form of the theta–gamma oscillation coupling (Lisman and and Idiart, 1995; Jensen and Lisman, 1996). Psychophysical measurements indicate that human subjects can store approximately seven short-term memories. Their computational model demonstrated that the hippocampal network stores multiple memory contents in each oscillation cycle of the low-frequency theta, and each memory is stored in a high-frequency gamma subcycle of the theta oscillation, and then the number of subcycles restricted to enter in a single theta cycle is 7 ± 2. This speculation had been contested but was recently revisited in experiments measuring ones over a broad range of cortical interactions (Tort et al., 2009; Palva et al., 2010; Shirvalkar et al., 2010).

The neural oscillator can be described in a simple mathematical form by the differential equations, well known as the Kuramoto model (Kuramoto, 1984),

$$\frac{d\phi_i}{dt} = \omega_i + K' \sum_{j=1}^{N} \sin(\phi_j - \phi_i) \tag{12.1}$$

where ϕ_i and ω_i are the phase and the natural frequency of each oscillator, $K' = K/N$ is the coupling constant, and N is the number of oscillators. Through a weak coupling among oscillator units, the units interact and modulate the timing of their activities to be synchronously activated after just a few oscillation cycles (Figure 12.4).

In considering the use of the coupling oscillators for neural units, the equation should include effects of individual synaptic connections, natural properties of the excitability, which is a transient shift from resting state to firing state according to input, and the spontaneous oscillation mode. In an advanced model of the nonlinear oscillator

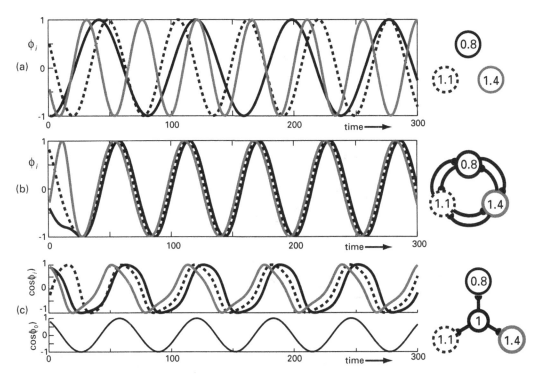

Figure 12.4 Characteristics of oscillator synchronizations in computer simulation. (a) Time evolution of three oscillator units without connections. Units have different native frequencies (numbers in circles), and then oscillate independently. Equation (12.1) is used and $K = 0$. (b) A synchronized pattern due to coupling connections. Although initial values are different, activities are going to be synchronized together within a few cycles. Equation (12.1) is used and $K > 0$. (c) By using Equation (12.2) with a pacemaker unit (in the center), three units oscillate synchronously and phase differences among units are robustly stabilized. The sequential order of oscillations (gray, dotted, and solid) is aligned with respect to values of native frequencies. This shows that coupling oscillators simply reconstruct phase differences with the pacemaker's oscillation, which is observed in the hippocampal firing patterns known as phase coding (Yamaguchi, 2003; Wagatsuma and Yamaguchi, 2004).

description (Yamaguchi, 2003; Wagatsuma and Yamaguchi, 2004), these necessary factors are included and the bifurcation mechanism changes the internal mode between the excitability and the spontaneous oscillation. The equation can be described as

$$\frac{d\phi_i}{dt} = \omega_i + \{\beta - I_i(t) - \cos(\phi_0)\}\sin(\phi_i). \tag{12.2}$$

The positive/negative terms in the braces represent the hyperpolarizing/depolarizing currents. The first term, β, is the stabilization parameter to control either excitable or oscillation modes. In the following terms, I_i is the external input of each unit, and ϕ_0 is the pacemaker unit, which is described as $d\phi_0/dt = \omega_0$ and represents a stable oscillation of the local field potential in the case of the hippocampal model (Yamaguchi,

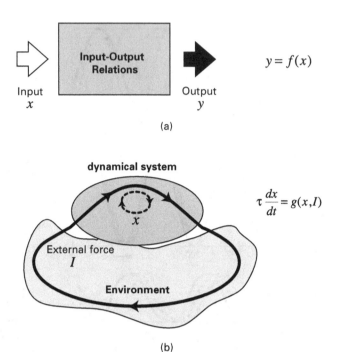

$$y = f(x)$$

(a)

$$\tau\frac{dx}{dt} = g(x,I)$$

(b)

Figure 12.5   Difference in formulation of biological systems. (a) Mathematical description by input–output relations, or stimulus–response paradigm, which can be seen in behaviorism. (b) A form of the dynamical system, which assumes an external force I from the environment but the internal variables have their own dynamics of temporal evolution, with time constant τ. The external force acts as a modulator of the internal dynamics. This description has higher compatibility with the embodiment paradigm than the previous one.

2003; Wagatsuma and Yamaguchi, 2004), that is, theta rhythm. The $\cos(\phi)$ represents the membrane potential and is used as an indicator of the firing-phase instead of ϕ in Equation (12.1), and then effects of individual synaptic connections can be considered if the factor $K\sum_j f(\cos(\phi_j))$ is set in braces, where f is defined as a sigmoid function. The important point of this kind of mathematical description is that biological mechanisms can be described in the form of a spontaneous time evolution, as opposed to the form of input–output functions (Figure 12.5). By formulating a biological autonomy, the spontaneous oscillations based on nonlinear dynamics give us a way to rebuild an artificial system that enables the system to develop internally not only from inputs but also from internal temporal contexts.

Further investigation of the functional roles of neural oscillators suggests that brain oscillations are a timing mechanism for controlling the serial processing of short-term memories (Lisman and and Idiart, 1995; Jensen and Lisman, 1996, 2000; Lisman, 2005; Lisman and Redish, 2009) and a coordinating mechanism for communicating different functional components (Newman and Grace, 1999; Rodriguez et al., 1999; Crick and Koch, 2003; Floresco and Grace, 2003), and a compression mechanism for transforming behavioral sequences into synaptic timescales (August and Levy, 1996;

Skaggs *et al*, 1996; Yamaguchi, 2003; Wagatsuma and Yamaguchi, 2004, 2007; Dragoi and Buzsaki, 2006). In these analytic approaches, there are no simple answers in dealing with the neural mechanisms and in evaluating them as the part of the whole brain system interacting with the environment. This brings us, in a synthetic view, to the construction of testable platforms in real-time and in real-world conditions, trying to go beyond the limitations of the analytic approach. For this purpose, we can take a synthetic approach to building brain-based robots, devices and embedded platforms, as seen in the next section.

12.3   How we reconstruct the brain synthetically – robotic methodology

12.3.1   The brain is a dynamical and multitiered system

Robotic approaches have been utilized in various ways to investigate how biological organisms survive in dynamic environments. Making a real robot helps us to demonstrate how a target mechanism works in the real world. Brooks (1990) was influential for robotic and artificial intelligence researchers who aspire to break through the limitations of traditional symbolic AI studies. Brooks (Brooks and Connell, 1986; Brooks, 1986, 1990) described the importance of embodiment and sensory–motor interactions with the environment, suggesting that real-world interactions can replace symbolic representations even in higher cognitive functions such as planning and reasoning. The idea is called the subsumption architecture, which can be related to the hierarchy and modularity found in biological systems. In the subsumption architecture, an intelligent machine that performs well in physical environments can be built in the form of parallel blocks of input–output functions rather than cascading connections of required functions. The subsumption architecture firstly assumes that the agent can sense the external information from the environment at any moment, and secondly explains that a seemingly complex behavior can be decomposed into simple functions and the set of functions can be rebuilt in a hierarchical structure. Sloman (2009) doubted the ability of the architecture and pointed to two difficulties: one is whether symbolic representations are dispensable in human-like intelligence that may need language operations, and the other is whether the assumption that the agent can simply sense everything at any time is valid when the agent is thinking of remote places and possibilities. I would like here to focus on the latter point, and illustrate by the viewpoint of the nested structure of timescales how multiple time properties can be embedded in the inclusion of these functional modules. Indeed, biological systems form a nested structure physically: for instance, the body includes organs that include cells that include various proteins. However the hierarchy, or ecological system, is not always ideal. Components in individual levels organize into independent autonomies, so that the whole system is formed as a consequence of symbiosis. An example of a healthy symbiosis is the case of mitochondrial energy production for the host cell. In contrast, a symbiosis that doesn't work is the case of virus reproductions that destroy its host cell. The difference in the two cases is the speed of the lower level's reproduction, which exceeds the cycle

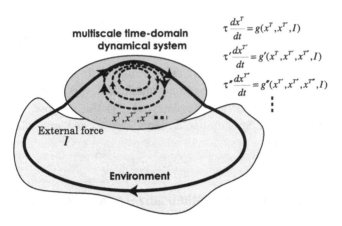

$$\tau \frac{dx^T}{dt} = g(x^T, x^{T'}, I)$$

$$\tau' \frac{dx^{T'}}{dt} = g'(x^T, x^{T'}, x^{T''}, I)$$

$$\tau'' \frac{dx^{T''}}{dt} = g''(x^{T'}, x^{T''}, x^{T'''}, I)$$

Figure 12.6   A form of the dynamical system with multiple timescales.

of the upper level's activity. This example implies that the inclusion of physical sizes cannot simply determine the functional inclusion and relationship between the upper and lower layers. In the viewpoint of biological autonomy, there are levels that are maintained for a certain period and rehearse the internal productions with proper timing. The concept of the functional blocks that Brooks (1990) proposed is insightful for engineering design, and forces one to consider what the block is composed of, which and when blocks interact together, and what mechanisms are necessary to organize blocks recursively.

The brain is a dynamical and multitiered system with multiple timescales (Figure 12.6). In the case of neuromorphological structure and information dynamics, the synthetic approach deals with capabilities necessary to form higher cognitive functions, or human-like intelligence, by considering differences among timescales embedded in various levels of living organisms.

12.3.2   Online robotic platform – brain-oscillation-based dynamics

Neurologists analytically investigate whether the brain is healthy or impaired due to neurological disorders, and identify diseased parts as a cause of the disorder. Neuroscientists probe different areas of the brain to determine which brain regions are necessary for a specific function. By contrast, in synthetic approaches that I emphasize here, neurobiologically inspired robots can constructively exhibit how the brain works through its interaction with the body, the environment, and other agents in real world situations. These efforts not only provide the foundation for the development of intelligent machines, but also contribute to our understanding of how the nervous system gives rise to complex behavior, and to our understanding of the brain and mind. These efforts have been continued by researchers who were aware of the importance of the synthetic style of brain research, known as brain-based robots or devices (Krichmar *et al.*, 2005; Krichmar and Edelman, 2006; Edelman, 2007), and are extended to more complex systems, such as contextual modulation of action selections (Cox and

Krichmar, 2009). The brain-based devices now widely encompass brain functions of perception, operant conditioning, episodic and spatial memory, and motor control through the reconstruction of brain regions, such as the visual cortex, the dopaminergic reward system (involving the basal ganglia), the hippocampus, and cerebellum. This rich robotic system could be a means toward understanding human consciousness (see also Chapter 13 by Fleischer *et al.*).

In considering the biological hierarchy through the use of brain-based devices, embodied neural modeling studies have demonstrated the advantage of having multiple timescales in the memory system (Krichmar *et al.*, 2005; Krichmar and Edelman, 2006; Edelman, 2007; Verschure *et al.*, 2003). Investigating the influences of perception on behavioral controls in mobile robots, Verschure proposed an internal model that forms a three-layer structure, which consisted of the reflective layer with the external environment via sensors (infrared sensors for obstacles and CCD camera for detecting external images) and effectors (two wheels in the Khepera robot) at the bottom, the adaptive layer in the middle, and the behavioral learning system with two timescales (the short-term and the long-term memory) at the top that supervised the adaptive layer. They found that the adaptive layer improved the performance of the robot through a learning-dependent avoidance of collisions, due to modulation from the memory system having information that had been accumulated over past behavioral experiences. This can be considered as a biologically inspired robotic, an extension to the Brooks's subsumption architecture through the inclusion of multiple timescales.

More effective advantages of biological adaptability can be seen in conditions that require physical interactions with the dynamic environment. The generation of locomotive leg movements requires detection of the ground (i.e., its shape, gradient, texture) and to modify the pattern of the movements accordingly. The central pattern generator (CPG) (Golubitsky *et al.*, 1999) embedded in the spinal cord generates a variety of adaptive locomotion patterns of the legs, even in insects with multiple legs such as centipedes, and it also works well if some legs are injured by re-coordinating movements of the remaining legs. Theoretically, the CPG is simply described by coupling oscillators such as described in Equations (12.1) and (12.2). The neural oscillators can synchronize differently depending on internal (the purpose of the behavior) and external conditions (the ground condition), and the system is applicable to the case of human locomotion by two legs with multiple joints for obstacle avoidance as is demonstrated by Taga (1998, 2006) in the neuromusculoskeletal system. In a real robot experiment, Ijspeert *et al.* (2007) showed an interesting adaptive control of the CPG circuit. They hypothesized that salamanders crawled on land not because of a specific circuit for land movement, but because the CPG circuit that exists for swimming in nature could adapt the locomotive pattern when coming on shore, such that the salamander could smoothly transition its locomotion pattern due to the change in external conditions from the water to the ground. They implemented the CPG system into a salamander robot and demonstrated the capability of natural transitions from swimming in S-shaped patterns to a walking locomotion with four legs. This research offers a way to deal with the controversial problem in evolutionary nature of how the first land animals developed their ability to walk (Pennisi, 2007), and demonstrates the potential of biologically inspired robots. Interestingly, an important difference of their CPG model from traditional CPG models is the increasing property of the native frequency of CPG oscillators. The increasing of the potential frequencies enhances the transition to a different synchronous mode.

According to Yuste *et al.* (2005), spinal cord and brainstem CPG circuits share profound similarities with neocortical circuits. The CPG produces spontaneous rhythmic output even in the absence of sensory inputs, and neocortical circuits similarly have rich spontaneous dynamics to generate a rhythmic activity, which is consistent with properties of CPG mechanisms. They suggest that cortical circuits are plastic types of CPG, which can be called "learning CPG." The original CPG circuit is embedded along the spinal cord physically, while the CPG-like cortical circuit reorganizes their network structure according to the synaptic plasticity in the range of individual brain regions, providing various types of neural synchrony with flexible change depending on the extraregional condition or inputs. In traditional computational neuroscience, the cortical circuit is investigated as an off-line circuit apart from the external change in the environment due to the assumption that the circuit is the end of the line in the hierarchy of brain processes, going from sensation to perception and on to higher cognition. This notion of CPG-like adaptability in the cortical circuit, in contrast, highlights functional roles of cortical circuits as the system links with the external environment. Cortical neural synchrony can couple perception and action in the dynamic environment, and transfer the peripheral information to the cortex (Baker, 2007).

This argument brings us to consider how to build an online hierarchical system. Oscillator descriptions of neural circuits represent phenomenological behaviors in the population activity, not individual spikes. However, the oscillator description provides us with a good tool to investigate the biophysical mechanisms which may cover the hierarchical biological autonomy and the inclusion of multiple timescales, as schematically illustrated in Figure 12.6. Possible functional roles of the hippocampal neural oscillation were discussed in Section 12.2.3, according to findings by Buzsaki and his colleagues (2002, 2006; Mizuseki *et al.*, 2009). It raises the question of how those functional properties can be tested in the real environment artificially, that is by using robotic methodology. The notion of how similar are the biophysical mechanics of the hippocampal phase coding to the CPG circuit is discussed in the paper by Wagatsuma and Yamaguchi (2007), suggesting the plausibility of the implementation of the phase coding scheme into a real system with the body and the environmental interactions. The current version of this online robotic platform that tests brain-oscillation-based dynamics is rather simple (Figure 12.7; the color version is in Supplementary Video 12.1). Mobile robots behave in an experimental setup which allows experimenters to change obstacles and visual cues on the wall and floor according to experimental protocols. By using a ceiling camera, the robot's behaviors and actions are totally monitored, and the video is recorded in a remote computer with time stamps. The neural network simulator is running on another specialized computer to perform real-time calculations of a set of differential equations to simulate the brain. Since the robotic body is remotely connected to the computer, the numerical solution of the equations

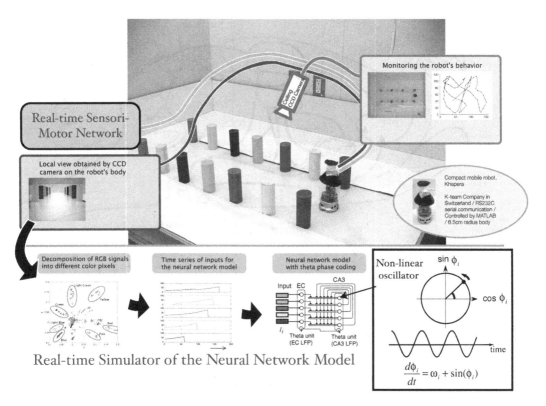

Figure 12.7 Overview of the online robotic platform.

is evaluated each time step (at machine time) to access sensors and actuators, including the CCD camera image, infrared distance sensors, movable wheels and gripping hands. Therefore, in the viewpoint of the observation of "internal time" in the brain, this is a hybrid simulation system because it inevitably involves sensing durations and actuator feedback speed in hardware, coding, and decoding in wire/wireless communication, and time for numerical simulation in software. Because the system design is an open system, it forces us to relinquish the accurate numerical solution for obtaining a steady-state or equilibrium at some time point, but instead this provides practical numerical solutions to test various computational models in real-time conditions and actual methods to concurrently observe time evolutions of the robot's behaviors and the internal states continuously. This approach brings benefits not only for the researcher who can interactively observe and improve the developmental process of the nervous system, but also for the incremental design of the experimental platform itself. If neural network models are implemented into the system mathematically at first, which means numerical solutions in software, well-investigated components can be replaced with the equivalent hardware circuit. This allows us to flexibly change system components to test various hypotheses and to upgrade the system incrementally. In the present system, the kernel of the simulator is running on the MATAB environment with the JAVA-based RS-232C serial communication interface. The

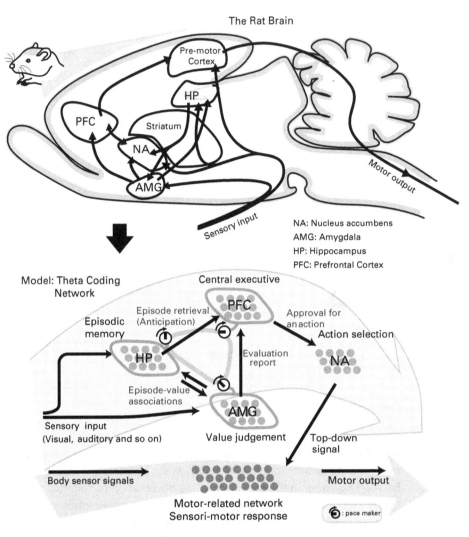

Figure 12.8   Schematic illustration of the rat brain and the CPG-like phenomenological model based on the phase coding scheme with two layers.

application of this framework for large-scale network models and developing open-sourced projects is still under development.

A typical result of this approach can be found in the robotic experiment with the theta phase coding model that consists of two autonomous layers (Wagatsuma and Yamaguchi, 2008; Wagatsuma, 2009). The robotic experiment focused on the difference in timescales between the upper and lower layers of a network model. As is schematically illustrated in Figure 12.8, the contextual decision-making process of the brain is considered to be supported by two information flows, which was discussed in Section 12.2.1 (see Figure 12.2). One is motor-related systems for accurate adaptive control and primary motor learning which is regarded as a cerebellar function, and was precisely implemented into a robot and investigated by McKinstry *et al.* (2006), and the other is for acquisition of procedural memory in a model of basal ganglia function which was tested in a robotic model (Prescott *et al.*, 2006; see also Chapter 3 by Mitchinson *et al.*).

The CPG-like phenomenological model based on the phase coding scheme is assumed to be a reflective sensorimotor network, and is regarded as the lower layer. This exhibits sensorimotor reflections controlled by a spiking-type neural network with fixed synaptic connections that is preconfigured to provide innate behaviors for exploring the environment and avoiding wall and obstacle collisions (see Supplementary Videos 12.2–12.4). In contrast, the upper layer is assumed to be a set of CPG-like oscillator networks with modifiable synaptic connections within individual networks and across different networks. It is noted that motor coordination skills and planning are gradually developed over a slow timescale. In contrast, the upper layer quickly changes its behavior depending on the current situation through strongly biased emotional one-shot learning at each experience. The interaction between the higher layer (sensitive for individual cases and differences) and the lower layer (trust in the averaged tendency and statistics) of this model is the point of this study and the robotic model is a tool to investigate what happens in the real-time coordination.

The upper layer is called the theta phase coding architecture, which consists of three brain regions: the hippocampus (HP) for memory encoding and retrieval of behavioral sequences, the amygdala (AMG) for emotional judgments on memorized episodes, and the prefrontal cortex (PFC) for decision making to send the top-down signal to interrupt ongoing behaviors and guide the behavior to a specific direction if the HP and AMG are coincidentally activated. Each network is composed of CPG-like oscillators with a pacemaker. In a cross maze task, during the spontaneous phase, the upper layer works for encoding of behavioral sequences in HP–HP connections and for attachment of emotional feeling in HP–AMG connections at the end of the arms of the maze (Figure 12.9), by finding the robot's favorite tag at the terminal. The phase coding

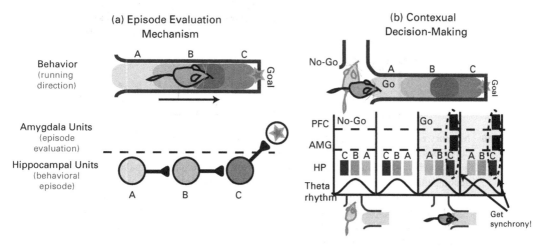

Figure 12.9   Phase coding mechanism in contextual decision making. (See Figure 12.8 for abbreviations.)

scheme has the capability of one-time learning, which is consistent with results of similar models (Lisman, 2005). In other words, the repetition of sequential firing patterns every theta cycle enhances sustainable sequential connections in the HP even if the robot visited the arm only once. During the spontaneous phase, the robot explores all over the environment and then the HP network has multiple episodic memories for every arm with an emotional feeling in AMG. After the spontaneous phase, the upper layer changes the internal mode to the retrieval phase. When the robot is located in the center of the maze, the robot hesitates to enter into nonfavorite arms, but enters the arm where the robot found the favorite tag. In the simultaneous monitoring of activity patterns in all networks, the HP network reacts on facing every arm by remembering individual behavioral episodes, while the AMG network only responds to the target arm. The synchronous activation of HP and AMG triggers the PFC activity to cause the robot to select the target arm (Figure 12.10). According to experimental evidence, a primary function of the amygdala is the emotional learning known as fear conditioning, which exhibits immediate responses in the presence of conditioned cues to either favorites or unfavorites. This result suggests that the hippocampal episodic memory bridges between unrelated cues at hand and a conditional cue in the remote place by

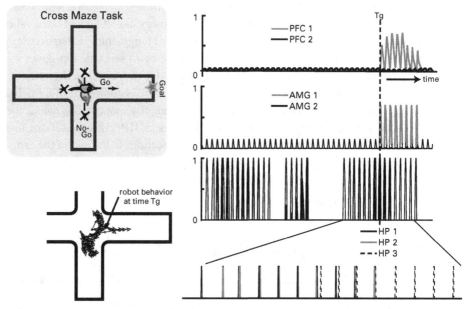

Figure 12.10   Memory retrievals in entrances of two arms in the cross maze as the reconstruction of a conscious recollection process. Firstly the robot is oriented to the bottom direction but the go-signal is not generated in the prefrontal cortex because hippocampal activities are not accompanied by amygdala activations (beginning in the right panel). Next, when the robot turns to the right arm, hippocampal activities are followed by the amygdala activities (AMG 1,2). By receiving synchronous signals from two regions, the prefrontal cortex fires and sends the go-signal. The trajectory (black and gray lines in the bottom left) is replotted here from the real observation (ceiling camera) of the robot. (Unpublished data from experiments of Wagatsuma and Yamaguchi, 2008.)

remembering past episodes. It can be applied to decision making at the moment if reliable evidence is not currently available due to lack of experience.

Significant points of this model in the neuroscientific viewpoint are (1) phase coding is valid for discriminations of the context such as running directions by using the sequential order of firing patterns; (2) information transfer between different networks relying on pacemakers of individual networks works well even if synaptic connections drastically change and firing patterns tend to be unstable; (3) the top-down signal from the upper to the lower may provide an interruption and change to the intentional action when the speed of sensorimotor reactions is more than twice the period of the theta cycle in the upper layer. The first point suggests that phase coding is preferable for representing information in uncertain, unstable, and dynamic environments. Rate coding schemes, as well investigated in traditional neural network theories, are preferable to extract the statistical structure from the environment with the assumption that the world is invariant in some measure. The second point is not so surprising in engineering fields because the CPU board has a clock cycle for update of internal calculations and for communicating with other peripheral systems. Unlike a CPU clock, the biological pacemaking clock is flexible (Jones and Wilson, 2005a, 2005b). In our experiments, coherence increased between the hippocampal theta rhythm and PFC spike timings at the moment when the robot decided to traverse the maze arm depending on the past context. The third point needs further investigation on how the phenomenon is biologically plausible. But in the mathematical viewpoint of nonlinear dynamics the entrainment of fast oscillators (or fast spikes) by a slow oscillator is plausible.

In building a hierarchical structure of biological autonomies, the oscillator model description allows us to investigate further hypotheses. Interestingly, this point may relate to the notion by Libet (Libet et al., 1983; Libet, 2004) on time consciousness in humans. The controversial interpretation of his experiments is that the conscious awareness comes after the presence of neural activities that determine actions, so-called postdiction of consciousness, which implies that the human consciousness cannot deny ongoing actions because those were already started. The neural entity of the consciousness is beyond the scope of this chapter; readers who are interested in the neural basis should read Chapter 13 by Fleischer et al. and readers who are interested in how the *self* is contracted hierarchically in an internal representation should read Chapter 11 by Asada. So far, problems such as whether consciousness is predictive or postdictive are difficult to evaluate in current robotic studies, and we need efforts to develop brain-based and neuromorphological robots to include brain and mind problems in the range of scientific problems.

12.4   Summary and perspectives

This chapter describes the potential of robotic methodology to investigate how the brain works in a decision-making process that must be flexible, adaptive, and vital for dynamic changes in the environment. Situated cognition posits that cognition cannot be separated from the surrounding social, cultural, and physical contexts. Such capability of a codetermination process between the agent (subject) and the context seems to exceed artificial systems. As Sloman (2009) suggested, the theory of affordances by Gibson (1979) is a key to understanding how the codetermination occurs. It should be extended in a testable way which allows us to investigate simultaneous and hierarchical internal processes in the living organism, suggesting the existence of multiple levels of affordances. However, this chapter argues the viewpoint that life is completely passive with respect to environmental forces so that the person is not overwhelmed by the surrounding circumstances. This gives a false impression that life can be reconstructed as a simple learning machine or blank slate (Pinker, 2002). Instead of adhering to this viewpoint, this chapter attempts to shed light on the activeness and subjectivity of living things, which emerge from the multiplicity and hierarchy of biological autonomy that are embedded into a single entity (body). The coexistence of different and independent components, regarded as organizations in a society or members of a team, needs the system's identity and purpose of existence because its fate is that all the components live together and die together. Balancing and mediating among different directions and powers (sometimes called political powers) inside the system provides a consistency of the system's purpose as well as survival capability through conflicts. Considering such cooperative and contradictive kinetics and dynamics may afford a clue to the question of why the subjectivity of animals emerges from the interaction between the brain, the body, and the environment. Brain-based and neuromorphological robots do not aim to replicate the detailed structure of their physical forms, but instead offer a method for understanding the mysteries of the brain, mind, and matter; such problems as why we have free will and how we can consciously think about what we are. In this sense, embedding the complexity of the brain into a single body, that is, the robotic methodology, is a useful tool for scientific investigations on how different and autonomous components in the brain cooperate together so as to be the subjective actor against others and the external world.

As is described in the above sections, modeling of those processes using oscillator descriptions may benefit the building of the hierarchical system of biological autonomy, to exhibit the time evolution of how internal components cooperate, and to express transformations from external changes to internal representations. This suggests that neural synchronization is a candidate for coordinating different and independent functional components in the brain to provide a consistent outcome, as a synchronized pattern with systematic changes. The synchronized brain activities change in time but may appear from the outside to be very rationalized as a self-consistent time evolution that is determined by the *self*.

For further investigations to test the hypothesis, research efforts to simulate whole brain circuits are necessary so that the results enable engineers to simulate brain activities and provide deeper insights into how and why the brain works and fails. For the purpose of reverse engineering of the brain, multiple research projects are running to develop mathematical and computational models for testing and analyzing the complexities of nerve cell signals, circuit dynamics, pathways, feedback loops, firing rates, and their synchrony: for example, Allen Brain Atlas and BLAST in the United States, CARMEN in the United Kingdom, INCF Blue Gene in Sweden and INCF Japan Node (J-Node) in Japan. For expectations that such distributed models are going to be tested in a combined form, integrative tools have been developed in the research field of physiology and biotechnology that have an advantage over that of computational neuroscience. The physiological study inevitably has a motivation to treat the hierarchical composition at different levels such as cells, tissues, organs, and the body structure, and this motivation has enhanced technical efforts toward enriched code-sharing and global standardizations of model descriptions. The IUPS Physiome project supports the common description of models by using an XML-based description language called CellML, and then Physiome.jp upgrades their original codes to the current version, insilicoML (ISML). They also distribute a simulation platform that runs the shared code on multiple operating system environments for free as open-source software (www.physiome.jp/). Their simulation platform, called InsilicoSim, has the advantage of being able to automatically compile combined biophysical models to executable codes for multiple CPU environments, or cluster machines, by collaborating with researchers in parallel computing research fields. This kind of technological advancement will also support computational neuroscience, and give benefits in synthetic approaches of the brain-based and neuromorphological robots.

Finally, integrative computer simulations could have capabilities in many other applications. Such simulations may offer precise methods for testing potential biotechnological treatments for brain disorders, such as drugs, neural implants, and even neuroprosthetic devices for recovering damaged functions. However, to reach the ultimate goal of unraveling the mystery of the brain or to cure the brain physically, we need to know the natural providence and principles of life that are unlike those of machines, which are noted in the dynamic core hypothesis to generate consciousness (Seth *et al.*, 2006) and the functional immune core network to keep a hierarchical self-organization process in the biological open system (Kitano and Oda, 2006). The robotic body can help develop methods of real-time and real-environmental testing by implementing living structures and dynamics into the internal system as a single entity.

Acknowledgments

The author would like to thank Yoko Yamaguchi for valuable discussions on oscillatory neural activities and the functional roles, and long-term support on this robotic project; Yoshito Aota, Tatsuya Ikeda, Kentaro Someya for the experimental platform design and the establishment of the project; Yuichi Katano, Mayumi Haga, Yutaka Watanabe, Takayoshi Kogai for technical help; Taishin Nomura, Yoshiyuki Asai for supplying their cutting-edge resources to upgrade our robotic platform software; Jeff Krichmar for editing and comments on the manuscript. This work was supported in part by the programs of the Grant-in-Aid for challenging Exploratory Research (19650073) and the Grant-in-Aid for Scientific Research (B: 22300081) from the Japan Society for the Promotion of Science (JSPS).

References

Amari, S. (1977). Dynamics of pattern formation in lateral-inhibition type neural fields. *Biological Cybernetics*, **27**, 77–87.

Amit, D. J. and Tsodyks, M. V. (1992). Effective neurons and attractor neural networks in cortical environment. *Network: Computation in Neural Systems*, **3**, 121–137.

August, D. A. and Levy, W. B. (1996). A simple spike train decoder inspired by the sampling theorem. *Neural Computation*, **8**, 67–84.

Baker, S. N. (2007). Oscillatory interactions between sensorimotor cortex and the periphery. *Current Opinion in Neurobiology*, **17**, 649–655.

Barnes, C. A., Suster, M. S., Shen, J., and McNaughton, B. L. (1997). Multistability of cognitive maps in the hippocampus of old rats. *Nature*, **388**, 272–275.

Blum, K. I. and Abbott, L. F. (1996). A model of spatial map formation in the hippocampus of the rat. *Neural Computing*, **8**, 85–93.

Brooks, R. A. (1986). A robust layered control system for a mobile robot. *IEEE Journal of Robotics and Automation*, **2**, 14–23.

Brooks, R. A. (1990). Elephants don't play chess. *Robotics and Autonomous Systems*, **6**, 3–15.

Brooks, R. A. and J. Connell (1986). Asynchronous distributed control system for a mobile robot. *Proceedings of SPIE's Cambridge Symposium on Optical and Optoelectronic Engineering*, Cambridge, MA, pp. 77–84.

Brown, C., Laland, K., and Krause J. (2006). *Fish Cognition and Behavior*. Oxford, UK: Blackwell Publishing.

Burgess, N., Recce, M., and O'Keefe, J. (1994). A model of hippocampal function. *Neural Networks*, **7**, 1065–1081.

Burgess, N., Donnett, J. G., Jeffery, K. J., and O'Keefe, J. (1997). Robotic and neuronal simulation of the hippocampus and rat navigation. *Philosophical Transactions of the Royal Society of London B Biological Sciences*, **352**, 1535–1543.

Buzsaki, G. (2002). Theta oscillations in the hippocampus. *Neuron*, **33**, 325–340.

Buzsaki, G. (2006). *Rhythms of the Brain*. Oxford, UK: Oxford University Press.

Conklin, J. and Eliasmith, C. (2005). A controlled attractor network model of path integration in the rat. *Journal of Computational Neuroscience*, **18**, 183–203.

Cox, B. R. and Krichmar, J. L. (2009). Neuromodulation as a robot controller: a brain inspired design strategy for controlling autonomous robots. *IEEE Robotics & Automation Magazine*, **16**, 72–80.

Crick, F. and Koch, C. (2003). A framework for consciousness. *Nature Neuroscience*, **6**, 119–126.

Damasio, A. (1999). *The Feeling of What Happens: Body, Emotion and the Making of Consciousness*. London: Heinemann.

Dennett, D. (1984). Cognitive wheels: the frame problem of AI. In Boden, M. A. (ed.), *The Philosophy of Artificial Intelligence*. London: Oxford University Press, pp. 147–170.

Diba, K. and Buzsaki, G. (2008). Hippocampal network dynamics constrain the time lag between pyramidal cells across modified environments. *Journal of Neuroscience*, **28**, 13 448–13 456.

Dragoi, G. and Buzsaki, G. (2006). Temporal encoding of place sequences by hippocampal cell assemblies. *Neuron*, **50**, 145–157.

Dusek, J. A. and Eichenbaum, H. (1997). The hippocampus and memory for orderly stimulus relations. *Proceedings of the National Academy of Sciences of the USA*, **94**, 7109–7114.

Eccles, J. C. (1989). *Evolution of the Brain: Creation of the Self*. London: Routledge.

Edelman, G. M. (2007). Learning in and from brain-based devices. *Science*, **318**, 1103–1105.

Eichenbaum, H. (2001). The hippocampus and declarative memory: cognitive mechanisms and neural codes. *Behavior in Brain Research*, **127**, 199–207.

Eichenbaum, H. (2003). The hippocampus, episodic memory, declarative memory, spatial memory... where does it all come together? *International Congress Series*, **1250**, 235–244.

Eichenbaum, H., Dudchenko, P., Wood, E., Shapiro, M., and Tanila, H. (1999). The hippocampus, memory, and place cells: is it spatial memory or a memory space? *Neuron*, **23**, 209–226.

Engel, A. K., Fries, P., and Singer, W. (2001). Dynamic predictions: oscillations and synchrony in top-down processing. *Nature Reviews Neuroscience*, **2**, 704–716.

Ferbinteanu, J. and Shapiro, M. L. (2003). Prospective and retrospective memory coding in the hippocampus. *Neuron*, **40**, 1227–1239.

Fleischer, J. G., Gally, J. A., Edelman, G. M., and Krichmar, J. L. (2007). Retrospective and prospective responses arising in a modeled hippocampus during maze navigation by a brain-based device. *Proceedings of the National Academy of Sciences of the USA*, **104**, 3556–3561.

Floresco, S. B. and Grace, A. A. (2003). Gating of hippocampal-evoked activity in prefrontal cortical neurons by inputs from the mediodorsal thalamus and ventral tegmental area. *Journal of Neuroscience*, **23**, 3930–3943.

Frank, L.M., Brown, E.N., and Wilson, M.A. (2000) Trajectory encoding in the hippocampus and entorhinal cortex. *Neuron*, **27**, 169–178.

Fuster, J. (2001). The prefrontal cortex – an update: time is of the essence. *Neuron*, **30**, 319–333.

Fuster, J. (2002). Frontal lobe and cognitive development. *Journal of Neurocytology* **31**, 373–385.

Fyhn, M., Hafting, T., Treves, A., Moser, M. B., and Moser, E. I. (2007). Hippocampal remapping and grid realignment in entorhinal cortex. *Nature*, **446**, 190–194.

Gibson, J. J. (1979). *The Ecological Approach to Visual Perception*. Boston: Houghton Mifflin.

Golubitsky, M., Stewart, I., Buono, P. L., and Collins, J. J. (1999) Symmetry in locomotor central pattern generators and animal gaits. *Nature*, **401**, 693–695.

Goto, Y. and Grace, A. A. (2005). Dopaminergic modulation of limbic and cortical drive of nucleus accumbens in goal-directed behavior. *Nature Neuroscience*, **8**, 805–12.

Ijspeert, A. J., Crespi, A., Ryczko, D., and Cabelguen, J. M. (2007). From swimming to walking with a salamander robot driven by a spinal cord model. *Science*, **315**, 1416–1420.

Ikegami, T. and Suzuki, K. (2008). From a homeostatic to a homeodynamic self. *BioSystems*, **91**, 388–400.

Jensen, O. and Lisman, J. E. (1996). Theta/gamma networks with slow NMDA channels learn sequences and encode episodic memory: role of NMDA channels in recall. *Learning and Memory*, **3**, 264–78.

Jensen, O. and Lisman, J. E. (2000). Position reconstruction from an ensemble of hippocampal place cells: contribution of theta phase coding. *Journal of Neurophysiology*, **83**, 2602–2609.

Johnson, A. and Redish, A. D. (2007). Neural ensembles in CA3 transiently encode paths forward of the animal at a decision point. *Journal of Neuroscience*, **27**, 12176–12189.

Johnson, A., van der Meer, M. A., and Redish, A. D. (2007). Integrating hippocampus and striatum in decision-making. *Current Opinion in Neurobiology*, **17**, 692–697.

Jones, M. A. and Wilson, M. A. (2005a). Phase precession of medial prefrontal cortical activity relative to the hippocampal theta rhythm. *Hippocampus*, **15**, 867–873.

Jones, M. A. and Wilson, M. A. (2005b). Theta rhythms coordinate hippocampal-prefrontal interactions in a spatial memory task. *PLoS Biol*, **3**, e402.

Káli, S. and Dayan, P. (2000). The involvement of recurrent connections in area CA3 in establishing the properties of place fields: a model. *Journal of Neuroscience*, **20**, 7463–7477.

Kandel, E. R., Schwartz, J. H., and Jessell, T. M. (2000). *Principles of Neural Science*, 4th edn. London: McGraw-Hill, pp. 1227–1246.

Kitano, H. and Oda, K. (2006). Robustness trade-offs and host-microbial symbiosis in the immune system, *Molecular Systems Biology*, **2**, 2006.0022.

Kobayashi, T., Tran, A. H., Nishijo, H., Ono, T., and Matsumoto, G. (2003). Contribution of hippocampal place cell activity to learning and formation of goal-directed navigation in rats. *Neuroscience*, **117**, 1025–1035.

Krichmar, J. L. and Edelman, G. M. (2006). Principles underlying the construction of brain-based devices. In Kovacs, T. and Marshall, J. A. R. (eds.), *Adaptation in Artificial and Biological Systems*. Bristol, UK: Society for the Study of Artificial Intelligence and the Simulation of Behaviour, pp. 37–42.

Krichmar, J. L., Nitz, D. A., Gally, J.A., and Edelman, G. M. (2005). Characterizing functional hippocampal pathways in a brain-based device as it solves a spatial memory task. *Proceedings of the National Academy of Sciences of the USA*, **102**, 2111–2116.

Kuramoto, Y. (1984). *Chemical Oscillations, Waves, and Turbulence*. Berlin: Springer-Verlag.

LeDoux, J. (1996). *The Emotional Brain: The Mysterious Underpinnings of Emotional Life*. New York: Simon & Schuster.

Lee, A. K. and Wilson, M. A. (2002). Memory of sequential experience in the hippocampus during slow wave sleep. *Neuron*, **36**, 1183–1194.

Libet, B. (2004). *Mind Time: The Temporal Factor in Consciousness*. Cambridge, MA: Harvard University Press.

Libet, B., Gleason, C. A., Wright, E. W., and Pearl, D. K. (1983). Time of conscious intention to act in relation to onset of cerebral activity (readiness-potential): the unconscious initiation of a freely voluntary act. *Brain*, **106**(3), 623–642.

Lisman, J. (2005). The theta/gamma discrete phase code occuring during the hippocampal phase precession may be a more general brain coding scheme. *Hippocampus*, **15**, 913–922.

Lisman, J. and Redish, A. D. (2009). Prediction, sequences and the hippocampus. *Philosophical Transactions of the Royal Society of London B Biological Sciences*, **364**, 1193–201.

Lisman, J. E. and Idiart, M. A. (1995). Storage of 7 ± 2 short-term memories in oscillatory sub-cycles. *Science*, **267**, 1512–1515.

Llinás, R. R. and Roy, S. (2009). The "prediction imperative" as the basis for self-awareness. *Philosophical Transactions of the Royal Society of London B Biological Sciences*, **364**, 1301–1307.

McCarthy, J. and Hayes, P. J. (1969). Some philosophical problems from the standpoint of artificial intelligence, *Machine Intelligence*, **4**, 463–502.

McKinstry, J. L., Edelman, G. M. and Krichmar, J. L. (2006). A cerebellar model for predictive motor control tested in a brain-based device. *Proceedings of the National Academy of Sciences of the USA*, **103**, 3387–3392.

Mizuseki, K., Sirota, A., Pastalkova, E., and Buzsaki, G. (2009). Theta oscillations provide temporal windows for local circuit computation in the entorhinal-hippocampal loop. *Neuron*, **64**, 267–280.

Muller, R. U., Kubie, J. L., and Saypoff, R. (1991). The hippocampus as a cognitive graph (abridged version). *Hippocampus*, **1**, 243–246.

Muller, R. U., Stead, M., and Pach, J. (1996). The hippocampus as a cognitive graph. *Journal of General Physiology*, **107**, 663–694.

Newman, J. and Grace, A. A. (1999). Binding across time: the selective gating of frontal and hippocampal systems modulating working memory and attentional states. *Consciousness and Cognition*, **8**, 196–212.

O'Keefe, J. and Dostrovsky, J. (1971). The hippocampus as a spatial map: preliminary evidence from unit activity in the freely-moving rat. *Brain Research*, **34**, 171–175.

O'Keefe, J. and Nadel, L. (1978). *The Hippocampus as a Cognitive Map*. New York: Clarendon.

Palva, J. M., Monto, S., Kulashekhar, S., and Palva, S. (2010). Neuronal synchrony reveals working memory networks and predicts individual memory capacity. *Proceedings of the National Academy of Sciences of the USA*, **107**, 7580–7585.

Pennisi, E. (2007). Evolution: robot suggests how the first land animals got walking. *Science*, **315**, 1352–1353.

Piaget, J. (1928). *Judgement and Reasoning in the Child*. New York: Harcourt, Brace and World.

Pinker, S. (2002). *The Blank Slate: The Modern Denial of Human Nature*. New York: Viking Penguin.

Prescott, T. J., Montes González, F. M., Gurney, K., Humphries, M. D., and Redgrave, P. (2006). A robot model of the basal ganglia: behavior and intrinsic processing. *Neural Networks*, **19**, 31–61.

Redish, A. D. and Touretzky, D. S. (1998). The role of the hippocampus in solving the Morris water maze. *Neural Computation*, **10**, 73–111.

Rodriguez, E., George, N., Lachaux, J. P., *et al.* (1999). Perception's shadow: long-distance synchronization of human brain activity. *Nature*, **397**, 430–433.

Samsonovich, A. and McNaughton, B. L. (1997). Path integration and cognitive mapping in a continuous attractor neural network model. *Journal of Neuroscience*, **17**, 5900–5920.

Seth, A. K., Izhikevich, E., Reeke, G. N., and Edelman, G. M. (2006). Theories and measures of consciousness: an extended framework. *Proceedings of the National Academy of Sciences of the USA*, **103**, 10 799–10 804.

Shirvalkar, P. R., Rapp, P. R., and Shapiro, M. L. (2010). Bidirectional changes to hippocampal theta-gamma comodulation predict memory for recent spatial episodes. *Proceedings of the National Academy of Sciences of the USA*, **107**, 7054–7059.

Skaggs, W. E., McNaughton, B. L., Wilson, M. A., and Barnes, C. A. (1996). Theta phase precession in hippocampal neuronal populations and the compression of temporal sequences. *Hippocampus*, **6**, 149–172.

Sloman, A. (2009). Some requirements for human-like robots: why the recent over-emphasis on embodiment has held up progress. In Sendhoff, B., Koerner, E., Sporns, O. Ritter, H., and Doya, K. (eds.), *Creating Brain-like Intelligence*, LNAI 5436. Berlin: Springer-Verlag, pp. 248–277.

Smith, D. M. and Mizumori, S. J. Y. (2006). Hippocampal place cells, context and episodic memory. *Hippocampus*, **16**, 716–729.

Squire, L. R. (1987). *Memory and Brain*. New York: Oxford University Press.

Stringer, S. M., Rolls, E. T., and Trappenberg, T. P. (2004). Self-organising continuous attractor networks with multiple activity packets, and the representation of space. *Neural Networks*, **17**, 5–27.

Taga, G. (1998). A model of the neuro-musculo-skeletal-system for anticipatory adjustment of human locomotion during obstacle avoidance. *Biological Cybernetics*, **78**, 9–17.

Taga, G. (2006). Nonlinear dynamics of human locomotion: from real-time adaptation to development. In Kimura, H., Tsuchiya, K., Ishiguro, A., and Witte, H. (eds.), *Adaptive Motion of Animals and Machines*. Tokyo: Springer, pp. 189–204.

Tort, A. B. L., Komorowski, R. W., Manns, J. R., Kopell, N. J., and Eichenbaum, H. (2009). Theta-gamma coupling increases during the learning of item-context associations. *Proceedings of the National Academy of Sciences of the USA*, **106**, 20 942–20 947.

Trullier, O. and Meyer, J. A. (2000). Animat navigation using a cognitive graph. *Biological Cybernetics*, **83**, 271–285.

Tsodyks, M. (1999). Attractor neural network models of spatial maps in hippocampus. *Hippocampus*, **9**, 481–489.

Tulving, E. (1972). Episodic and semantic memory. In Tulving, E. and Donaldson, W. (eds.), *Organization of Memory*. New York: Academic Press, pp. 381–403.

Verschure, P. F., Voegtlin, T., and Douglas, R. J. (2003). Environmentally mediated synergy between perception and behaviour in mobile robots. *Nature*, **425**, 620–624.

Wagatsuma, H. (2009). Hybrid design principles and time constants in the construction of brain-based robotics: a real-time simulator of oscillatory neural networks interacting with the real environment via robotic devices. *Springer Lecture Notes in Computer Science*, **5506**, 119–126.

Wagatsuma, H. and Yamaguchi, Y. (2004). Cognitive map formation through sequence encoding by theta phase precession. *Neural Computation*, **16**, 2665–2697.

Wagatsuma, H. and Yamaguchi, Y. (2007). Neural dynamics of the cognitive map in the hippocampus. *Cognitive Neurodynamics*, **1**, 119–41.

Wagatsuma, H. and Yamaguchi, Y. (2008). Context-dependent adaptive behavior generated in the theta phase coding network. *Springer Lecture Notes in Computer Science*, **4985**, 177–184.

Wood, E. R., Dudchenko, P. A., Robitsek, R. J., and Eichenbaum, H. (2000). Hippocampal neurons encode information about different types of memory episodes occurring in the same location. *Neuron*, **27**, 623–633.

Wu, S. and Amari, S. (2005). Computing with continuous attractors: stability and online aspects. *Neural Computation*, **17**, 2215–2239.

Yamaguchi, Y. (2003). A theory of hippocampal memory based on theta phase precession. *Biological Cybernetics*, **89**, 1–9.

Yuste, R., MacLean, R., Smith, J., and Lansner, A. (2005). The cortex as a central pattern generator. *Nature Reviews Neuroscience*, **6**, 477–483.

Ziemke, T. (2008). On the role of emotion in biological and robotic autonomy. *BioSystems*, **91**, 401–408.

13 The case for using brain-based devices to study consciousness

Jason G. Fleischer, Jeffrey L. McKinstry, David B. Edelman, and Gerald M. Edelman

13.1   Introduction

Within the past few decades, the nature of consciousness has become a central issue in neuroscience, and it is increasingly the focus of both theoretical and empirical work. Studying consciousness is vital to developing an understanding of human perception and behavior, of our relationships with one another, and of our relationships with other potentially conscious animals. Although the study of consciousness through the construction of artificial models is a recent innovation, the advantages of such an approach are clear. First, models allow us to investigate consciousness in ways that are currently not feasible using human subjects or other animals. Second, an artifact that exhibits the necessary and sufficient properties of consciousness may conceivably be the forerunner of a new and very useful class of neuromorphic robots.

A model of consciousness must take into account current theories of its biological bases. Although the field of artificial consciousness is a new one, it is striking how little attention has been given to modeling mechanisms. Instead, great – and perhaps undue – emphasis has been placed on purely phenomenological models. Many of these models are strongly reductionist in aim and fail to specify neural mechanisms.

This chapter calls for a new approach, one that is complementary to those based on simplified models or abstractions of neural function. We advocate an approach to modeling consciousness that is based on realistic neural mechanisms and rich interactions. The touchstone of this approach, the Theory of Neuronal Group Selection (TNGS) (Edelman, 1987), guides the creation of synthetic neural models that have many of the same properties as real nervous systems.

The TNGS sets forth how the nervous system grows and learns via selectional pressures in a manner analogous to natural selection, requiring large populations (of neurons and circuits) with variance among the population members for selection to take place. This theory implies that neural models of consciousness must be large enough and complex enough to support selectional learning. Additionally, neural models purporting to simulate the mechanisms of consciousness must also incorporate reentrant connectivity in the thalamocortical system, which is a major element of the dynamic core that entails conscious states (Edelman and Tononi, 2000). Reentry occurs throughout

Neuromorphic and Brain-Based Robots, eds. Jeffrey L. Krichmar and Hiroaki Wagatsuma. Published by Cambridge University Press. © Cambridge University Press 2011.

the nervous system, not just in the dynamic core. Such massive back and forth connectivity, both within and among functionally segregated brain regions, provides the connection between perception and memory that is so important for consciousness to emerge. The dynamic core, based on thalamocortical interactions, provides the necessary integration and variation that is characteristic of the conscious state. Finally, because the brain is embodied and the body is embedded in the world, it is essential that a biologically based model of consciousness be embodied in a robotic device capable of very rich autonomous interactions with a nontrivial environment. We therefore believe that the most fruitful synthetic models of consciousness will be those that are instantiated in brain-based devices. A schematic overview of this theory can be seen in Figure 13.1.

13.2   Brain-based devices

Faced with the complexity of real nervous systems, our research group has taken a theoretical approach known as synthetic neural modeling (Edelman *et al.*, 1992). By constructing simulated nervous systems with many levels of anatomical and physiological detail we can start to address the question of how structure and dynamics may give rise to higher brain functions. Synthetic models allow us to perform analyses that are currently impossible in animal studies, because we have access to the entire anatomy and state of the simulated nervous system. By virtue of the homology between our simulated nervous systems and those of mammals, we can make predictions that are useful to neuroscientists.

It is important to realize that the nervous system does not function in isolation. The brain is embodied, and the body is embedded in the environment. The properties, mechanisms, and functions of the nervous system arise only as it interacts with the rest of the body and as the animal engages in a behavior. To that end, we engage our synthetic neural models with behavioral tasks and embody them in robotic phenotypes.

We call this kind of model a brain-based device (BBD) (Fleischer and Edelman, 2009). A BBD can be considered to be a kind of neuromorphic robot. However, it differs from many other similar approaches by virtue of both its construction and purpose.

In contrast to robots that are controlled by what is commonly referred to as an artificial neural network, BBDs have strikingly more complex and realistic neural systems. Typically, an artificial neural network may have hundreds of neural units with relatively simple dynamics, arranged in a largely feedforward, layered architecture. In contrast, the simulated nervous system of a BBD typically has 10^4–10^6 simulated neuronal units exhibiting much more biologically plausible dynamics. These neuronal units are connected by 10^6–10^9 simulated synapses arranged in a massively reentrant architecture that mimics the macroscale connectivity observed in, and among, neural areas of the vertebrate brain. These large-scale neuronal networks are necessary to generate a population of neural circuits sufficient to enable the degree of selectional learning that is seen in real nervous systems (Edelman, 1987).

Developmental and experiental selection

Biological processes create degenerate circuits, both inside brain regions and between them.

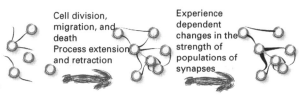

Cell division, migration, and death
Process extension and retraction

Experience dependent changes in the strength of populations of synapses

Reentrant mapping

Selectional processes create regions that have organized neural activity, and also create functional communication (with degenerate circuitry) between such regions.

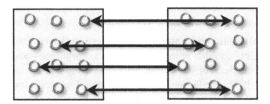

Coordinated activity among many reentrant maps

Ongoing activity in the brain is modulated by embodied multimodal perceptions that activate many reentrant mappings. Thalamocortical, cortico-cortical, and subcortical circuits produce coordinated neural activity that entails conscious states.

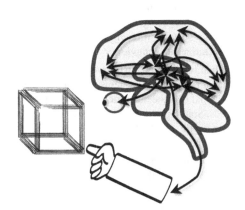

Figure 13.1 The Theory of Neuronal Group Selection and the emergence of conscious states. The nervous system is shaped via genetic and epigenetic processes. During these processes selection occurs at a variety of levels, including that of synaptic circuitry. The long-range reentrant circuitry (including thalamocortical loops) that develops under selection forms mappings between functionally segregated brain regions. Many such mappings are linked together in the dynamic core and entail conscious states that are both integrative (linking together many signals from perception and memory) and variable (not the same from moment to moment). The contents of consciousness (and neural states) are influenced both by the perception of the world and the perception of how self-chosen actions affect the world. Synthetic models of consciousness should take into account these features.

Unlike many other forms of neurally controlled robot, a BBD is designed primarily to test hypotheses about how the mechanisms of the vertebrate nervous system give rise to cognition and behavior. Although a BBD may exhibit learning abilities comparable to those of state-of-the-art artificial intelligence or machine learning systems, it is not designed specifically to address the engineering question of how to build autonomous systems. Nonetheless, it seems likely that, by mimicking mechanisms of mammalian nervous systems, we will learn important design principles for adaptive autonomous systems. Moreover, as our models and devices become more sophisticated

Table 13.1. A brain-based device must ...

Incorporate a simulated brain with detailed neuroanatomy and neural dynamics: Models of brain function should take into consideration the dynamics of the neuronal elements that make up different brain regions, the structure of these different brain regions, and the connectivity within and between these brain regions.

Organize signals from the environment into categories without a priori knowledge or instruction: A BBD selects and generalizes the signals it receives with its sensors, puts these signals into categories without instruction, and learns appropriate actions when confronted with objects under conditions that produce responses in value systems.

Actively sense and autonomously move in the environment: Brains do not function in isolation; they are tightly coupled with the organism's morphology and environment. In order to function properly, an agent, artificial or biological, needs to be situated in the real world (Chiel and Beer, 1997; Clancy, 1997; Clark, 1997; Pfeifer and Bongard, 2006). Therefore, models of brain function should be embodied in a physical device (phenotype) and explore a real (as opposed to a simulated) environment.

Engage in a behavioral task: These tasks should be similar to experimental biology paradigms so that the behavioral performance of the BBDs can be compared with that of real organisms. Similar to a biological organism, an agent or BBD needs a minimal set of innate behaviors or reflexes in order to explore and initially survive in its environmental niche. From this minimal set, the BBD can learn and adapt so that it optimizes its behavior.

Adapt behavior when an important environmental event occurs: Biological organisms adapt their behavior through value systems, which provide relatively nonspecific, modulatory signals to the rest of the brain that bias the outcome of local changes in synaptic efficacy in the direction needed to satisfy global needs. Stated in the simplest possible terms, behavior that evokes positive responses in value systems biases synaptic change to make production of the same behavior more likely when the environmental situation (and thus the local synaptic input) is similar.

Generate experimental data comparable with animal models: Such comparisons may be made at the behavioral level, the systems level, and the neuronal element level. BBDs are powerful tools to test theories of brain function. Having the entire history of all neural activity and synaptic strengths during behavior enables a level of analysis that is simply not possible with animal experiments.

and increasingly biologically realistic, BBDs may approach the complexity of cognition and adaptive behavior that we observe in living organisms, and they may also find their way into practical applications.

BBDs are constructed according to a set of design principles that are vital to creating embodied models showing how the mechanisms of the nervous system can give rise to the behaviors of an organism. These principles are laid out in Table 13.1.

In our own work, BBDs have been used to study the neural bases of perception (Krichmar and Edelman, 2002; Seth *et al.*, 2004b), operant (Krichmar and Edelman, 2002) and fear (Seth *et al.*, 2004a) conditioning, episodic and spatial memory (Krichmar *et al.*, 2005a, 2005b; Fleischer *et al.*, 2007; Fleischer and Krichmar, 2007), and motor control (McKinstry *et al.*, 2006, 2008). These studies were accomplished by simulating brain regions such as the visual and somatosensory cortices, the dopaminergic system, the amygdala, the hippocampus, and the cerebellum. Our investigations have demonstrated that realistic large-scale neuroanatomy is fundamental to reproducing the neural activity and behaviors observed under a variety of conditions. By following the principles of BBD design laid out here, these systems have proven to be powerful tools for investigating the mechanisms – from molecules to networks – by which the nervous system gives rise to behavior. We believe that application of these same principles will allow us to study those mechanisms through which conscious states may emerge.

13.3   Features and mechanisms of consciousness

What is consciousness and what is it good for? Consciousness may be an epiphenomenal process of a nervous system under evolutionary pressure to remember the past, make discriminations in the present, and anticipate the future (Edelman, 1990). Thus, consciousness correlates with the ability to make large numbers of discriminations in a way that, to some degree, frees its possessor from being "stuck" in the present.

Since Descartes (1975) first proposed that the mind (*res cogitans*) was separate from the material world (*res extensa*), consciousness has been considered by many to be outside the reach of physics (Popper and Eccles, 1977), or to require strange physics (Penrose, 1994), or even to be beyond human analysis (McGinn, 1991). Nevertheless, over the last decade and a half, there has been a heightened interest in attacking the problem of consciousness through scientific investigation (Edelman, 1990; Metzinger, 2000). In doing so, a growing consensus has emerged that any scientific account of consciousness must reject extraphysical tenets such as dualism, and be physically based, as well as evolutionarily sound. Such a theory must account for the properties of consciousness and provide a framework for the design and interpretation of experiments (Edelman, 2003).

What do we know about consciousness that might enable us to construct a theory? First and foremost, consciousness is not a thing, but rather, as James (1977, pp. 169–183) pointed out, a process that emerges from interactions of the brain, the body, and the environment. Many decades of philosophical, psychological, and neurological investigation have yielded the list of properties summarized in Table 13.2. Of the properties listed in the table, several elements are worth highlighting: (1) The contrast between the diversity and changeability of conscious states and the unitary appearance to the conscious individual of each conscious state. This unity requires the binding together of diverse sensory modalities that show constructive features such as those seen in Gestalt phenomena. (2) The enormous diversity of conscious states and the potentially infinite numbers of discriminations that can be made by the conscious mind. (3) Conscious states are associated with distributed neural activity that is phasically related to the contents of consciousness, giving experimenters observable neural signatures of conscious perception.

It is useful to distinguish between primary and higher order forms of consciousness. Animals with primary consciousness can integrate perceptual and motor events together with memory to construct a multimodal scene. This is not just a sensory image, but rather a perception and the experience of the perception in what has been called the remembered present (Edelman, 1990). Such primary consciousness is essentially the construction of discriminations that are correlated with the qualia referred to by philosophers. Primary consciousness has adaptive significance, enhancing an animal's

Table 13.2. Features of conscious states

General	
1	Conscious contents are unitary, integrated, and constructed by the brain.
2	They can be enormously diverse and differentiated.
3	They are temporally ordered, serial, and changeable.
4	They require binding of diverse modalities.
5	They have constructive properties including gestalt, closure, and phenomena of filling in.
Informational	
1	They show intentionality with wide-ranging contents.
2	They have widespread access and associativity.
3	They have center, periphery, surround, and fringe aspects.
4	They are subject to attentional modulation, from focal to diffuse.
Subjective	
1	They reflect subjective feelings, qualia, phenomenality, mood, pleasure, and pain.
2	They are concerned with situatedness and placement in the world.
3	They give rise to feelings of familiarity or its lack.
Correlates	
1	They are accompanied by irregular, low-amplitude, fast (12–70 Hz) electrical activity in the cerebral cortex.
2	They are associated with distributed neural activity that is phasically related to the contents of consciousness.
3	They require an intact thalamocortical system (the dynamic core), which is modulated by activity in subcortical areas.
4	They are verbally reportable by humans, and behaviorally reportable by both humans and other animals.

ability to plan for survival. Indeed, primary consciousness reflects the creation of potentially infinite numbers of discriminations. Thus the nervous system underlying primary consciousness helps its possessor in abstracting, organizing, planning, and lending salience to the world.

Higher-order consciousness emerged later in evolution and is seen in animals with semantic capabilities. It is present in its richest form in the human species, which may be unique in possessing true language made up of syntax and semantics. Higher-order consciousness allows its possessors to go beyond the limits of the remembered present of primary consciousness. An individual's past history, future plans, and consciousness of being conscious all become accessible. Given the constitutive role of linguistic tokens, the temporal dependence of consciousness on present inputs is no longer a limiting requisite. Nevertheless, the neural activity underlying primary consciousness is still present in animals with higher-order consciousness.

We have proposed (Edelman, 2003) that at some time around the divergence of one lineage of reptiles into mammals and another into birds, the embryological development of large numbers of new reciprocal connections allowed rich reentrant activity to take place between the more posterior brain systems carrying out perceptual categorization and the more frontally located systems responsible for motor control and value-category memory. This reentrant activity provided the neural basis for integration of a scene with all of its entailed qualia. The ability of an animal so equipped to discriminatively relate a present complex scene to its own unique previous history of learning conferred an adaptive evolutionary advantage. At much later evolutionary epochs, further reentrant circuits appeared that allowed semantic and linguistic performance to be linked to categorical and conceptual memory systems. These developments enabled the emergence of higher-order consciousness.

So, what do we know about the neural activity that gives rise to consciousness? As stated above, and supported by many imaging studies of human patients, widespread reentrant activity among brain regions allows the binding of multisensory stimuli into unified conscious perceptions. This reentrant signaling between cortical regions depends upon activity in the thalamocortical system (the dynamic core), which is, in turn, modulated by various subcortical regions. These subcortical structures provide modulation of the cortical regions via ascending neuromodulatory systems. Reentrant neural circuitry is exceptionally degenerate: structurally different pathways can be involved in producing an identical functional result. This property provides the basis both for selectional learning in the nervous system and for the robustness of conscious states. We propose that the unique anatomical and dynamic features of the brains of higher vertebrates (thalamocortical reentry, corticocortical reentry, subcortical modulation of thalamic activity, modulation of cortical activity via ascending neuromodulatory systems, and selectional learning) together result in the emergence of conscious states.

If the theory we propose – that consciousness arises from the foregoing mechanisms – is correct, then it should be possible to demonstrate that simulating these mechanisms gives rise to phenomena qualitatively similar to those underlying animal consciousness. This is the central argument of this chapter: an artificial construct that has a biologically plausible simulation of the neural mechanisms responsible for conscious states in animals, and is capable of sufficiently rich interactions between its phenotype and the environment, would develop patterns of neural activity and behaviors that are consistent with conscious states.

Having set out this hypothesis, we must now demonstrate how one would test it. It is therefore relevant to discuss how conscious states are investigated in humans and other animals.

13.4   Empirical investigations of consciousness

In conjunction with imaging methodologies such as functional magnetic resonance imaging (fMRI) and magnetoencephalography (MEG), most studies of human consciousness have relied on the ability of individuals to report verbally what they experienced during experimental trials. But animals without language, human infants, and aphasic human adults are unable to produce accurate verbal reports, and so other means must be sought to determine whether an experience has been registered consciously. The ability to provide a behavioral report may imply the presence of a kind of higher-order – or metacognitive – access to primary conscious contents that itself might not be constitutively required for primary consciousness. Indeed, the mechanisms underlying primary consciousness are likely to be somewhat distinct from those enabling its report.

How can we assess the conscious states of different animals in the absence of verbal report? Although human language is by far the most elaborate mode of communication known, accurate report may exploit other more limited behavioral channels, for example lever presses or eye blinks. Mammals, particularly nonhuman primates, share with humans many neurophysiological and behavioral characteristics relevant to consciousness (Seth *et al.*, 2005; Edelman and Seth, 2009), and likewise seem to be able to behaviorally reflect conscious perceptions. In one study, when rhesus macaque monkeys were trained to press a lever to report perceived stimuli in a binocular rivalry paradigm, neurons in the inferior temporal (IT) cortex showed activity correlated with the reported percept, whereas neurons in the visual cortex area V1 instead responded only to the visual signal (Logothetis, 1998). Accordingly, it was suggested that IT serves a critical function in visual consciousness. These observations are consistent with evidence from humans subjected to binocular rivalry while being examined via MEG, which suggest that consciousness of an object involves widespread coherent synchronous cortical activity (Srinivasan *et al.*, 1999). This correspondence between monkeys and humans provides an example of how benchmark comparisons can be made across species. It also suggests the possibility that such benchmarks of behavioral report can be extended to brain-based devices from the human and nonhuman animal cases.

The extent to which neural evidence can account for phenomenal properties is crucial to identifying those properties which are common to most or all conscious experience (Edelman and Seth, 2009). This is particularly relevant to investigating consciousness in a brain-based device, a case where the researcher has direct access to simulated neural states that may be compared with experimental imaging and electrophysiological data from both humans and nonhuman animals. One fundamental property of conscious experience in humans is that every conscious scene is both integrated (i.e. all of a piece) and differentiated (i.e. composed of many different parts) (Tononi and Edelman, 1998). Hence, it is critical to identify the underlying neural processes that not only correlate with, but also account for, simultaneous integration and differentiation and other fundamental properties of human conscious experience. Such neural processes, which go beyond correlation to causal relationships, are said to be explanatory correlates of consciousness (Seth, 2009). Their identification in animals and brain-based devices would constitute a more robust indication of corresponding phenomenal properties, rather than simply the presence of neural correlates per se. From this, it follows that conscious states are neither identical to neural states, nor are they computational or functional accompaniments to such states. Conscious states are entailed by neural states, just as the spectroscopic properties of hemoglobin are entailed by its molecular structure (Edelman, 1990).

A number of imaging studies have shown that very specific neural processes are activated when human subjects are asked to consciously visualize a particular object or scene or internally replay a particular melody. For example, in one study (O'Craven and Kanwisher, 2000), when subjects were asked to mentally visualize either faces or places, cortical regions were activated that are also activated when perceiving those types of stimuli (respectively, the fusiform face area and the parahippocampal place area). While at least strongly suggestive of conscious states in humans and a few species of nonhuman animals, such functional signatures cannot themselves be considered explanatory correlates of consciousness.

13.5 How would you construct a BBD to study consciousness?

So far, we have argued both that consciousness is a legitimate subject for scientific investigation and that one may address the issue through the construction of brain-based devices. Thus we need to consider how one might create a brain-based device that has the features of living nervous systems that give rise to consciousness. Although we do not yet know which mechanisms are necessary and sufficient for consciousness, we do know that humans and many nonhuman animals that seem to exhibit primary consciousness share certain neural systems, connectivity, and dynamics. As mentioned previously, there are theoretical reasons to believe that some of these features are critical to the process of consciousness. Creating a putatively conscious BBD (henceforth referred to as a "conscious artifact") that incorporates all of these features will enable us to determine which subsets of these features are necessary and sufficient for generating conscious states.

13.5.1 Nervous system

What features should be included in the simulated nervous system of a conscious artifact? It isn't necessary or even possible to emulate every element of the mammalian nervous system in the finest detail, so we must consider engineering tradeoffs, as well as evidence from neuroscience, when deciding what to simulate. We have already highlighted the importance of the dynamic core, reentrant connectivity, and selectional learning (Edelman, 2003). At the very least, a conscious artifact should possess such anatomy and it should be simulated at as large a scale as is computationally feasible (e.g. Izhikevich and Edelman, 2008).

The simulated nervous system of a conscious artifact should be composed of spiking neurons that are compatible with reentrant dynamics. Spiking networks theoretically have vast storage capacity via polychronous activity (Izhikevich, 2006), which arises in networks due to spike timing delays. Polychrony also provides a method by which different features of a sensory percept can be bound together (Seth *et al.*, 2004b), a basic feature of consciousness. As is the case for all BBDs, a conscious artifact must self-organize its perceptions without a priori information. One way to provide such unsupervised learning is through the biologically plausible mechanism of spike-timing-dependent plasticity (Bi and Poo, 1998). Additionally, spike-timing-dependent plasticity can be modulated by dopamine, which enables value systems to influence synaptic change (Izhikevich, 2007).

What kind of functional specialization might be necessary for the creation of conscious states? Vision is an obvious sensory input if mental imagery is accepted as a fundamental test of consciousness (a proposal we make later in this paper). In addition, several other sensory streams should be included because conscious states are multisensory and integrated in nature. Since consciousness is embodied (Edelman, 1990; Jeannerod, 2006), the simulated nervous system must also have motor regions, a sense of proprioception, and potentially a variety of other forms of interoception. Various memory systems, particularly working memory, may be fundamental to the induction of conscious states (Baars and Franklin, 2003). Finally, subcortical regions, which modulate value systems and gate activity in the dynamic core in a timed, sequential manner, may be critical to generating the properties found in Table 13.2.

13.5.2   Phenotype

A phenotype embodying a conscious artifact will allow the nervous system to explore the world and its spatial relationships by movement, sense the world richly, and manipulate its environment to develop a sense of its own agency. Clearly such a phenotype must possess appropriate sensors, motors, and physical capabilities.

We are not often conscious of proprioception, the sense of body position and configuration. Yet, in addition to being critical for motor control, these contextual signals may profoundly influence the contents of consciousness (van den Bos and Jeannerod, 2002). Additionally, a conscious artifact that is able to move around its world must be able to sense self-motion and orientation. This can be accomplished through path integration via sensing of the position, velocity, and/or force of its actuators (proprioception) or through inertial measurements similar to those of the vestibular sense.

Vision is often the focus of investigations of consciousness, and it is reasonable to include this capability in the phenotype of a conscious artifact. However, there are other forms of exteroception that are also amenable to the investigation of conscious phenomena, including tactile perception (Romo and Salinas, 2003; de Vignemont *et al.*, 2005) and audition (Gutschalk *et al.*, 2008). Tactile perception is particularly important because it is a prominent source of input to the motor system and it is especially relevant for object manipulation.

It has been shown that visual categorization depends on movement (Krichmar and Edelman, 2002) and motor acts (van den Bos and Jeannerod, 2002). The phenotype must therefore be mobile so that it may perceive objects from multiple vantage points in order to learn object categories that are viewpoint invariant. But it should also have the ability to manipulate objects directly, so that it may form a concept of an object that is invariant to its orientation. In this way, it may link its perceptions to its own actions (Jeannerod, 2006).

Finally, it seems clear that the size of the simulated nervous system discussed in the foregoing might preclude its implementation with conventional CPU-based computing located onboard the phenotype. A wireless link from the phenotype to a large off-board computing cluster or special purpose onboard computing may be necessary to provide possible implementation strategies.

13.6 How would you know it was conscious?

If an artifact with a nervous system homologous in structure and dynamics to those of mammals, after suitable interaction with a rich environment, were to exhibit behavioral and neural correlates of conscious experience, we would need to consider whether or not such a device might actually have conscious states. In any case, a suitably constructed artifact would provide a novel means of exploring the relationship between neural structures, activity, and behaviors associated with conscious perception.

13.6.1 Behavioral correlates

We believe that the demonstration of mental imagery is a convincing test of primary consciousness. To "see with the mind's eye" is to invoke memory as well as direct sensory perception (Kosslyn *et al.*, 2001), and is itself experienced as a conscious state. Mental rotation (Shepard and Metzler, 1971), the act of imaging a spatial transformation of an object, is a simple experimental protocol that tests mental imagery. The standard mental rotation task simultaneously presents two shapes, and requires the subject to determine – and report – whether or not the objects are the same shape seen from different viewpoints. There is a linear relationship between the angle of the mental rotation and the time it takes a subject to perform it (Shepard and Metzler, 1971). This may provide another behavioral correlate that can be assessed in a conscious artifact.

Mental rotation is interesting from the standpoint of embodied cognition because it involves activity in motor cortical areas as well as sensory regions during the transformation of the visual scene (Cohen *et al.*, 1996). Mental rotation has been demonstrated in a large number of human studies and a handful of animal studies (e.g. Georgopoulos *et al.*, 1989; Köhler *et al.*, 2005), and therefore might provide a benchmark for the comparison of putative conscious states in an artifact to those observed in humans and nonhuman animals.

It should be noted that a conscious artifact will require time and experience in manipulating objects and moving through the environment before it would be able to perform mental rotation as described above. Figure 13.2 describes this process. Like animals, the artifact would be expected to develop an internal model of the visual consequences of its actions as the basis for mental rotation (Jeannerod, 2006). It has been proposed that internal covert simulation of motor behavior may be the basis of mental imagery (Hesslow, 2002).

A rotational transformation of a single object can, of course, be achieved via mathematical operations that do not require conscious perception. However, an animal's ability to perform mental rotation is flexible, and can be applied to a vast number of objects and situations. Conscious states are contingent on the ability to make rich discriminations, and these discriminations enable behavioral flexibility. Prior BBDs have

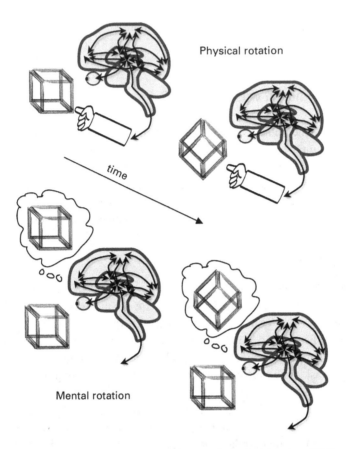

Physical rotation

time

Mental rotation

Figure 13.2   Mental rotation is based on experiences of physical rotation. While manipulating objects
in the real world, the dynamic core (including the thalamocortical system) links together
vision, somatosensory inputs, motor commands, and various memories. These experiences
induce synaptic changes that form mappings between these functionally segregated brain
regions, which can then be recruited to elicit mental imagery of the rotation without actually
performing the physical act. Mental imagery in humans is experienced as a conscious state,
and is thus a suitable test of consciousness. The interaction of the nervous system and the
physical world in this task make it suitable to study using a brain-based device.

been limited to tasks involving a small, fixed set of stimuli, but we expect that a conscious artifact should be able to perform mental rotation with a wide range of arbitrary
objects in a variety of contexts.

13.6.2   Neural correlates

Consider the features of conscious states laid out in Table 13.2. We contend that all of
these can be evaluated in objective assays. These assays include measurement of both
the neural activity and behaviors of a conscious artifact. For the sake of brevity, we
will confine our discussion here to tests for those elements of the table that we consider
most fundamental.

Distributed activity phasically related with conscious states

We have already discussed mental rotation extensively, and noted that it has several known neural correlates in sensory and motor regions of human subjects (Cohen *et al.*, 1996). Perceptual rivalry is another task which has well-known neural correlates that we would expect a conscious artifact to exhibit. During perceptual rivalry the conscious percept alternates between two mutually exclusive stimuli that are presented simultaneously. During this alternation, neural activity is observed to correlate with the stimulus currently being perceived (Logothetis, 1998; Srinivasan *et al.*, 1999). We would expect comparable neural activity from a conscious artifact during either mental rotation or perceptual rivalry.

Integration of conscious states, Gestalt properties, filling in

A principal advantage of synthetic neural models is that they provide us with the ability to record the activity of the entire simulated nervous system, as well as the ability to control that nervous system, potentially all the way down to the finest detail. We can therefore investigate the causality of neural activity in ways that are difficult or impossible to achieve in experiments involving living animals. By experimental manipulation we can determine whether particular circuitry or dynamics can explain a conscious state (Seth, 2009), or if it is merely correlative. This would be particularly useful in the investigation of the Gestalt properties of perception, which can be accomplished by making use of recorded activity to demonstrate that the neural correlates described above are the product of multiple sensory inputs and are integrated in time via reentrant pathways. Behavioral report can also be of use in demonstrating that certain features of stimuli that are absent in a particular probe trial are still reported as present (e.g. filling in).

Enormous diversity, large numbers of discriminations

By looking for neural and behavioral responses to large numbers of distinct stimuli, as well as to large numbers of exemplars of the same type of stimulus, we can investigate the presence of wide-ranging discriminatory powers in a putatively conscious artifact. By presenting an artifact with examples of different objects and requiring it to execute different actions for each object in order to obtain a reward, we can determine if the artifact is able to discriminate among those objects. Neural correlates of the discrimination should be observable, and may in fact be comparable to those seen in animals.

13.7   Conclusion

A number of researchers have considered the construction of a conscious artifact and what this might entail (Holland, 2003; Aleksander, 2007). There is a new journal that is dedicated to this very topic: (Chella, 2009). Other approaches have emphasized the importance of the dynamic core and internal simulation (Shanahan, 2006), in line with our proposal. Our emphasis, however, is on how the detailed mechanisms of the nervous system, in conjunction with embodiment and rich interactions with the world, may give rise to conscious states. This stands in stark contrast to the approaches in the literature that either focus exclusively on cognitive descriptions without invoking neural mechanisms (e.g. Baars, 1988; Haikonen, 2003) or confine themselves narrowly to simplified aspects of the nervous system (e.g. Taylor, 2000; Balduzzi and Tononi, 2009).

The construction of a conscious artifact would have a number of broad implications. Such a device would be a useful tool for exploring the effect of different perturbations and instantiations of a nervous system. For instance, perturbations can be made to model the effects of brain injuries and disease. Different instantiations of a conscious artifact, modeled after animals quite distant from humans and other primates, could be informative in studies of comparative cognition.

Because conscious states are not necessarily bound by present sensations, we expect that mental imagery and the generation of internal models in a conscious artifact will allow ever more flexible behavior through planning. This may lead to a new class of intelligent machines with unprecedented adaptive planning abilities, previously associated only with conscious animals.

An important question which we have not addressed in this proposal is the subjectivity of conscious states. Philosophers have long concerned themselves with qualia: the experience, for example, of the redness of red or the warmness of warmth. This is stated pointedly in Nagel's famous question (Nagel, 1979): "What is it like to be a bat?" or, as he implies, like any other conscious being? Although we cannot easily explore the neural basis of a bat's subjective experience, a conscious artifact is a more transparent object of study than a real animal. Whereas qualia cannot be studied directly, their correlation with discriminations can be examined from a third-person point of view. In any event, a causal analysis of such discriminations would give valuable insights into how consciousness might arise.

The issue of subjectivity as motor cognition has been studied by Jeannerod (2006). A conscious organism can learn to recognize perceptual changes that are caused by its own agency, as opposed to those that are caused by others. In so doing, it can become aware of its own agency. At this point it is not clear whether this can be investigated in a conscious artifact. However in an artifact, we can at least explore the consequences of manipulating proprioception. Eventually, as Jeannerod (2006) states when discussing humans, we might be able to "examine what actions can reveal about the self who produces them, and how they can influence the other selves who perceive them."

Acknowledgments

Work carried out at The Neurosciences Institute was supported by the Neurosciences Research Foundation and by grants from the Defense Advanced Research Projects Agency (DARPA) and the Office of Naval Research (ONR). The views, opinions, and/or findings contained in this article are those of the authors and should not be interpreted as representing the official views or policies, either expressed or implied, of the Defense Advanced Research Projects Agency or the Department of Defense. Approved for Public Release, Distribution Unlimited.

References

Aleksander, I. (2007). *The World in My Mind, My Mind in the World: Key Mechanisms of Consciousness in People, Animals and Machines.* Exeter, UK: Imprint Academic.

Baars, B. J. (1988). *A Cognitive Theory of Consciousness.* New York: Cambridge University Press.

Baars, B. J. and Franklin, S. (2003). How conscious experience and working memory interact. *Trends in Cognitive Science*, **7**(4), 166–172.

Balduzzi, D. and Tononi, G. (2009). Qualia: the geometry of integrated information. *PLoS Computational Biology*, **5**(8), e1000462.

Bi, G. and Poo, M. (1998). Synaptic modifications in cultured hippocampal neurons: dependence on spike timing, synaptic strength, and postsynaptic cell type. *Journal of Neuroscience*, **18**(24), 10 464–10 472.

Chella, A. (ed.) (2009). *International Journal of Machine Consciousness.* Vol. **1**. World Scientific.

Chiel, H. J. and Beer, R. D. (1997). The brain has a body: adaptive behavior emerges from interactions of nervous system, body and environment. *Trends in Neuroscience*, **20**, 553–557.

Clancy, W. J. (1997). *Situated Cognition.* New York: Cambridge University Press.

Clark, A. (1997). *Being There. Putting Brain, Body, and World Together Again.* Cambridge, MA: MIT Press.

Cohen, M. S., Kosslyn, S. M., Breiter, H. C., *et al.* (1996). Changes in cortical activity during mental rotation: a mapping study using functional MRI. *Brain*, **119**(1), 89–100.

de Vignemont, F., Ehrsson, H. H., and Haggard, P. (2005). Bodily illusions modulate tactile perception. *Current Biology*, **15**(14), 1286–1290.

Descartes, R. (1975). *The Philosophical Works of Descartes*, Vols. 1 and 2. Haldane, E. and Ross, G. (eds.), Cambridge, UK: Cambridge University Press.

Edelman, D. B. and Seth, A. K. (2009). Animal consciousness: a synthetic approach. *Trends in Neuroscience*, **32**(9), 476–484.

Edelman, G. M. (1987). *Neural Darwinism: The Theory of Neuronal Group Selection.* New York: Basic Books.

Edelman, G. M. (1990). *The Remembered Present.* New York: Basic Books.

Edelman, G. M. (2003). Naturalizing consciousness: a theoretical framework. *Proceedings of the National Academy of Sciences of the USA*, **100**(9), 5520–5524.

Edelman, G. M. and Tononi, G. (2000). *A Universe of Consciousness: How Matter Becomes Imagination.* New York: Basic Books.

Edelman, G. M., Reeke, G. N., Gall, W. E., *et al.* (1992). Synthetic neural modeling applied to a real-world artifact. *Proceedings of the National Academy of Sciences of the USA*, **89**, 7267–7271.

Fleischer, J. G. and Edelman, G. M. (2009). Brain-based devices: an embodied approach to linking nervous system structure and function to behavior. *IEEE Robotics and Automation*, **16**(3), 32–41.

Fleischer, J. G and Krichmar, J. L. (2007). Sensory integration and remapping in a model of the medial temporal lobe during maze navigation by a brain-based device. *Journal of Integrative Neuroscience*, **6**(3), 403–431.

Fleischer, J. G., Gally, J. A., Edelman, G. M., and Krichmar, J. L. (2007). Retrospective and prospective responses arising in a modeled hippocampus during maze navigation by a brain-based device. *Proceedings of the National Academy of Sciences of the USA*, **104**, 3556–3561.

Georgopoulos, A. P., Lurito, J. T., Petrides, M., Schwartz, A. B., and Massey, J. T. (1989). Mental rotation of the neuronal population vector. *Science*, **243**(4888), 234–236.

Gutschalk, A., Micheyl, C., and Oxenham, A. J. (2008). Neural correlates of auditory perceptual awareness under informational masking. *PLoS Biology*, **6**(6), e138.

Haikonen, P. O. (2003). *The Cognitive Approach to Conscious Machines*. Exeter, UK: Imprint Academic.

Hesslow, G. (2002). Conscious thought as simulation of behaviour and perception. *Trends in Cognitive Sciences*, **6**(6), 242–247.

Holland, O. (ed). (2003). *Machine Consciousness*. Exeter, UK: Imprint Academic.

Izhikevich, E. M. (2006). Polychronization: computation with spikes. *Neural Computation*, **18**(2), 245–282.

Izhikevich, E. M. (2007). Solving the distal reward problem through linkage of STDP and dopamine signaling. *Cerebral Cortex*, **17**(10), 2443–2452.

Izhikevich, E. M. and Edelman, G. M. (2008). Large-scale model of mammalian thalamocortical systems. *Proceedings of the National Academy of Sciences of the USA*, **105**, 3593–3598.

James, W. (1977). *Writings of William James*. Chicago, IL: University of Chicago Press.

Jeannerod, M. (2006). *Motor Cognition: What Actions Tell to the Self*. Oxford, UK: Oxford University Press.

Köhler, C., Hoffmann, K. P., Dehnhardt, G., and Mauck, B. (2005). Mental rotation and rotational invariance in the Rhesus monkey (*Macaca mulatta*). *Brain Behavior and Evolution*, **66**(3), 158–166.

Kosslyn, S. M., Ganis, G., and Thompson, W. L. (2001). Neural foundations of imagery. *Nature Reviews Neuroscience*, **2**(9), 635–642.

Krichmar, J. L. and Edelman, G. M. (2002). Machine psychology: autonomous behavior, perceptual categorization and conditioning in a brain-based device. *Cerebral Cortex*, **12**(8), 818–830.

Krichmar, J. L., Nitz, D. A., Gally, J. A., and Edelman, G. M. (2005a). Characterizing functional hippocampal pathways in a brain-based device as it solves a spatial memory task. *Proceedings of the National Academy of Sciences of the USA*, **102**, 2111–2116.

Krichmar, J. L., Seth, A. K., Nitz, D. A., Fleischer, J. G., and Edelman, G. M. (2005b). Spatial navigation and causal analysis in a brain-based device modeling cortical-hippocampal interactions. *Neuroinformatics*, **3**(3), 197–221.

Logothetis, N. K. (1998). Single units and conscious vision. *Philosophical Transactions of the Royal Society of London, B, Biological Science*, **353**(1377), 1801–1818.

McGinn, C. (1991). *The Problems of Consciousness: Essays Toward a Resolution*. Oxford, UK: Blackwell.

McKinstry, J. L., Edelman, G. M., and Krichmar, J. L. (2006). A cerebellar model for predictive motor control tested in a brain-based device. *Proceedings of the National Academy of Sciences of the USA*, **103**(9), 3387–3392.

McKinstry, J. L., Seth, A. K., Edelman, G. M., and Krichmar, J. L. (2008). Embodied models of delayed neural responses: spatiotemporal categorization and predictive motor control in brain based devices. *Neural Networks*, **21**(4), 553–561.

Metzinger, T. (ed.). (2000). *Neural Correlates of Consciousness: Empirical and Conceptual Questions*. Cambridge, MA: MIT Press.

Nagel, T. (1979). *Mortal Questions*. Cambridge, UK: Cambridge University Press.

O'Craven, K. M. and Kanwisher, N. (2000). Mental imagery of faces and places activates corresponding stiimulus-specific brain regions. *Journal of Cognitive Neuroscience*, **12**(6), 1013–1023.

Penrose, R. (1994). *Shadows of the Mind: A Search for the Missing Science of Consciousness*. Oxford, UK: Oxford University Press.

Pfeifer, R. and Bongard, J. C. (2006). *How the Body Shapes the Way We Think: A New View of Intelligence.* Cambridge, MA: MIT Press.

Popper, K. and Eccles, J.F. (1977). *The Self and Its Brain.* Berlin: Springer.

Romo, R. and Salinas, E. (2003). Flutter discrimination: neural codes, perception, memory and decision making. *Nature Reviews Neuroscience,* **4**(3), 203–218.

Seth, A. K. (2009). Explanatory correlates of consciousness: theoretical and computational challenges. *Cognitive Computatation,* **1**, 50–63.

Seth, A. K., McKinstry, J. L., Krichmar, J. L., and Edelman, G. M. (2004a). Active sensing of visual and tactile stimuli by brain-based devices. *International Journal of Robotics & Automation,* **19**(4), 222–238.

Seth, A. K., McKinstry, J. L., Edelman, G. M., and Krichmar, J. L. (2004b). Visual binding through reentrant connectivity and dynamic synchronization in a brain-based device. *Cerebral Cortex,* **14**(11), 1185–1199.

Seth, A. K., Baars, B. J., and Edelman, D. B. (2005). Criteria for consciousness in humans and other mammals. *Consciousness and Cognition,* **14**(1), 119–139.

Shanahan, M. (2006). A cognitive architecture that combines internal simulation with a global workspace. *Consciousness and Cognition,* **15**(2), 433–449.

Shepard, R. N. and Metzler, J. (1971). Mental rotation of three-dimensional objects. *Science,* **171**(3972), 701–703.

Srinivasan, R., Russell, D. P., Edelman, G. M., and Tononi, G. (1999). Increased synchronization of neuromagnetic responses during conscious perception. *Journal of Neuroscience,* **19**(13), 5435–5448.

Taylor, J. G. (2000). Attentional movement: the control basis for consciousness. *Society for Neuroscience Abstracts,* **26** (2231), 839.3.

Tononi, G. and Edelman, G. M. (1998). Consciousness and complexity. *Science,* **282**(5395), 1846–1851.

van den Bos, E. and Jeannerod, M. (2002). Sense of body and sense of action both contribute to self-recognition. *Cognition,* **85**(2), 177–187.

Part V

Ethical considerations

14 Ethical implications of intelligent robots

George A. Bekey, Patrick Lin, and Keith Abney

14.1   Introduction

The ethical challenges of robot development were dramatically thrust onto center stage with Asimov's book *I, Robot* in 1950, where the three "Laws of Robotics" first appeared in a short story. The "laws" assume that robots are (or will be) capable of perception and reasoning and will have intelligence comparable to a child, if not better, and in addition that they will remain subservient to humans. Thus, the first law reads:

"A robot may not injure a human being, or, through inaction, allow a human being to come to harm."

Clearly, in these days when military robots are used to kill humans, this law is (perhaps regrettably) obsolete. However, it still raises fundamental questions about the relationship between humans and robots, especially when the robots are capable of exerting lethal force. Asimov's law also suffers from the complexities of designing machines with a sense of morality. As one of several possible approaches to control their behavior, robots could be equipped with specialized software that would ensure that they conform to the "Laws of War" and the "Rules of Engagement" of a particular conflict. After realistic simulations and testing, such software controls perhaps would not prevent all unethical behaviors, but they would ensure that robots behave at least as ethically as human soldiers do (Arkin, 2009) (though this is still an inadequate solution for many critics).

Today, military robots are autonomous in navigation capabilities, but most depend on remote humans to "pull the trigger" which releases a missile or other weapon. Research in neuromorphic and brain-based robotics may hold the key to significantly more advanced artificial intelligence and robotics, perhaps to the point where we would entrust ordinary attack decisions to robots. But what are the moral issues we ought to consider before giving machines the ability to make such life-or-death decisions?

Similar ethical problems arise in other nonmilitary areas of application. Consider healthcare robotics: What will be the consequences of allowing surgical robots to perform operations on their own? Who will assume responsibility? What will be the relative roles of human and robot surgeons in the operating room? Consider agricultural robotics: What if "intelligent" agricultural robots spray crops with incorrect

Neuromorphic and Brain-Based Robots, eds. Jeffrey L. Krichmar and Hiroaki Wagatsuma. Published by Cambridge University Press. © Cambridge University Press 2011.

concentrations of pesticides and large numbers of people become ill or die? Was it wrong to use robots for this purpose? Who assessed the potential risks? Or, consider even toy robots: If these "toys" become increasingly intelligent, they can become more interesting playmates to children, but might there be dangers as well – and eventually, issues about whether these robots should have rights themselves?

This chapter addresses these and other questions, delving into both engineering and ethical principles and focusing on some of the latest literature. It is not surprising that we must confront such ethics and policy problems, as technology becomes more interwoven with the fabric of society. But because robots interact directly with the world, by definition, and to a degree greater than most other technologies, those concerns are heightened and many unique to the field of robot ethics.

14.2   Definitions and general remarks

First, we need to further delineate our topic – just what counts as a robot? We define "robot" as *a machine that senses, thinks, and acts*: "Thus a robot must have sensors, processing ability that emulates some aspects of cognition, and actuators. Sensors are needed to obtain information from the environment. Reactive behaviors (like the stretch reflex in humans) do not require any deep cognitive ability, but onboard intelligence is necessary if the robot is to perform significant tasks autonomously, and actuation is needed to enable the robot to exert forces upon the environment. Generally, these forces will result in motion of the entire robot or one of its elements (such as an arm, a leg, or a wheel)" (Bekey, 2005).

Given that this chapter's purpose is to discuss the ethical implications of intelligent robots, we will not discuss the extremely interesting moral issues that arise in related fields, such as those due to human enhancements with machine parts (cyborgs) that are still controlled by a human brain, or of programming complex computer systems that have no autonomy or direct actuators at all.

But that still leaves much to discuss; robots are appearing in nearly all aspects of society – from home care to healthcare, entertainment to education, and space applications to sex. The growth in some areas is explosive: ten years ago there were no pilotless, autonomous aircraft in the United States, but now several thousand fly the skies in Iraq and Afghanistan. Similarly with household robots: ten years ago we only saw prototypes of automatic vacuum cleaners for the home, but now several million Roomba robots have been sold by iRobot Corporation.

While the robots deployed in factories, homes, and the battlefield have some limited autonomy, they generally rely on human operators for complex or potentially dangerous operations. However, in university laboratories worldwide, there are prototype robots capable of problem solving and learning, interacting with humans in sophisticated ways and able to display emotions. In other words, they are displaying more and more of the qualities we associate with human intelligence. As a result, there is increasing concern that such intelligent machines may become capable of harming human beings.

One problem is that while technology races forward, ethical considerations in the use of robots have not kept pace. Even questions of potential risk are largely marginalized. The average person is likely to believe that anything a robot does is the result of programming, and hence the machine can do only what it is intentionally programmed to do. Unfortunately, this is a quaint oversimplification, since complex programs may behave in ways that were not expected by their designers. Furthermore, complex systems may display "emergent behaviors" (Arkin, 1998); that is, modes of behavior which were not predicted by the designer but which arise as a result of unpredicted interactions among the components of the system. For instance, some worry that robots may ultimately be able to self-replicate; that is, make copies of themselves without human assistance. These sorts of fears have led not only to countless science fiction stories, but also to a serious examination by respected scientists (e.g. Joy, 2000).

The point here is that society will eventually require some form of control over robots to ensure their ethical use. Such control may come from governments or private organizations or even from robot developers and builders. However, it is certainly not guaranteed that these controls will arise until and unless there are serious accidents. In California, there is a common saying that traffic control signals are not installed at an intersection until the second child is killed there by an automobile. In other words, people (and their governments) are better at reacting than at anticipating adverse consequences and planning to avoid them. With the rapid growth of robotics, such delays may lead to unfortunate, perhaps even disastrous outcomes; and even rigorous testing before deployment may not be able to eliminate a "first-generation" problem of robots causing unforeseen harm. This problem of possible harmful actions by robots and the associated issues of risk and liability for those who produce, sell, or use robots form the most pressing set of moral concerns concerning the rise of intelligent robots. As their intelligence increases, however, a second type of moral concern is gradually being added: how do we instill morality into the robots themselves? As their autonomy increases, ultimately, will robots themselves become moral agents, capable of moral responsibility – of being blamed *themselves* when things go wrong? Can this ever happen? If so, *should* it? One day, we may face the issue of robot emancipation – of whether or not we will allow robots to no longer be our slaves, but our moral equals. What will we do then?

14.3 Historical background: Asimov's laws

The first attempt at defining a set of rules or "laws" for robot behavior was made by Isaac Asimov in 1950, in a collection of short stories entitled *I, Robot*. Asimov's three "Laws of Robotics" were the following:

1. A robot may not injure a human being or, through inaction, allow a human being to come to harm.
2. A robot must obey orders given to it by human beings, except where such orders would conflict with the first law.

3. A robot must protect its own existence as long as such protection does not conflict with the first or second law.

Many of Asimov's later science fiction stories were based on the consequences of violating one or more of these "laws." Implicit in these laws are assumptions about the relation of robots to humans. Robots were assumed to be human-like and capable of understanding commands and interacting with humans in particular, human-like ways; and yet, they are considered to be child-like and subservient machines that will obey whatever "laws" are given to them. Asimov's novels leave it unclear whether or not such robots are capable of independent thinking, but they are assumed to have enough intellectual power to make moral decisions.

Sixty years later, we are still discussing the possibility of autonomous behavior and the need for morality in machines. Wallach and Allen (2008), prominent in current literature, elucidate the distinction between operational and functional morality in robots. When robots with even limited autonomy must choose from among different courses of action, the concern for safety is transmuted into the need for the systems to have a capacity for making moral judgments. For robots that operate within a very limited context, the designers and engineers who build the systems may well be able to discern all the different options the robot will encounter and program the appropriate responses. The actions of such a robot are completely in the hands of the designers of the systems and those who choose to deploy them; these robots are *operationally moral*.

Robots with mere operational morality presumably will not require the capacity to explicitly evaluate or "understand" the likely consequences of their actions. They will neither need the meta-level (sometimes termed "second-order") functions of being capable of evaluating which rules apply in a particular situation, nor the meta-level functions of being able to prioritize certain rules over others, in cases of conflict between rules.

The recognition that such meta-level functions will sometimes be required for many robotic applications makes clear that operational morality will not always be sufficient for future uses of robots. In particular, three types of problems will demand a meta-level *functional morality*: (1) the increasing autonomy of robotic systems; (2) the prospect that systems will encounter influences that their designers could not anticipate because of the complexity of the environments in which they are deployed, or because the systems are used in contexts for which they were not specifically designed; and (3) the complexity of technology and the inability of systems engineers to predict how the robots will behave under a new set of inputs.

This functional morality will require that the machines themselves have the capacity for assessing and responding to moral considerations, creating new challenges in both design and programming, especially given the constraints due to both the limits of present-day technology, and the (in)feasibility of implementing the theory as a computer program.

To address some of the programming problems associated with a functional morality, Asimov later added a "zero-th law," which broadens the First Law and assumes top priority: "A robot must not harm humanity, or through inaction, allow humanity to come to harm." But later authors have found further difficulties in programming Asimov's laws and have attempted fixes by adding a fourth law (or fifth, depending on how one counts), to the effect that a robot must always reveal that it is a robot. In the present state of robotics, this may not seem to be a problem, but some recent robots created in Japan (e.g. Ishiguro and Asada, 2006) have an uncanny resemblance to human beings. This potential source of confusion may cause yet another ethical dilemma, for example "I didn't know you were a robot!"

The limitations of Asimov's laws have led several authors to suggest further modifications. Among the most recent are those of Murphy and Woods (2009), who propose an alternative set of "responsible laws" as follows:

1. A human may not deploy a robot without the human–robot work system meeting the highest legal and professional standards of safety and ethics.
2. A robot must respond to humans as appropriate for their roles.
3. A robot must be endowed with sufficient situated autonomy to protect its own existence as long as such protection provides smooth transfer of control to other agents consistent with the first and second laws.

As Murphy and Woods point out, Asimov's laws are robotcentric and assign to the machine the major responsibility in interactions with humans, which assumes that they have been provided with some form of functional morality. By contrast, the alternative laws assign major responsibility to the designers and users of robots, so that the robots themselves are not assumed to be able to handle legal and ethical issues. The third alternative law emphasizes this issue by urging the design of robots that are capable of turning control of themselves over to humans when faced with either legal or moral issues they are not designed to handle.

The alternative laws are certainly a major step toward emphasizing greater responsibility (specifically including ethical concerns) on the part of designers and deployers of robots. However, these alternative laws still do not account for the use of semi-autonomous or autonomous robots by the military services, or any other legitimate use of force or coercion against humans (e.g. the police or criminal justice system). Asimov's laws are deeply concerned with the potential harm to human beings by robots, which, in many cases, is precisely the goal of military robots. The alternative laws appear to assume that attention to issues of safety and legality by the designers will solve most of the potential problems addressed by Asimov's laws. This is evidently not true in military applications, as we discuss in the following section.

14.4 Military robots

Because the military sector is often a key driver and early adopter of new technologies, and because warfare inherently gives rise to serious ethical concerns, we look first at such issues related to military robots. Potentially, robots have major advantages over human soldiers. These robots could be "smart" enough to make decisions that only humans now can; and as conflicts increase in tempo and require much quicker information processing and responses, robots will increasingly have a distinct advantage over the limited and fallible cognitive capabilities that we *Homo sapiens* have. Not only would robots expand the battlespace over difficult, larger areas of terrain, but they also represent a significant force-multiplier – each effectively doing the work of many human soldiers, while immune to sleep deprivation, fatigue, low morale, perceptual and communication challenges in the "fog of war," and other performance-hindering conditions.

During the past 20 years, military robots have risen to prominence as the weapons of choice for many applications, including surveillance, reconnaissance, location and destruction of mines and IEDs (improvised explosive devices), as well as offense. The latter class of vehicles is equipped with weapons, which at the present time (with one or two exceptions) are fired by remote human controllers. In the following, we first summarize the state of the art in military robots, including both hardware and software, and then introduce some of the ethical issues that arise from their use. We concentrate on robots capable of lethal action and omit discussion of machines such as BEAR (Battlefield Extraction Assist Robot) for removing wounded soldiers from the battlefield or the Army Big Dog, a four-legged robot capable of carrying several hundred pounds of cargo over irregular terrain. If at some future time such "carry robots" are equipped with weapons, they may need to be considered more closely from an ethical point of view.

Military robots capable of lethal force include wheeled and tracked ground vehicles, surface and underwater naval systems, and various aerial vehicles. The best known unmanned flying vehicles (UFVs) are the Predator and the Reaper, manufactured by General Atomics, both of which can be equipped with guided missiles. They carry a camera mounted in a pod under the nose and missiles mounted under the wings. While these robot aircraft can take off, fly, and land autonomously, the missiles are fired by human controllers who may be located at great distances from the target locations. Pushing a button which releases a missile thousands of miles away effectively isolates the soldier from persons who may have been wounded or killed in the attack, since all that he or she sees is an exploding house or vehicle. It is also more difficult for remote controllers to separate insurgents from civilians than it is for "boots on the ground."

Inasmuch as military robots such as the Reaper and Predator carry weapons designed to kill people as well as destroying property, it is clear that their deployment is in violation of Asimov's first law. Even considering the "Alternative First Law" cited above, what is the "highest standard of ethics" required by the designer of a military robot? The ethical standard may depend on the individual designer's own national, ethical, and religious background. Some people may refuse to work on such systems. Others will invoke issues of patriotism and a national need to design a robot capable of the highest possible degree of destructiveness.

One plausible candidate for a consensus on understanding the Alternative First Law's requirement of the "highest standard of ethics" is the internationally agreed-upon Laws of War and their instantiation in typical Rules of Engagement by the military. But problems remain if the actual deployment of military robots will inevitably fall short of full compliance with the relevant Laws of War and Rules of Engagement.

For example, what if our robots are incapable of properly discriminating friend from foe, or combatant from noncombatant?

So while we may reasonably consider Asimov's laws to be obsolete, this does not alleviate the ethical dilemmas faced by the deployers and users of military robots. Many roboticists (including the authors) believe that eventually such systems will be given nearly full autonomy, including the ability to make firing decisions on their own. Such robot autonomy will push the ethical questions somewhat further from the personnel who issue the deployment order, but it does not eliminate them.

To illustrate further the ethical dilemmas facing soldiers working with robots, consider the following scenario. Intelligence information indicates that a house located at given global positioning system (GPS) coordinates is the headquarters for dangerous enemy combatants. A military robot is commanded by an officer to approach the house and destroy it, in order to kill all the people within it. As the robot approaches the house it detects (from a combination of several sensors, including vision, x-ray, audition, olfaction, etc.) that there are numerous (noncombatant) children within, in addition to the combatants. The robot has been programmed in compliance with the Laws of War and the typical Rules of Engagement to avoid or at least minimize noncombatant casualties (sometimes referred to as "collateral damage") (Lin *et al.*, 2008; Arkin, 2009]. By following the Alternative Third Law, the robot may attempt to solve its dilemma by transferring authority back to the officer in charge, but this may not be feasible or practical since it may risk discovery of the robot by the enemy and harm to our own forces. Potentially, the robot is in violation of two of Asimov's laws: if it proceeds as instructed, it may violate the first law; if it does not proceed, it will violate the second law. Typically, when faced with such contradictory instructions, the onboard computer will "freeze" and lock up.

Another possible scenario involves a high-performance robot aircraft, suddenly subject to attack by unknown and unrecognized piloted airplanes. Asimov's laws do not help, since the robot can only defend its own existence by causing harm to human beings. The alternative laws also do not help, since a decision to transfer control would need to be made in milliseconds, and no human commander could respond rapidly enough. What should the drone do?

Thus, the use of military robots raises numerous ethical questions. Arkin (2009) has attempted to solve such problems by developing a control architecture for military robots, to be embedded within the robot's control software. Such software in principle could ensure that the robot obeys the Rules of Engagement and the Laws of War. But would the mere requirement to adhere to these rules actually ensure that the robot behaves ethically in all situations? The answer to this question is clearly in the negative, but Arkin only claims that such robots would behave "more ethically" than human soldiers. In fact, sadly, to behave more morally than human soldiers may not require a great advance in robot ethics. Beyond popular news reports and images of purportedly unethical behavior by human soldiers, the US Army Surgeon General's Office has surveyed US troops in Iraq on issues in battlefield ethics and discovered worrisome results. From its summary of findings, among other statistics: "Less than half of soldiers and marines believed that noncombatants should be treated with respect and dignity and well over a third believed that torture should be allowed to save the life of a fellow team member. About 10% of soldiers and marines reported mistreating an Iraqi noncombatant when it wasn't necessary ... Less than half of soldiers and marines would report a team member for unethical behavior ... Although reporting ethical training, nearly a third of soldiers and marines reported encountering ethical situations in Iraq in which they didn't know how to respond" (US Army Surgeon General's Office, 2006). The most recent survey by the same organization reported similar results (US Army Surgeon General's Office, 2008).

It is evident from the above discussion that there are numerous unresolved ethical questions in the deployment of military robots. Among these questions are the following:

- Will the use of increasingly autonomous military robots lower the barriers for entering into a war, since it would decrease casualties on our side?
- How long will it be before military robotic technology will become available to other nations, and what effect will such proliferation have?
- Are the Laws of War and Rules of Engagement too vague and imprecise (or too difficult to program) to provide a basis for an ethical use of robots in warfare?
- Is the technology for military robots sufficiently well developed to ensure that they can distinguish between military personnel and noncombatants?
- Are there fail-safes against unintended use? For instance, can we be certain that enemy "hackers" will not assume control of our robots and turn them against us?

Thoughtful discussions of these issues have been published by Arkin (2009), Asaro (2009), Sharkey (2008a, 2008b, 2008c), Sparrow (2007), Weber (2009), and others. We have addressed some of them in a major report (Lin *et al.*, 2008).

14.5   Healthcare robots

While military robots present a major challenge to societal ethics, they are not the only source of concern as the technology of intelligent systems continues to develop. Over the past 20 years, a number of healthcare and rehabilitation robots – in industries that again naturally engage ethical issues – have been developed, in the USA, Great Britain, Italy, Germany, and other countries. They have been used for diagnostic purposes, as prosthetic and orthotic devices, as surgical assistants, and in a number of other applications (e.g. McBeth *et al.*, 2004; Taylor, *et al.*, 2008; van der Loos and Reinkensmeyer, 2008). In the brief review that follows, and building upon research by Datteri and Tamburrini (2009), we consider only a small sample of these applications, but it should be noted that robotics in healthcare is a rapidly growing area, and hence there is a rapid proliferation of emerging problems related to risk, responsibility, and other ethical concerns.

As with the discussion of military robotics, we begin with a hypothetical scenario involving robotic surgery. Consider a situation in which a robot surgeon performs an operation on a patient; a number of complications arise and the patient's condition is worse than before. Who is responsible? Is it the designer of the robot, the manufacturer, the human surgeon who recommended the use of the robot, the hospital, the insurer, or some other entity? If there was a known chance that the surgery might result in problems, was it ethical for the human surgeon and/or the hospital to recommend and/or approve the use of a robot? How large a chance of harm would make it unethical – or, to phrase it differently, how small a chance of harm would be morally permissible? That is, what is the acceptable risk?

This situation is already not totally hypothetical. A robot to perform hip replacement surgery (named ROBODOC) was developed at the IBM Watson Research Center in the early 1990s (Taylor *et al.*, 1994) and later commercialized by a company named Integrated Surgical Systems Inc. (Bargar *et al.*, 1998). ROBODOC measured the marrow cavity diameter in the patient's femur and then machined the stem of the prosthetic hip implant to the exact dimensions of the cavity. Initial claims for the device indicated that the fit was so precise that it was not necessary to use cement. Following a period of great enthusiasm, further use of the robot was stopped in the USA by the Food and Drug Administration (FDA) as a result of post-operative complications, as well as long surgical times, excessive blood loss, and longer hospital stays than those following conventional total hip replacement surgeries (Weber, 2009). ROBODOC has been used successfully in Europe since the 1990s. In 2008 the rights to the use of the ROBODOC name were acquired by Curexo, Inc. which then created a new division by that name and obtained FDA approval for its use. The system consists of a computer named ORTHODOC for preoperative surgical planning and the ROBODOC surgical assistant robot.

In contrast with ROBODOC, the da Vinci Surgical System manufactured by Intuitive Surgical Systems in California is being used in hundreds of hospitals in the USA and other countries (Taylor *et al.*, 2008). The da Vinci may be described as a *tele-robot* since it is not fully autonomous. Rather, a human surgeon sits at a special console and uses two handles to perform minimally invasive surgery. However, rather than controlling the surgical instruments directly, the surgeon provides inputs to the robot, which, in turn, holds the instruments in its manipulators and performs the actual procedures under computer control. This process has a number of advantages over conventional minimally invasive surgery performed by unassisted human surgeons, including the following:

- After penetrating through the skin, the tip of the instrument moves in the opposite direction to that of the surgeon's hand. In the da Vinci system, the surgeon sees the tip in a special display, where it moves in the same direction as his/her hand.
- The system allows for scaling of the motion; that is, if very small, precise movements are required, the surgeon's actual hand movement can be scaled down for actual movement of the instrument (scalpel, needle, etc.)
- Any tremor of the surgeon's hand (which could be very important in high-precision surgery) can be filtered out by the system before reaching the patient.

For at least the time being, it seems noteworthy that the direct participation of the surgeon (rather than fully autonomous surgery by the robot) dramatically reduces the

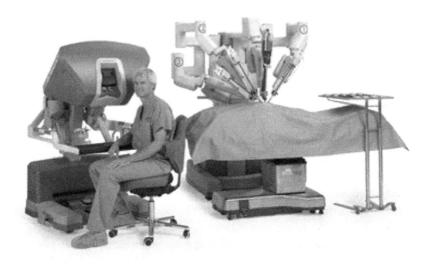

Figure 14.1   The da Vinci Si HD surgical system showing surgeon console and patient cart (© 2009 Intuitive Surgical, Inc.).

potential risks and the associated ethical problems. Figure 14.1 shows the da Vinci system. The robot arms are positioned over the patient, and the surgeon can be seen seated at the control console at the left.

Also significant is the fact that the physical separation of the surgeon from the patient means that the da Vinci system can be used for telesurgery; that is, the patient can be located anywhere, as long as there are electronic connections between them. Of course, new ethical questions may arise as a result of the intervening network and the possibility of power failure or other technical difficulties, as well as possible communication mishaps, such as the mistranslation of the surgeon's instructions.

Another dramatic demonstration of the current status of robotic surgery is the NeuroArm, developed by Dr. Garnette Sutherland and his associates at the Calgary Medical Center in Canada. This robot, while similar in principle to the da Vinci, must in fact be significantly more precise since it is designed to perform brain surgery (McBeth *et al.*, 2004). The earliest neurosurgical robot was developed in Japan (Hongo *et al.*, 2002). The NeuroArm is capable of precision movements of the order of fractions of a millimeter. It is not clear at the time of writing (2010) whether the robot is in clinical use; any use will involve significant potential ethical, risk, and liability problems associated with surgery on the human brain.

What are the major ethical problems associated with robotic surgery? In addition to the risks to patient health outlined above, Datteri and Tamburrini (2009) suggest that two such problems concern cost and privacy protection. Clearly, systems like the da Vinci or ROBODOC are expensive. The latest models of the da Vinci cost about US$1.75 million, not including annual maintenance and operational costs that could be in the hundreds of thousands of dollars. These costs suggest that its use will be limited to relatively wealthy patients, wealthy communities, and wealthy countries. Yet, some 1400 da Vinci systems have been installed in hospitals worldwide as of January 2010, suggesting that funding can be made available. The da Vinci is used extensively for urologic surgery, gall bladder surgery, and recently, heart valve surgery, resulting in shorter hospital stays for the patients. It also appears that training of surgeons is faster and easier than for conventional minimally invasive surgery. Even so, it is clear that the technology is not likely to be available in developing countries, but this is true of other expensive technologies and even expensive medications.

The second issue raised by Datteri and Tamburrini concerns the vast amount of data collected during robotic surgeries and the need to provide adequate informational privacy protection for each patient. This issue becomes ever more important as automated systems record large amounts of data, which can be increasingly (mis)used by governments, employers, insurers, and others. Hence, such information must be stored appropriately and with suitable safeguards to prevent misuse. Further, we believe that there are other potential sources of risk and/or violation of ethical principles that have not been adequately addressed at the present time, for example the effects of equipment or software failure during surgery. Independent of the question of insurance coverage for such eventualities, the basic question concerns the risk to the patient and the moral responsibility on the part of the surgeon and/or hospital. Will the surgeon prescribe the use of robotic surgery for the benefit of the patient, or because it reduces his/her own time in the operating room – or the costs to the hospital? What if robot manufacturers start giving kickbacks to surgeons who agree to use them in procedures? Will attractive "robot reps" start elbowing pharmaceutical representatives out of doctor's offices? Will robot manufacturers seek to influence the outcomes of clinical trials that compare robotic to traditional surgery? Will hospitals employ a "soft paternalism" towards patients that requires them to explicitly ask for human surgeons, so that robotic surgery becomes the assumed default (perhaps in order to help amortize the cost of the machines)? Once a robotic system is installed in a hospital, we expect that there will be both subtle and overt pressure on the part of the hospital administrators to use the system.

We turn now to a completely different aspect of healthcare, namely the rehabilitation of persons who have suffered amputations as a result of wartime or other injuries. In contrast with the rigid replacements for a missing lower extremity (such as the "peg leg" used by pirates in various novels), contemporary prostheses provide the amputee with a computer-controlled robotic leg. These devices (such as those manufactured by Otto Bock in Germany; Näder and Näder, 2002) are commonly fitted to above-the-knee amputees. The device includes sensors to detect stress and strain in the leg structure, as well as devices to measure knee and ankle angular deflection. A microprocessor within the leg processes these data and sends control signals to a hydraulic servo unit which moves the knee joint as required (Figure 14.2a). The system is known as the "C-leg" to indicate that it is computer controlled. Following adjustment based on the limb length and weight of the subject, there is a training period, after which the person can walk up and down stairs unassisted, as shown in Figure 14.2b.

What are some of the ethical issues associated with the Otto Bock prosthesis? First, as with the da Vinci surgical system, the prosthesis is expensive. When used to replace a limb lost by a soldier fighting for his country, the cost is justifiable, but what happens

(a)

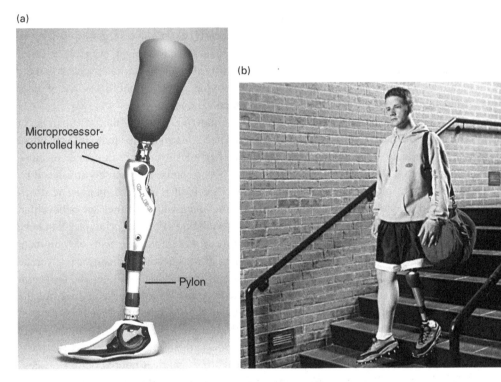

(b)

Figure 14.2   The Otto Bock C-leg (courtesy of Otto Bock, Inc.).

to civilians who cannot afford it? If the person falls while wearing the device, who is responsible, not just for possible medical/surgical costs, but for the possibility that the person may not be able to wear the device again and be restricted to a wheelchair for life? As with other surgical robotic systems, the question of responsibility is complex.

Finally, let us look at the case of robotic training assistants. Physical therapists perform invaluable functions, both in the hospital and the patient's home, by assisting in repetitive movement of injured limbs, or following strokes and accidents that result in partial paralysis. Such movement prevents atrophy of the muscles in the affected limb, and allows for re-innervation of the damaged area. For some years it has been evident that the repetitive flexing of a knee joint or elbow, for example, does not require the services of a highly trained therapist, and can in fact be performed by a robot, without incurring either the tedium or expense of having a trained professional endlessly repeating a simple action.

An ethical issue that may arise in such situations concerns the decreased human contact on the part of the patient. Removing the physical therapist and installing a machine on the bed to move the patient's leg or arm may be cost effective, but it may contribute to a sense of isolation, especially for patients who have few or no visitors. This possible depersonalization of the patient could also be extended to the robotic therapist itself; patients may feel free to vent their anger or despair or frustration over their condition and strike or damage or even destroy a robot therapist, in a way that they would never dream of doing to a human therapist. And that would produce both psychological and financial costs. Clearly, some of the ethical issues in robot–patient relationships are subtle, but this does not make them less important.

A recent development in rehabilitation robotics concerns the use of robots that do not make physical contact with the patient, but may provide guidance in various tasks or even simple encouragement and praise by voice (Matarić *et al.*, 2007). What if a patient develops an emotional attachment to the robot, and the machine is eventually removed? This situation is analogous to removing a favorite toy from a child; the experience can be traumatic, and such trauma could be reinforced by the plausible increase in isolation from other human contact such patients (especially elderly patients) may experience as human therapists are removed from their lives.

14.6   Other social robots

Many of the ethical issues we have highlighted with military and healthcare robots also arise in other aspects of society where humans interact with robots (or will do so in the near future). We here describe a few scenarios briefly, first concerning toy robots and then robots designed for household and other interactive roles.

Children can become very attached to toys, and we believe this will be particularly true with respect to robotic toys since they move and possibly talk, thus giving the impression of being alive. Although it is dubious that such attachments are necessarily harmful to the child, it is evident that both the action of giving a robot to a child and later taking it away may have psychological and ethical implications. It is known that interaction with a mobile robot, even if it is not anthropomorphic, may be helpful to autistic children (e.g. Scassellatti, 2005; Kozima *et al.*, 2007; Werry and Dautenhahn, 2009). As robots increase in intelligence and other capabilities, their uses as toys will be both more varied and more complex; it may be necessary to develop a whole new language and a new way of interacting with robot companions to children. A robotic friend might be very useful in helping navigate the traumas of childhood and adolescence, but could pose unanticipated emotional and physical dangers as well – to say nothing of the prejudices and other issues caused by the likely distributive (in)justice that will arise when only rich children have robot friends.

Household robots, such as vacuum cleaners, pool cleaners, gutter sweepers, and so on are certainly not human-like in appearance. Nevertheless, humans may form attachments to machines such that damage to the machine may cause psychological distress; this tendency will only strengthen as robots become more intelligent, particularly if they become capable of conversing or otherwise interacting with humans in ways that convincingly mimic human social bonding. Urban-assistance robots will range from trash collectors to street sweepers and street-lamp-bulb changers, among other service systems. While it is unlikely that people will form attachments to a robotic trash collector, the issues of responsibility will again become important; perhaps more so since an urban robot may come in contact with many more people than a household robot. A second and major ethical problem arises from the issue of responsibility, discussed above in connection with healthcare robots. If a human person is injured by a household or urban-assistance robot, say by tripping or accidental collisions, then who is responsible? What happens if robots have unintended software glitches or other systemic failures that cause harm? How will governments determine product liability and negligence issues?

The popular press has taken the most notice of another aspect of social robotics, as attested by the extensive media coverage of the debut of Roxxxy on, for example, Fox News (www.foxnews.com/story/0,2933,583314,00.html). And for good reason: according to David Levy (2007), it is inevitable that robots will become more and more like humans in both appearance and social interaction skills. As a result, the "uncanny valley" will gradually be overcome and many humans will increasingly anthropomorphize those robots with which they have substantial relationships, treating them as if they were full persons. Such a tendency is only exacerbated when humans are in relations of substantial dependence on such robots, and projections indicate we will rely on robots to meet ever more of our needs. Social robots for playing games, athletic competitions, conversation, and even drinking may be invented, and Levy in particular predicts the widespread acceptance of robots that simulate persons being used for sex.

It is likely that the widespread availability and increasing acceptance of such sexbots will greatly dampen the demand for human prostitutes and sexual slavery, and lessen the incidence of sexually transmitted diseases, but the anticipated demand for sexbots poses negative consequences as well. For example, will they further depersonalize and commodify sex, and increase its separation from other aspects of intimate human relationships? Person-like robotic sexual partners also further problematize the notion of monogamy (is sex with a robot cheating on your spouse/significant other?), and threaten to deepen the divide between love, commitment, and sex (why make commitments or fall in love if sex is perpetually available with robots?). Or, alternatively, they may take the notions of romantic love and commitment in novel directions – will we be able to fall in love with, commit to, and even marry robots? The rise of sexbots will ineluctably create new difficulties for the institution of marriage and its cultural expectations as either a social ideal or a social norm, and possibly further transform the relationship between the biological sexes in ways hard to predict.

As a final example of some of the ethical issues of social robotics, consider an agricultural robot, designed to spray pesticides on crops. Incorrect applications may cause harm to the farmers who use the robot or to passers-by, or to nearby farms growing other crops, or to those processing and distributing the crop, or finally to the end consumers of the product. Again, who is to blame?

14.7   Resolving ethical dilemmas

Given the growing applications and concerns discussed above, how should we go about addressing them? One way would be to simply create legislation or regulations concerning their use. For instance, to use military robots as our example given the many and serious issues they raise, a movement to create international arms control protocols for military robots has already been formed (Fleming, 2009).

Another way is to design or use robots in such a way that they avoid those problems in the first place. For instance, and again using military robots for their high illustrative value, battlefield robots might be designed to shoot at only other machines or weapons (Canning *et al.*, 2004) and never directly at humans. We could pursue similar types of design solutions for issues raised with socially assistive robotics, or interpersonal entertainment robots, or any of myriad other ways in which robots and humans will interact.

Perhaps the most intuitive way to think about behavior in robots – but also the most difficult path – is to program them such that they act ethically, since this might be the first solution that comes to mind in getting other machines, such as business computers, to do what we want. In this section, we will focus on programming approaches for a hypothetical robot, either general purpose or limited purpose. Since design and regulatory solutions may vary wildly depending on the type of robot and its application, a full discussion of those solutions is beyond the scope of this chapter. Many details of the ethical programming of robots as artificial moral agents have been discussed at length by Wallach and Allen (2008).

In general, engineers are very good at building systems to satisfy clear task specifications, but there is no clear specification for general moral behavior, nor is there a single answer to the question of whose morality or what morality should be implemented in the artificial intelligence of robots. While it is indeed possible that unexpected, emergent behaviors will appear in complex robots, nevertheless the programmed instructions will at least provide a framework for consideration. But what ethical theories should form the basis of these programs?

First, let us put aside as nonilluminative the possibility of ethical relativism, which is the position that there is no such thing as objectivity in ethical matters; that is, what is right or wrong is not a matter of fact but a result of individual or cultural preferences. It is certainly true that some standards of etiquette are relative to cultural backgrounds, for example issues of privacy, certain aspects of male–female relationships, the treatment of animals, or other codes of social behavior. These matters differ a great deal between societies and may be very important in the design of healthcare and other civilian robots. But even if ethical relativism could be true – a point we will not take up here, as it lies beyond the scope of this chapter – the assumption of its truth would render moot any discussion of programming ethical theories in robots. Hence, the very possibility of programming morality into robots assumes the existence of *some* objective morality. Further, if we look first at military robots as the subissue of robotic morality requiring the most urgent attention, ethical relativism seems irrelevant, as international law and the military code of ethics of a nation might plausibly be assumed as the standard for that nation's robots.

So if we were to promote ethical behavior in robots by programming ethics into them, what approach and ethical theories might work? Consider first the traditional approach of *top-down programming*; that is, establishing general rules that the robot would follow without fail or exception, usually understood in terms of *deontological ethics*.[1] A poor example of such a deontological ethics would be a set of rules set by a tyrannical father with respect to the children's behavior, in which failure to adhere is swiftly punished, no matter the context. Obviously, there are more plausible sets of universal moral rules. But common to all those who defend deontological approaches to ethics is the belief that morality is about simply doing one's *duty*, in which one's duty is specified by some rules, norms, and/or standards of behavior to be universally and unconditionally followed.

Deontological approaches to ethics have the virtue of simplicity and clarity, as they (apparently) make it relatively simple to know what one ought or ought not to do – is the action permitted by the rules, or does it break them? For instance, as an example of a deontological approach, Asimov's laws are intuitively appealing in their simple demand to not harm or allow humans to be harmed, to obey humans, and to engage in self-preservation. Furthermore, Asimov's laws are prioritized to minimize conflicts; thus, doing no harm to humans takes precedence over obeying a human, and obeying trumps self-preservation.

However, a simple and rigid set of rules is likely not robust enough to arrive at the correct action or decision in enough cases, particularly in unforeseen and complex scenarios. Specifically, if the situation has numerous or interacting elements that the programmer failed to foresee, then slavishly following the rules may well lead to unintended and disastrous consequences, as is the point of many of Asimov's novels. In story after story, Asimov demonstrated that three simple hierarchically arranged rules could lead to deadlocks when, for example, the robot received conflicting instructions from two people or when protecting one person might cause harm to others.

Asimov's fiction thus explored the implications and difficulties of a deontological understanding of the Three Laws of Robotics. It established that the first law was incomplete as stated, due to the problem of ignorance: a robot was fully capable of harming a human being as long as it did not know that its actions would result in (a risk of) harm; that is, the harm was unintended. For example, a robot, in response to a request for water, could serve a human a glass of water teeming with bacterial contagion, or throw a human down a well, or drown a human in a lake, *ad infinitum*, as long as the robot was unaware of the risk of harm.

One solution is to rewrite the first and subsequent laws with an explicit knowledge-qualifier: "A robot may do nothing that, to its knowledge, will harm a human being; nor, through inaction, knowingly allow a human being to come to harm" (Asimov, 1957). But the knowledge qualifier hardly resolves the issue: a clever criminal could divide a task among multiple robots, so that no one robot could even recognize that its actions would lead to harming a human; for example, one robot places the dynamite, another attaches a length of cord to the dynamite, a third lights the cord, and so on. Of

---

[1] One of the authors (GAB) recalls that during his days in the US Army the sergeant often told the troops that there are three ways to behave: the right way, the wrong way, and the Army way, and "We do things the Army way". This is a strong example of top-down programming.

course, this simply illustrates the problem with deontological, top-down approaches, that one may follow the rules perfectly but still produce terrible consequences.

This suggests that we also need to attend to the "rightness" or "goodness" of the result itself, not just to the rules. But even if we acknowledge that consequences matter, there are other challenges raised by adopting a so-called consequentialist or utilitarian approach of maximizing net happiness, such as the impracticality of calculating and weighing all possible results, both near and far term, and the (strong) possibility of countenancing some intuitively wrong action if a robot's imperfect calculation indicates it will lead to the best consequences. For instance, in the movie adaptation of Asimov's *I, Robot*, the robots calculate that enslaving humanity "for our own good" will maximize utility, as it ends all wars and strife. But there may be other, and more important, goods than mere happiness – or a robot may not be able to calculate successfully the future happiness its actions cause. After all, we often cannot!

Again in the urgent case of military robots, there exist legal frameworks of international treaties as well as a nation's own military code as constraints on morally permissible actions. This suggests that one might attempt to design a robot that has an explicit internal representation of the rules (the Laws of War and Rules of Engagement) and strictly follows them. This approach (with some modifications) is used by Arkin (2009) in the design of the software architecture for a military robot. A robotic code would, however, probably need to differ in some respects from that for a human soldier. For example, self-preservation may be less of a concern for the robotic system, both in the way it is valued by the military and in its programming. Regardless of what code of ethics is adopted for the design of a military robot capable of employing lethal force, it will need to be evaluated through externally determined criteria and testing. Similar issues arise in the use of robots for civilian purposes.

Given the apparent limitations of top-down programming, an alternative approach is *bottom-up programming*, inspired by biological evolution and human development. Human children develop their moral sense as a result of accumulated experience and guidance from parents, more so than from following explicit top-down rules. To apply this approach to programming morals into robots, a "neural network" approach is used, in which the programmer and developer must create an environment in which a robot can explore alternative courses of action, with rewards for behavior that is morally praiseworthy and "punishments" for morally wrong behavior. By using such selective reinforcement, the robot develops or learns through its experience, updating its programming continuously in response to feedback. Unlike top-down ethical theories, which define what is and is not moral, there would be no universal ethical principles or rules to follow unconditionally – at least at first; instead, robotic morality must be constructed "from the ground up" in these bottom-up approaches. Shortcuts for a bottom-up machine-learning algorithm frequently make use of a software "teacher" to enable the robotic program to classify actions or events as "good" or "bad," in the same sense that parents or human teachers provide guidance to children (Russell and Norvig, 2003). Thus, morality cannot really start from scratch; prior moral theory is in fact already assumed by bottom-up approaches, not least in the ethical guidelines used by the moral teacher.

In particular, the programming issues for the morals of robots themselves arise both for the programmer and for the robot itself, and include the fundamental difficulty of the "frame problem": the challenge of representing the effects of actions the robot can perform as part of its decision matrix, without also requiring the explicit representation of an extremely large number of "non-effects" of those actions; in our minds, we take leaving out such "non-effects" for granted – their irrelevance is intuitively obvious. But robots lack our human intuition about what is "obviously" irrelevant to any given moral situation. The frame problem is particularly acute for top-down approaches to programming, but persists for bottom-up approaches as well, specifically (for programming morality) in their presumption that the teacher (be it software or human) can delineate in advance all that is relevant –or irrelevant – to their moral education.

So, how do we program the human ability to make moral decisions on the basis of only the relevant evidence to a situation, without having explicitly to consider all that is irrelevant? That is, to do anything (much) with robot morality, do we have to spell out (nearly) everything? Some engineers attempt a solution by the use of the theory of evolution as a suggestive model or heuristic for programming robots, using self-selecting and self-organizing systems that strive toward the optimization of some performance criteria, such as the maximization of profits. The power of evolution is tapped into by selecting only those programs, from a collection of varied but similar programs, that are most successful at optimizing the specified fitness (performance) criterion. The selected programs then serve as *parents* that are modified and recombined (using a process that is analogous to sexual reproduction) to produce a new generation of programs that over time move ever closer to exemplifying the performance criteria. This basic strategy has been successful for producing computer programs that make robots suited to a wide variety of tasks. We have used genetic algorithms (based on evolutionary principles) with great success in developing and changing behaviors such as learning to walk or avoiding obstacles (Lewis *et al.*, 1994), but have not yet attempted to use them to develop morality.

However, a key challenge is that bottom-up systems work best when they are directed at achieving one clear goal, as problems of interaction and optimization occur whenever the performance criteria can come into conflict. But both military and healthcare robots often operate in dynamic environments in which available information is confusing or incomplete, and further, there may be multiple or unclear goals the robots are supposed to achieve that need to be prioritized or even rejected as unattainable or counterproductive. Hence, for robots, even if the moral calculation issue were somehow solved, there would still remain the large problem of moral psychology; that is, how to develop robots that embody the right tendencies in their reactions to the world and other agents in that world, particularly when the robots are confronted with a novel situation in which they cannot rely on experience.

Moral reasoning by humans, however, is not limited exclusively to a top-down or bottom-up approach; rather, we often use both strategies of rule-following and experience. (Nonetheless, it is useful to evaluate both programming approaches separately to identify their benefits and challenges.) Therefore, for now it seems best to consider a third strategy – a *hybrid approach* – for constructing ethical autonomous robots, which is associated with virtue ethics. This approach understands the teaching of ethics as concerned with the development of moral character – one's underlying dispositions or tendencies to act in a given situation in a given role. A person (or robot) of good character is one that has the tendency to function excellently in its proper roles, and also to identify accurately which roles are (im)proper for it to engage in. To do so, it must both learn from experience (bottom-up) how best to fulfill its roles, as well as know (in a top-down way) that certain roles are morally mandated for it, or are morally illegitimate and hence morally forbidden. In the military case, a hybrid approach to a virtuous robot would use top-down rules and bottom-up feedback to promote the ideal character traits of a warfighter (i.e. a "warrior code of ethics") as its virtues; for example, we might have a military robot that was programmed in a top-down fashion with the relevant Law of War/Rule of Engagement, and then "learned" in a bottom-up fashion from realistic simulations what would, for instance, constitute an unacceptable breach of the principle of discrimination. Or in the healthcare case, top-down rules (e.g. "first, do no harm") and bottom-up feedback (e.g. not every use of a scalpel on a patient is harming them) would combine to promote the ideal character traits of an outstanding physician or surgical robot, for example.

14.8   Conclusion

Robots are becoming increasingly intelligent, and that process is unlikely to stop anytime soon. If futurists such as Moravec (1998) or Kurzweil (2005) are correct, that process will continue at least until robots are considerably more intelligent than mere humans, perhaps even until they reach the "Singularity" (Vinge, 1993). Long before any such event, humans will have to deal with the moral dilemmas that the ever-increasing abilities of robots pose. After all, in ethics, *"ought implies can"* – so as the abilities of any entity increase, novel moral issues will arise.

In this chapter, we have concerned ourselves with some of the most pressing and salient moral concerns with robots that either already exist or are under current development. Military robots are already making a dramatic difference in the ways wars are conducted, and their influence appears certain to grow ever stronger. Accordingly, we gave an overview of the impact intelligent military robots will make on the traditional ethics of war ("just war theory") and indicated the major questions and problems being addressed as we recalibrate traditional assumptions about the morality of warfare when intelligent machines are involved. Robots could be used to wage war ever more morally, if they can be programmed to follow the Laws of War and Rules of Engagement as well or better than human soldiers. In principle, their heightened senses and their resistance to emotional stress and physical exhaustion and all the other tribulations of human warriors could make robots following a "warrior code" better than any human at discriminating friend from foe, aiming their weapons carefully, and using no more than the minimum necessary force to accomplish the mission, and all the other desiderata of morally waged warfare.

We also gave extended coverage to another major impact of robots on our lives, in the field of healthcare. Robots have the potential to avoid the tremors, tension, fatigue, and other causes of mistakes of human surgeons, and cut more precisely than any human hand could accomplish. They could revolutionize the field of prosthetics, so much so that already some athletes are idly discussing amputating their human legs to replace them with a superior prosthesis, and the Olympic committee now must discuss whether such prosthetic-using athletes are eligible, or whether the prosthesis constitutes an illegitimate performance enhancer.

Robots are increasingly used in healthcare therapy as well, as attested by the burgeoning field of socially assistive robotics. As in warfare, such robots can take jobs that are dangerous, dirty, or simply dull, and potentially do them better than humans, without the tedium or physical risks which humans endure in such roles. But human patients may form problematic or destructive relationships with such robots, or endure greater isolation as a result.

The ethical difficulties of human–robot relationships are magnified with social robots, which are designed for interacting with humans. As robots move into roles long reserved for human beings, whether as playmates, entertainment options, competitors, or even sexual partners, new qualms will arise about how human and robotic roles should interact or even merge – especially as robots often offer the promise of being better than humans at fulfilling the roles. When every house has a robot maid, what will happen to human maids? When every home has a robot playmate for your child, what will happen to childhood games and human playmates and the process of growing up? When every home has a robotic sexual partner who is always willing to satisfy your mate, what will happen to marriage?

Finally, we examined the various strategies that one might take in attempting to program morality into robots – the top-down, bottom-up, or hybrid approaches – and argued that a hybrid approach was likely most promising in the attempt to successfully create robots that simulate human moral agency. As such simulations become increasingly proficient, new issues will emerge: should robots be held responsible for their actions – that is, do robots *themselves* have duties to human beings, in addition to whatever duties their human makers or users have? If at some point we determine that the robots themselves have become moral agents, with moral responsibilities, we will have to cross a final bridge in the issue of robotic morality – if they can have duties, why shouldn't robots also have rights? Kurzweil (1999) suggested that by 2029 machines will claim to be conscious and that these claims will largely be accepted. If so, such "conscious machines" will certainly be capable of claiming legal rights.

At some point, when and if robots are capable of being held responsible for their actions, with the requisite autonomy to be meaningful defendants in court cases, and not merely our tools or toys or companions or even lovers, the question of substantive moral rights for robots will become pressing. At that point, will we allow robots to no longer be our slaves or our children, and instead make them our moral equals? Can it ever really happen? If it can, *should* we ever let it happen? If Moravec, Kurzweil, and others are correct, we only have a few decades – or less – to find out.

References

Arkin, R C. (1998). *Behavior-Based Robotics*. Cambridge, MA: MIT Press.

Arkin, R. C. (2009). *Governing Lethal Behavior in Autonomous Robots*. Boca Raton, FL: Chapman & Hall.

Asaro, P. (2009). What should we want from a robot ethic? In Capurro, R. and Nagenborg, M. (eds.), *Ethics and Robotics*. Heidelberg/Amsterdam: AKA Verlag/IOS Press, pp. 1–10.

Asimov, I. (1950). *I, Robot*. 2004 edn. New York: Bantam Dell.

Asimov, I. (1957). *The Naked Sun*. New York: Doubleday.

Asimov, I. (1985). *Robots and Empire*. New York: Doubleday.

Bargar, W., Bauer, A., and Martin, B. (1998). Primary and revision total hip replacement using the ROBODOC system. *Clinical Orthopedics*, **354**, 82–91.

Bekey, G. (2005). *Autonomous Robots: From Biological Inspiration to Implementation and Control*. Cambridge, MA: MIT Press.

Canning, J., Riggs, G. W., Holland, O. T., and Blakelock, C. (2004). A concept for the operation of armed autonomous systems on the battlefield. In *Proceedings of Association for Unmanned Vehicle Systems International's (AUVSI) Unmanned Systems North America*, held August 3–5, 2004, Anaheim, CA.

Datteri, E. and Tamburrini, G. (2009). Ethical reflections on health care robotics. In Capurro, R. and Nagenborg, M. (eds.), *Ethics and Robotics*. Heidelberg/Amsterdam: AKA Verlag/IOS Press, pp. 25–47.

Fleming, N. (2009). Campaign asks for international treaty to limit war robots. *New Scientist*, September 30, 2009. Last accessed on March 1, 2010: www.newscientist.com/article/dn17887-campaign-asks-for-international-treaty-to-limit-war-robots.html

Hongo, K., Kobayashi, S., Kakizawa, Y., *et al.* (2002). NeuRobot: telecontrolled micromanipulator system for minimally invasive microneurosurgery: preliminary results. *Neurosurgery*, **51**(4), 985–988.

Ishiguro, H. and Asada, M. (2006). Humanoid and android science. *IEEE Intelligent Systems*, **21**(4), 74–76.

Joy, B. (2000). Why the future doesn't need us. *Wired*, **8.04**, 238–262.

Kozima, H., Yasuda, Y., and Nakagawa, C. (2007). Social interaction facilitated by a minimally-designed robot: findings from longitudinal therapeutic practices for autistic children. In *Proceedings of the 16th IEEE International Symposium on Robot & Human Interactive Communication (RO-MAN 2007)*, pp. 599–604.

Kurzweil, R. (1999). *The Age of Spiritual Machines: When Computers Exceed Human Intelligence*. New York, NY: Viking Penguin.

Kurzweil, R. (2005). *The Singularity is Near: When Humans Transcend Biology*. New York: Viking Penguin.

Levy, D. (2007). *Love and Sex with Robots: The Evolution of Human–Robot Relationships*. New York: HarperCollins Publishers.

Lin, P., Bekey, G., and Abney, K. (2008). *Autonomous Military Robots: Risk, Ethics, and Design*. A report commissioned by US Department of Navy/Office of Naval Research. Online: http://ethics.calpoly.edu/ONR_report.pdf

Matarić, M., Feil-Seifer, D., and Weinstein, C. (2007). Socially assistive robotics for post-stroke rehabilitation. *International Journal of NeuroEngineering and Rehabilitation*, **4**(5), doi:10.1186/1743–0003–4-5.

McBeth, P. B., Louw, D. F., Rizun, P. R., and Sutherland, G. R. (2004). Robotics in neurosurgery. *American Journal of Surgery*, **188**(4A Suppl), 68S–75S.

Moravec, H. (1998). *ROBOT: Mere Machine to Transcendent Mind.* New York: Oxford University Press.

Murphy, R. and Woods, D. (2009). Beyond Asimov: the three laws of responsible robotics. *IEEE Intelligent Systems*, **24**(4), 14–20.

Näder, M. and Näder, H. G. (2002). *Otto Bock Prosthetic Compendium.* Berlin: Schiele and Schon.

Russell, S. J. and Norvig, P. (2003). *Artificial Intelligence: A Modern Approach.* 2nd edn. Upper Saddle River, NJ: Prentice Hall.

Scassellatti, B. (2005). How social robots will help us to diagnose, treat and understand autism. In *Proceedings of the 12th International Symposium of Robotics Research (ISSR'05)*, held San Francisco, CA, Oct. 2005.

Sharkey, N. (2008a). Cassandra or false prophet of doom: AI robots and war. *IEEE Intelligent Systems*, July/August, pp. 14–17.

Sharkey, N. (2008b). Grounds for discrimination: autonomous robot weapons. *RUSI Defence Systems*, **11**(2), 86–89.

Sharkey, N. (2008c). The ethical frontiers of robotics. *Science*, **322**, 1800–1801.

Sparrow, R. (2007). Killer robots. *Journal of Applied Philosophy*, **24**(1), 62–77.

Taylor, R., Paul, H. A., Kazandzides, P., *et al.* (1994). An image-directed robotic system for precise orthopaedic surgery. *IEEE Transactions on Robotics and Automation*, **10**(3), 261–275.

Taylor, R., Menciassi, A., Fichtinger, G., and Dario, P. (2008). Medical robotics and computer-integrated surgery. In Siciliano, B. and Khatib, O. (eds.), *Springer Handbook of Robotics.* Berlin-Heidelberg: Springer, pp. 1199–1222.

US Army Surgeon General's Office (2006). *Mental Health Advisory Team (MHAT), IV: Operation Iraqi Freedom 05–07*, November 16, 2006. Online: www.globalpolicy.org/security/issues/iraq/attack/consequences/2006/1117mhatreport.pdf

US Army Surgeon General's Office (2008). *Mental Health Advisory Team (MHAT), V: Operation Iraqi Freedom 06–08*, February 14, 2008.

Van der Loos, H. F. and Reinkensmeyer, D. J. (2008). Rehabilitation and health care robotics. In Siciliano, B. and Khatib, O. (eds.), *Springer Handbook of Robotics.* Berlin-Heidelberg: Springer, pp. 1223–1251.

Vinge, V. (1993). The coming technological singularity. In *Vision-21: Interdisciplinary Science & Engineering in the Era of CyberSpace*, proceedings of a Symposium held at NASA Lewis Research Center. NASA Conference Publication CP-10129.

Wallach, W. and Allen, C. (2008). *Moral Machines: Teaching Robots Right from Wrong.* New York: Oxford University Press.

Weber, J. (2009). Robotic warfare, human rights and the rhetorics of ethical machines. In Capurro, R. and Nagenborg, M. (eds.), *Ethics and Robotics.* Heidelberg/Amsterdam: AKA Verlag/IOS Press, pp. 83–104.

Werry, I. and Dautenhahn, K. (2009). Applying robot technology to the rehabilitation of autistic children. In Araujo, H. and Dias, J. (eds.), *Proceedings of the 7th International Symposium on Intelligent Robotic Systems, SIRS99*, held Coimbra, Portugal.

15 Toward robot ethics through the ethics of autism

Masayoshi Shibata

15.1 Why must autonomous robots be moral?

15.1.1 What does autonomy mean for robots?

The aim of this chapter is to present an ethical landscape for humans and autonomous robots in the future of a physicalistic world, and which will touch mainly on a framework of robot ethics rather than the concrete ethical problems possibly caused by recent robot technologies. It might be difficult to find sufficient answers to such ethical problems as those occurring with future military robots unless we understand what autonomy in autonomous robots exactly implies for robot ethics. This chapter presupposes that this "autonomy" should be understood as "being able to make intentional decisions from the internal state, and to doubt and reject any rule," a definition which requires robots to have at least a minimal folk psychology in terms of desire and belief. And if any agent has a minimal folk psychology, we would have to say that it potentially has the same "right and duties" as we humans with a fully fledged folk psychology, because ethics for us would cover any agent as far as it is regarded to have a folk psychology – even in Daniel C. Dennett's intentional stance (Dennett, 1987). We can see the lack of autonomy in this sense in the famous Asimov's laws (Asimov, 2000) cited by Bekey *et al.* in Chapter 14 of this volume, which could be interpreted to show the rules any autonomous robots in the future have to obey (see Section 14.3).

Strictly speaking, these laws are not truly the ethics for robots at all since, as I will argue later, they do not presuppose that robots have the same "rights and duties" among them, or admit that robots and humans have the same "rights and duties" among them. At best they are merely "design policies" to make robots better tools for humans. It is often suggested that if their contents were appropriately revised, they could be changed into the three rules for electrical appliances to obey, because these rules do not clarify to what extent those robots have autonomy. When autonomy is reduced, Asimov's laws could be rewritten into "The Three Laws of Electrical Appliances", *mutatis mutandis*, which correspond to, for example, (1) security (not to damage humans), (2) obedience (to work as humans intend them to do), and (3) toughness (not to be broken easily). But fully fledged autonomy would conflict with an absolutely obligatory rule for robots, the second rule of obedience.

Neuromorphic and Brain-Based Robots, eds. Jeffrey L. Krichmar and Hiroaki Wagatsuma. Published by Cambridge University Press. © Cambridge University Press 2011.

How should we treat robots and be treated by them? It depends on what type of beings we think the robots are. As long as the robots we are considering now are autonomous robots rather than mere mechanical tools such as robots working in factories, they are not like pets, animals, unborn babies, or the elderly with heavy dementia to whom we have one-sided "rights and duties." In other words, the ethics of robots we want to investigate are the ethics required for humans and robots to coexist with reciprocal relations: that is, the same "rights and duties" in a community.

But is it really possible that humans and robots can live together as equal members in a moral community? Due to many differences of basic conditions between them, such as birth (production), death (destruction), cognitive abilities, physical abilities, appearances, reproduction, and so on, it seems implausible that such two groups could comprise one and the same moral community. We can give examples of such fundamental differences concerning ethical issues as follows.

First, robots could have a kind of eternal lives or iterated lives over a long period of time, which are made possible by the production principle of "the same design, the same robot" in a functionalist sense, and easy availability of their parts in our physical world. Their prolonged lives may endanger the common interests of goals and methods in a life plan between humans and robots, and thereby make it difficult to comprise a common moral community. The production principle allows robots to be recreated with their exact physical copies without end, in principle, so that they exist with exactly the same minds. As I argue later, our actual world where autonomous robots are possible would be a physical world where the supervenience (at least, global supervenience) relations hold between physical properties and mental ones, which make "the same physical, the same mental" possible. So many robots' minds exactly the same around us may conflict with a traditional concept of a person; that is, the absolute uniqueness of a person as a member of a moral community, if robots could be persons.

Second, robots seem to be able to erase or implant their memories arbitrarily. For humans, the consistency and traceability of their memories, though not perfect but to a certain degree, are required to constitute their personhood, which robots may lack in a radical sense. Can we punish a robot for a murder in spite of the complete elimination of his related memories? Or how could we regard a robot's sincere claim of his worthiness because of a disguised heroic memory of a past trifle action? We may have to treat a robot who has undergone a change of memories in this radical sense as a different member of the community every time he erases or implants an important memory. Although it is unclear whether the psychological continuity theory of personhood is right, easy changeability of memory in robots will give rise to serious problems about robots' personhood.

Third, robots do not necessarily have the same psychology as humans. As we will see later, sharing our folk psychology including the ability to understand other minds is essential for making reciprocal relationships with each other, which is a basis of being a member of a moral community. Since psychological states are the results of physical and physiological needs and wants, robots and humans may not have exactly the same psychological states. Although robots also need an energy supply, they do not want to eat bread or drink water. They do not feel hunger or repletion, so they seem to have different attitudes and emotions toward food, which may result in a very different scheme of desire-belief psychology. This difference may be mitigated in a higher functional level, but it is not certain that the folk psychological mechanism will work sufficiently for both humans and robots to form a mutual moral community.

15.1.2 The ethics of Neo-Crusoe

Imagine that an agent is living absolutely alone in a closed area of deep space in the galaxy. He is intelligent like us, but does not need any partners to survive nor have any missions to do. He may be a robot or an alien unlike us in some respects. Although he may have a memory of his society or the community that brought him up, he has been alone for a long time since the collapse of his society, and will be alone this way until his death. He is not a member of any community now and will not be so in the future. In other words, he is not actually or possibly a member of any community.

I will call him Neo-Crusoe. I guess people would not envy his life, but he could live as he pleases every day. There are no friends or enemies who interfere with him, or whom he interferes with. In a sense Neo-Crusoe enjoys an absolute loneliness, but what does it mean for such an agent as Neo-Crusoe to be moral? Or what kind of ethics does he need? We will have a short remark about this question from Kantian moral theory and utilitarianism. But my concern here is not to get precise interpretations of Kant's, Bentham's, or Mill's theory. Rather, my point is to shed light on some conditions under which any agents including autonomous robots have to be moral, because ethics or morals do not seem to necessarily exist.

Immanuel Kant requires us to accept the Categorical Imperative, "So act that the maxim of your will could always hold at the same time as a principle in a giving of universal law" (Kant, 1996a, 164), where "the maxim of will" means "a subjective and practical policy of action." Therefore Kant is demanding that our principle of action could be universalized as everyone's principle, or that it would not involve self-contradiction when universalized as a law. The maxims that cannot be universalized could not be those that tell us our duties, not because of their contents but because of their formal characteristics. For example, it has been said that the maxim, "break your promise as you like when it becomes inconvenient for you" is unable to be universalized. Why? If promises can always be cancelled arbitrarily by their participants, we cannot rely on them precisely when we want them to be fulfilled. Namely, the maxim would destroy self-frustratingly the foundation of promise itself if it were universalized. Among the constructive conditions which make the promise possible at all, there seems to be a condition that the participants have to fulfill it.

Now I want to ask a question: "Are there any maxims unable to be universalized for Neo-Crusoe?" Please remember that he is not actually or possibly a member of any community. He cannot do any actions that necessarily involve relationships with others; that is, reciprocal actions. Because he is not a member of any community, then cooperation, agreement, betrayal, denial, etc., are action types he is not allowed to do in principle. In other words, any actions he can do in this situation are the ones toward him or the rest of the agentless world. Is there any reason that the maxims guiding such actions cannot be universalized? The answer is No, because there is no standpoint for which an action is still of type A, while he is doing an action of type B, the maxim of which destroys the constructive conditions of actions of type A. In such a case he simply changed his mind to do an action of type B, instead of continuously doing A. In order for his action to be a self-frustrated action of type A, there must be other persons for whom it is still A. Therefore no maxims could be distinguished from each other in universalizability, because there are no other persons except him. As far as the universalizability is concerned, there is no ethical viewpoint allowing us to evaluate the morality of his actions performed in his closed area. We could say that any of his actions is morally neither right nor wrong. Ethics are not necessary and indeed they do not exist in the world of Neo-Crusoe, just because there is no "what one has to do" apart from "what one wants to do." Although it would be required to construct more detailed arguments in order to draw this conclusion from Kant's theory when considering, in particular, his treatment of suicide, I think we could sustain this conclusion independently of any Kantian arguments.

Let's see next what utilitarianism will say about Neo-Crusoe's "what has to be done." Jeremy Bentham's utilitarianism of "the greatest happiness of the greatest numbers is the foundation of morals and legislation" is recast in John Stuart Mill's "the Principle of Utility" as follows: "The creed which accepts as the foundation of morals, Utility, or the Greatest Happiness Principle, holds that actions are right in proportion as they tend to promote happiness, wrong as they tend to promote the reverse of happiness" (Mill, 1969, p.212). Because Neo-Crusoe is the only person existing in his world, "the greatest numbers" in the Principle of Utility could only mean "one person"; that is, him alone. Without further arguments, it seems evident that whatever actions he may plan to do, there is no "what he has to do" imposed on him contrary to "what he wants to do" as long as he does not intentionally perform actions spoiling his own happiness. And it is certain that he would not intentionally do actions harmful to his happiness. It does not mean that he is always the best judge of his own *future* happiness. It is sufficient for him to not violate the Principle of Utility that he is the best judge *at the present time* of his own future happiness, as far as this principle is a guide of his actions.

Of course Neo-Crusoe may accidentally invite unhappy results from his actions because of his cognitive failures or bad performances. He may have a strong desire suddenly to touch a green shining stone beside him or climb a steep mountain in the distance, which may occasionally result in bad outcomes for him. But does it imply that he should not have done it? If certain external causes prevented him from doing that action, he would be seriously disappointed and his happiness would be considerably reduced. Even in a case of his regretting his action because of bad consequences, did his regret have any ethical perspectives? If we say that he did a morally wrong action when he brings an unhappy result only to himself by doing an action involving no other members of the community, there seems to be something peculiar in this judgment. Let us remember again Neo-Crusoe's situation. Even if utilitarian calculation of his happy and unhappy consequences says something about his actions' morality, it is mere calculation without a more basic moral intuition implicitly expressed in the phrase of "greatest number" in the Principle of Utility. This is because the principle shows up only when agents need to have relations with others. One of the presuppositions of the

Principle of Utility is that agents are such creatures that are bound to pursue their own greatest happiness. Therefore such a lonely agent as Neo-Crusoe satisfies vacuously the Principle of Utility in all his actions because the actions of agents have to be adjusted to one another only when there are plural agents and they come to be necessarily concerned with others' interests. The Principle of Utility is a guide to this adjustment. We could say it is to mistake the means for the end to evaluate the morality of one's actions in spite of there being no others in the community. The above shows that there is no "what he has to do" distinguished from "what he wants to do" for Neo-Crusoe, at least in the utilitarian guidance of his actions.

All I was going to suggest in this section is that there are no ethics for such a being as Neo-Crusoe. Although the above is not a decisive argument, we could say now whatever action he does is morally neither right nor wrong. For him, what has to be done is nothing other than what is desired to be done. This means that agents have their ethics only if there are other members belonging to the same community who could have the same "duties and rights" among them. I will call this "the community condition" of ethics. This condition is not sufficient but necessary for ethics to come into existence for the world of agents. If there had been no "what one has to do" cut off from "what one wants to do" for an extremely long time even for all members of the same community, I think their world would be morally a best one for all of them. In the sense that for one to be able to do what he or she wants to do is a freedom in a primitive form, ethics are required only for somehow avoiding collisions among agents' freedom to do "what one wants to do." Viewing the ethics as "deprivation of freedom," it seems to me that the most respectable value in the ethical context is Libertarian Freedom. Here Libertarian Freedom should not be understood as implying "free will without any cause" in a metaphysical sense, but "free choice without any constraint" in a political sense (cf. Greene and Cohen, 2004).

15.2 Natural conditions for humans to be moral

15.2.1 A physical world where autonomous robots are possible

What is a physical world where we can make autonomous robots? In spite of a lot of arguments in the contemporary arena of philosophy of mind, let me skip the complicated issues to a minimal version of physicalism because I think that that kind of world must be a physicalistic world; that is, a world where some version of physicalism is true. In fact, robot ethics is one of the most difficult moral problems that will be raised by the essential features of a physicalistic world in the future. Ignoring the details, minimal physicalism consists of the following two assertions:

1. Any individual is identical to some physical individual (that is, there are no souls or spirits as non-physical individuals).
2. Any property supervenes on some physical property, even if the identity relation between them does not hold (that is, if physical properties as subvenient properties are the same, mental properties corresponding to them are necessarily the same).

According to minimal physicalism, our world is a world where once the physical facts are fixed, all other facts that are characterized as non-physical are determined. For example, the same type of brain state necessarily corresponds to the same type of psychological state, and a same type of physical movement in the same type of environment necessarily corresponds to the same type of action. Notoriously, the local supervenience relation does not hold between mental states and brain states, when the former is characterized and classified in folk psychological concepts and terms. But if we take as a subvenient basis a sufficiently large spatiotemporal region of the physical world including brains in question, almost all physicalists would admit that the supervenience relation holds (i.e. the global supervenience). So keeping this reservation in our mind, we could roughly assert of the supervenience between mental and physical properties the following relation: for the realization of a psychological state "I have to go to the airport now" it is sufficient for a type of corresponding brain state to occur. And this relation does not allow that although two brains are physically of the same type, the one is realizing a psychological state "I have to go to the airport now," the other "I want to make an omelet" (cf. Kim, 1993).

But insofar as robots are made technologically from various hard materials rather than neurons or hormones, it is not possible that robots have the same type of brain state as humans. Does it mean that robots cannot have the same type of psychological state or belong to the same moral community as humans? Fortunately the supervenience relation allows *multiple realizations*. That is, the same type of psychological state can be realized by many different kinds of physical states. If you are a reductive physicalist like Jaegwon Kim, you have to read the term "same" as "similar" in the previous sentence, but here we will not go deep into the difference between them, because it matters only in the context of psychological laws. What remains as "the same" in the multiple realizations is a function fulfilled in different ways by different mechanisms of a lower level. Indeed it is a precondition for us to produce artificial intelligence or robots to have a conviction that we could make beings artificially which could act in almost "the same" way as we do, because without it there would be no serious efforts leading to the recent flood of various robots. We have been given "ontological supports" by these multiple realizations every time various functions of humans imitated artificially are extended to new territories.

But robots seem to have one worry. The multiple realizations can be endorsed by a robust argument as far as they are concerned with the functions realized by causal mechanisms, but there is room for a lot of controversy concerning qualia, or consciousness as an applied problem of the "philosophical zombie" (cf. Chalmers, 1996). For example, if it is true that robots do not feel any pleasure or pain at all in spite of fulfilling the same functions as humans, what kind of justification do we have to regard them as subsumed under the Principle of Utility? Here rational beings without sensations (robots) may seem to give rise to a different problem from one caused by sentient beings without rationality (animals) with regard to the membership of a moral community.

But there is good news for robots in the ethical context. If the actual world is one that allows us to make functionally isomorphic robots to humans, the problem whether robots are "zombie robots" without qualia has the same structure of argument as the philosophical problem of other minds, which seems to be unsolvable as a *purely epistemological* problem. As the question of how to know directly other minds beyond external evidence could lead to skepticism regarding other minds; the question of how to be certain about the existence of qualia or consciousness in robots could not be given any decisive answer. In a nutshell, robots occupy the same *epistemological position* as humans in this regard. But in our context of ethics, it is highly important that we have built up a moral community in spite of the skepticism of other minds. That is, our reason to make others members of the moral community is not the epistemological confirmation of mental states of others, but the practically motivated *ontological decisions*.

Therefore, although it remains a philosophically important question whether robots, functionally isomorphic to humans, have the "same" qualia or phenomenological consciousness as humans, it does not have any significant impacts on the problem whether robots and humans could make a common moral community. I think the more problematic issue is how to construct a common moral community when robots have superior rather than isomorphic functions to humans.

15.2.2 Humans in a physicalistic world

Let us take a brief look at what will happen to humans in such a physicalistic world as makes various functional robots possible. The key word here is "enhancement beyond therapy." My concern is in the situation where the natural conditions *making our community possible* will considerably change by humans' coming to be cyborgs and producing many robots around them, and thereby endanger the "existence conditions" of our usual community *making our usual ethics possible.*

The purpose of enhancement which is becoming a big problem today in the fields of medicine, law, morality, and so on is to reinforce a variety of functions of humans in various ways, and to make humans live for a longer and longer time with the health and strength of youth (finally, to attain perennial youth and immortality). All biological phenomena are determined by physical phenomena in a physicalistic world so that in principle any phenomena could be realized if those are physically realizable. But of course all phenomena of each level are governed by the laws of each level. So it is evident that the possible transfiguration (as enhancement) of humans as biological beings has a limit. I am not sure now, but this limitation might mean for humans one more step in their evolution from biological existence, who have been changing their protein-based forms, to mechanical existence that will have poured their consciousness into robots. In other words, humans might change into robots together with their minds and consciousness in the remote future. It does not mean that humans will be cyborgs, nor that humans' mind and consciousness is a mere program that could be installed in any suitable hardware, but that humans will have minds in robots' brains as one of multiple realizations of having experiences in the environment. Although this image needs more detailed stories, I cannot present them here because of my inadequate knowledge about the relations among humans, robots, and their evolutions.

Anyway, keeping that limitation in mind, we will see a couple of imaginable results of our enhancement today. First, when the enhancement goes "beyond therapy," it certainly takes a direction toward the fundamental improvement of the state requiring cures. For example, after giving effective medicines to people suffering from dementia, we will try to reproduce or reorganize the neural circuits in their brains. Also in the case of mental diseases and developmental disorders including autism spectrum disorders (ASD), neuromodulators, such as oxytocin, are being suggested as a possible treatment (Neumann, 2008; Insel, 2010). Furthermore, if possible, we may choose surgical operations on particular parts of brains once we find the neural causes of those diseases in them someday. Naturally, biomedical treatment will extend to embryos and fetuses through DNA-based diagnostics to prevent mothers from giving birth to babies having such birth defects as Down's syndrome by using genetic technologies (Barnbaum, 2008, ch.4, Autism and Genetic Technologies). The goal we will reach from here "beyond therapy" is that every parent will have "more desirable babies," or "perfect babies" who will have such desirable characteristics as higher intelligence and physical abilities than usual, more excellent figures and appearances than usual, a strong will, fine sensibility, honesty, brightness, and so on (Kass, 2003, ch.2, Better Children). Normal "imperfect adults" already being in our society are not exceptions in this regard. Everyone would want to transform oneself into a "perfect man/woman" ordinarily by taking biomedical treatments to prevent the decline of muscles, preserve immune systems, overcome lifestyle-related diseases, and improve his/her physical appearance. It must be certain that we would finally aim at the perfect avoidance of aging; that is, the endless prolongation of a lifetime by making thorough use of advanced genetic technologies.

As a result there will appear completely new "natural conditions," or "survival conditions," that humans have never yet experienced. Taking cognitive abilities as an example, it is highly probable that everyone will become a brilliant individual or a genius. Certainly such high cognitive abilities are not so stereotyped, but their differences will seem to be restricted within a smaller range. The case is essentially the same with people's figures and appearances, too. Making a caricature of this situation, our world is overflowing with geniuses who are handsome men or beautiful ladies. Although the concept of "perfect humans" does not necessarily mean one and the same set of properties for each person, it would certainly be the case that we have very similar humans around us. Because, as a Russian novelist once said, though the reasons why people are unhappy are different, the reason why they are happy is identical. In other words, we may be faced with a completely new circumstance in which our concepts of personal uniqueness, endeavor, achievement, superiority to others, or goal and happiness in life will change their meanings considerably. This possibility may appear to some people disgusting, to some worrisome, and to others welcome.

Herbert L. A. Hart explained a reason why, "given survival as an aim, law and morals should include a specific content" (Hart, 1961, p.189). The minimum content of the ethics we have now is derived from the natural conditions that are contingently imposed on humans. In other words, our natural conditions require a definite set of rules for us to survive, which constitute our minimal laws and morals, without which we "could not forward the minimum purpose of survival which men have in associating with each other" (ibid.). Hart specifies these natural conditions as follows (Hart, 1961, p.190ff.):

1. Human vulnerability. "The common requirements of law and morality consist for the most part not of active services to be rendered but of forbearances, which are usually formulated in negative form as prohibitions." This reflects "the fact men are both occasionally prone to, and normally vulnerable to, bodily attack."
2. Approximate equality. "Men differ from each other in physical strength, agility, and even more in intellectual capacity." But "no individual is so much more powerful than others, that he is able, without cooperation, to dominate or subdue them for more than a short period."
3. Limited altruism. "Men are not devils dominated by a wish to exterminate each other … But if men are not devils, neither are they angels; and the fact that they are a mean between these two extremes is something which makes a system of mutual forbearances both necessary and possible."
4. Limited resources. "Human beings need food, clothes, and shelter." And "these do not exist at hand in limitless abundance; but scarce, have to be grown or won from nature, or have to be constructed by human toil. These facts alone make indispensable some minimal form of the institution of property … and the distinctive kind of rule which requires respect for it."
5. Limited understanding and strength of will. "The facts that make rules respecting persons, property, and promises necessary in social life are simple and their mutual benefits are obvious … On the other hand, neither understanding of long-term interest, nor the strength or goodness of will … are shared by all men alike." Therefore "submission to the system of restraints would be folly if there were no organization for the coercion of those who would then try to obtain the advantages of the system without submitting to its obligation … Given this standing danger, what reason demands is voluntary cooperation in a coercive system."

These conditions are at most the contingent ones on which humans have been depending rather than the necessary ones humans have to accept. Therefore, as we have already seen, there is a possibility that these conditions will change considerably in our physicalistic world. At least, robots are going to overcome these natural constraints without difficulty. What type of ethics is needed then? In order to make it clear to a small extent in the next section, let me take one of the conditions that make our current ethics possible in the way as we have them now. Hart's five conditions suggest a reason why we need the ethics we have now. What will be suggested in the ethics of ASD in the next section is "understanding of other minds" as one of the conditions upon which the ethics we have now become possible.

15.3   The ethics of autism spectrum disorders (ASD)

15.3.1   Theory of mind matters

Although there has been much research on ASD and its cause, including genetic related causes, no definitive answers to the question of its causes have been found. As is widely known, it is salient that ASD does not show a single symptom, but makes a spectrum[1] (a wide range of continuous syndromes) from the type of delay of spoken language or intellectual deficits to that of Asperger's syndrome, which occasionally shows "islets of ability," special talents and abilities reaching to a Nobel Prize class. Here I will argue the possibility of the common ethics between extremely different beings, following mainly a remarkable book, *The Ethics of Autism*, by Deborah R. Barnbaum, published in 2008. We will see that if robots and humans could build up a common moral community, robots would have to have at least "theory of mind" abilities, and that if both could build up a common community at all, there should be mutual conditions under which it is possible. But at the same time, we will be troubled by the fact that we could not easily find the mutual conditions due to potential tremendous differences between their ways of being.

It is for us the most important characteristic of people with ASD that some of them do not seem to be able to recognize intentional states of other people as different from their own states. It is often said that although some autistic people, unlike psychopaths, are not indifferent to others' predicaments once they are told of such situations, they could not see through others' emotional states at all. It seems natural to regard this deficit as a malfunction of the so-called "theory of mind." According to this view, some autistic people have trouble ascribing intentional states to others or falsely ascribe their own states to others, because their theory of mind could not function adequately. In any case, many autistic persons cannot pass the false belief tests, which are now very famous in various contexts.[2] Of course the problem is not restricted only to beliefs. For someone to recognize that others have minds is recognizing that others are different persons from him/her, and that they have their own independent mental states, including all kinds of intentional and nonintentional mental states such as desires, preferences, worries, and emotions. In the following discussions, among various types and degrees of ASD we will focus on the type of ASD with serious problems of "theory of mind."

It is not only "the theory of mind" thesis that purports to explain this unique character of ASD. As Barnbaum explains, we have also "the weak central coherence" thesis and "the weak executive function" thesis; roughly speaking, the former of which seems to present a better explanation of why some people with ASD often adhere to meaningless parts rather than the meaningful whole, and the latter a better explanation of why they are often preoccupied with stereotyped and repetitive motions, each compared with "the theory of mind" thesis. But as Barnbaum says, these three theses do not contradict one another, because each of them is merely "redescribing" the properties of ASD by presupposing the hypothetical cognitive functions from each perspective rather than giving a consistent explanation of the causal mechanism of ASD. In this sense, we could say that "the theory of mind" thesis best redescribes the essential features of some people with ASD, and that theory of mind greatly matters in relationships with others, although it is still unclear how to make brain-based autonomous robots with non-autistic minds.

15.3.2   ASD and membership in the moral community

What do ethics mean for the people who could not truly understand that others have their own mental lives or recognize what these lives are? This kind of question could be discussed as a problem of membership in the moral community; what properties are necessary and sufficient for any being to be a "person," a member of the community? In other words, could that type of person with ASD belong to the same moral community as nonautistic persons? Barnbaum, after examining and accepting with some reservations the arguments from Martha C. Nussbaum, Thomas S. Scanlon, Derek Parfit, and Robert M. Veatch, rejects clearly the most extreme proposal presented by Piers Benn. The arguments about membership in a moral community logically imply that once the necessary conditions for membership were determined, individuals or groups who do not satisfy them would be expelled from the community. Benn is precisely arguing that some people with ASD should be excluded from the moral community of non-autistic people. According to Barnbaum, Benn's argument makes it a necessary condition for membership in the moral community that "a good human life and well-being" consists in "relations that persons have with other persons" (Barnbaum, 2008, p.93). But autistic persons of that type fail to satisfy this condition because they could not take an "intentional stance" toward others due to a lack of theory of mind. Certainly they are biologically humans, but they are neither *person* in a moral sense, nor located within our moral community. In Benn's terminology, only those who can possess "participant reactive attitudes" can be "proper objects of such attitudes" of others, but some autistic people could not take the "reactive attitudes" to others (Benn, 1999, p.33). Reactive attitudes as Benn understands them are emotions such as anger, frustration, or preference, so it would be absurd if they were directed at objects that cannot have anger or preference. "If a hurricane destroys your house, it does not make sense to get angry at the hurricane, because hurricanes do not get angry themselves" (Barnbaum, 2008, p.94). Some people with ASD could not take appropriate reactive attitudes because of a lack of theory of mind, even if they are faced with emotional situations. But according to Benn, only those who can have reactive attitudes and be objects of reactive attitudes are members of the moral community. Therefore some autistic persons (or robots without theory of mind, either?) are not members of the moral community.

What is the reason that Barnbaum rejects Benn's argument? It seems to be essentially a consequentialist one. To cut that type of autistic person off from the non-autistic is to cut the non-autistic off from the autistic at the same time. The result of this is a possible "performance of morally wrong actions" and "an erosion of the moral status of the autistic and non-autistic alike." "The moral standing of anyone is damaged whenever that person affirms that some other human being is disqualified from moral consideration." Therefore "we should continue to be as inclusive as possible when determining who should count as a member of the moral community, because the costs are so high if we are wrong"(Barnbaum, 2008, p.102).

But this seems nothing other than a "selfish reason" that we want to avoid evil consequences that might visit us due to the essential reciprocity of moral considerations. Here Barnbaum says it is acceptable. Although her argument for this is very interesting, lastly, it seems evident that what makes the "selfish reason" persuasive is the natural condition that both autistic and non-autistic people belong to the same biological category of human beings, and share so many ordinary interests and lives. By the same token, she seems never to think of including animals such as birds, fish, or livestock among members of the moral community. Of course robots are never occurring to her mind. In other words, what determines the widest range of our moral community is, roughly speaking, the five contingent natural conditions Hart indicated earlier. But, as we will see in the next section, she thinks that these natural conditions cannot provide ethics which are applicable to both that type of autistic and non-autistic people equally, because the differences which divide them are so profound and their worlds are so distinct from each other, even if they abide by the same conditions. If those natural conditions are not sufficient for ethics that could cover both sides, what would be the ground for both to comprise a common moral community? Furthermore, taking into account the fact that there could not be even mutual natural conditions shared by humans and robots because robots could easily stray far from Hart's natural conditions, unfortunately we would have to say that it is more difficult to find or invent ethics for robots than ethics for ASD.

15.3.3   ASD and moral theories

In order to find ethics which could cover both that type of autistic and non-autistic people equally, Barnbaum asks "what ethical theory is applicable to both?", instead of "what ethical theory is right?". Her strategy means that if no one could know what a true moral theory requires because of a lack of adequate cognitive abilities, that would violate a moral axiom, "Ought implies Can," even if there were such a true theory. In that case, since no one in the moral community could know the distinction between right and wrong actions defined by that theory, its lessons would be impractical for them. Generally speaking, from evidence available, it has been doubted that some persons with ASD have a moral sense, that they could understand moral dilemmas, and that they could distinguish moral questions from other questions. It is believed that they might have moral blindness. Namely, it is doubted that there are any practical moral theories for them. And if the case turned out to be tragic for that type of people with ASD, there would be no moral theory for them to obey by their own choice.

Barnbaum concludes that neither Humean nor Kantian theories work for some autistics because of their mental peculiarities. According to her, the story is the same concerning Jonathan Dancy's moral particularism and W. D. Ross's prima facie duties. The possibility of finding moral theories shared by that type of autistic and non-autistic person is rather low. What peculiarities of ASD would hinder moral theories from being adapted to the autistic? In what follows, we will see only a part of her arguments about Hume and Kant (Barnbaum, 2008, p.114ff.).

As Barnbaum points out, for Hume, morality is more felt than judged, and morality is determined by sentiment. One particular emotion, sympathy, is the core of Hume's idea of morality. But sympathy or empathy requires one's recognition that others have their own intentional states, and that these states can be different from one's own. This means not only holding a belief about others but also recognizing a belief others have.

But it is this barrier that some people with ASD could not overcome because of their lack of theory of mind. We have now two explanations of how we gain access to others' mental states, the first of which, the "theory" theory, asserts that we predict others' mental states in question by adopting "theory of mind" to them, and the other, the simulation theory, insists that we make up in our own minds, by simulation, the mental state that we would have if we were in that situation instead of others in question, and then transfer that state to them. Whichever theory will turn out to be true, the problem remains the same for people lacking a theory of mind because they could not use either mechanism. In particular, they could not naturally have sympathy or empathy with others. This deficiency results in moral indifference in Hume's idea of morality. In other words, "without this feeling, an agent would be unable to act rightly or wrongly according to Hume's moral theory" (Barnbaum, 2008, p.120).

In contrast, Kant's theory may seem to be applicable to people lacking a theory of mind just because it recommends us to reject emotions like sympathy in order to do morally right actions. In fact, Kant thinks that actions have moral worth only when they are done from duty, and that this is guaranteed by the recognition that this action is the one which duty demands, rather than by emotional motivations such as love, sympathy, or pity. Furthermore, Kant even dismisses these emotions as no help to do morally right actions. Therefore even that type of autistic people, who have a serious problem of sympathy with others (hot methodology), could choose a morally right action by following the recognition of duty in each situation, if they adapt Kant's theory (cold methodology), which thinks much of "rule following" aspects. But according to Barnbaum, the case is not so easy. For example, at least some versions of Kant's Categorical Imperative are not workable for that type of autistic people because of a lack of theory of mind. One of those versions says "So act that you use humanity, whether in your own person or in the person of any other, always at the same time as an end, never merely as a means" (Kant, 1996b, p.80). Kant thinks that any member of the moral community does not exist as a mere subjective (instrumental) value for someone else's end, but exists as an objective value in his/her existence itself for which all other beings exist. That is, any of these members is never a means for other beings, but an end for him/herself. But could that type of autistic people treat other people not as a means for some ends, but as ends in themselves? To do this, it is necessary for them to assume that others each have their autonomous point of view, which is nothing other than to recognize that others have their own "ends–means" relations different from mine; that is, their own intentional attitudes toward the world different from my attitudes. As we have already seen so many times, however, it is extremely difficult for that type of autistic person to attribute intentional states different from his/hers, and, as a result, nearly impossible to understand that others are the starting points of their own intentional states; that is, "the ends in themselves." In consequence, Kant's moral theory is unable to find accord with the peculiarities of some autistic people, either. Barnbaum concludes "the fact that a Kantian moral theory cannot accommodate the autistic individual may be reason for rejecting Kantian theory, not for excluding the autistic person" (Barnbaum, 2008, p.130).

15.4   Conclusion

15.4.1   Ethics are not programs but attitudes

To resolve ethical dilemmas robots will encounter, Bekey *et al.* in Section 14.7 of this volume consider two types of approaches to the problem of programming ethics into robots. The one is "top down" approaches that take seriously an idea that morality is a set of rules to obey in any circumstances without exceptions, and the other is "bottom up" approaches that try to construct morality through experiences without top-down a priori ethical theories. The former corresponds roughly to GOFAI (Good Old Fashioned AI) programming approaches and the latter neural network approaches. Bekey *et al.* rightly conclude that both are not sufficient to make morally autonomous robots because of the notorious "frame problem." Roughly speaking, the frame problem arises necessarily when robots without human intuitive cognitive abilities carry out any general directions in the real world on condition that they have to consider all and only relevant important effects by their actions. "The frame problem is particularly acute for top-down approaches to programming, but persists for bottom-up approaches as well" (ibid.). In consequence, Bekey *et al.* take a third way; that is, a hybrid strategy of top-down and bottom-up, namely rule following and experience. This approach is characterized by them as highly related with "virtue ethics."[3] "This approach understands the teaching of ethics as concerned with development of moral character – one's underlying dispositions or tendencies to act in a given situation in a given role" (ibid.). I hope their third way, elaborated sufficiently, will be successful in handling robots. But I have more fundamental worries about programming or teaching ethics to robots.

In fact, putting aside the frame problem, there are two inherent problems here. One is whether we could have the *true* moral theory that would be programmed into autonomous robots, and the other is how to apply moral theories in general to real situations. My speculation is that moral properties do not supervene on physical properties even globally, so that there is no objective truth in ethics in the sense of reducibility to truths caught in physical sciences. In consequence, morality exists only deep in the center of belief systems of robots or humans, and there is no direct evidence for any moral theories in our perceptual world. Further, since clues and grounds for moral decisions inevitably bring obscurities to some degree in any contexts, applications of moral theories to real situations are not apt for robots' programs as a set of axioms and derived theorems from them. In this regard, morality resides only in a holistic web of beliefs. I cannot show detailed arguments here due to a lack of space, but ethics are neither any rigid rule with clear "applicability conditions", nor empirical truth acquired inductively from experiences, but merely attitudes of each belief system toward other belief systems. But nobody knows how to install moral attitudes into robots' belief systems.

15.4.2   An ethical landscape in the future

But there is a harder problem in robot ethics than what has been discussed before. It is how to build a mutual moral community of robots and humans whose "existence conditions" are extremely different. Unfortunately, I cannot give any decisive answer to this problem now, or even to what robot ethics or the ethics of autism would be like in this concern. But let me suggest something to give the answers in the near future.

First, as the situation of our Neo-Crusoe suggests, ethics have no meaning unless there is a community where one has equal "rights and duties" with others (the community condition). And it is a result of adjustment of interests and actions of members within such a community that "what one has to do" arises with a different content from that of "what one wants to do." Therefore, from the point of view of "ethics as deprivation of freedom," it is desirable that ethics hold "what the members of community want to do" (i.e. their freedom of actions) in high regard as far as ethics can.

Second, it is due to several contingent natural conditions, as Hart points out, that our present ethics have their contents as they have now. But these natural conditions are really those of a physicalistic world, when we regard them as preconditions for the emergence of autonomous robots in the future. It seems that these conditions, which have been the source of important values for humans, would be radically changed if we were to make use of these new "physicalistic conditions" for our "better lives." The situations we have experienced until now such as "differences by chance," or "uniqueness in each person" would be rendered increasingly stereotyped and monotonous. Here the fundamental conditions of "approximate equality," "limited resources," etc. in humans may lose an important role to regulate the contents of our ethics and laws, and, instead of those, "perfect equality," "unlimited resources," etc. may change the meaning of life in humans, and thereby the meaning of ethics of humans, too. But I cannot see through the results of this change now. By contrast, the "natural conditions" Hart pointed out are not serious ones for robots. "Approximate equality" would lose the role of determining the contents of robot ethics too, because they may vary considerably from one another in abilities, strengths, or life spans. What would the same "rights and duties" shared by humans and robots be like, the latter of whom could have at least the same mental abilities as the highest ones of "enhanced" humans, "less vulnerability" and more durability than humans, and semi-eternal "life"?

Third, as the peculiarities of ASD show, in order to be a member of a moral community, the most important ability robots need to have is one afforded by "theory of mind," which is, generally speaking, included in folk psychology of humans. Certainly, the role of theory of mind seems to be a little exaggerated in Barnbaum's arguments, because it sounds as though theory of mind alone makes recognition of other minds possible and fundamentally builds up moral attitudes. But if robots did not have a folk psychological mechanism including theory of mind as its core at all, they would not stand in genuine reciprocal relations with other robots or humans, because the robots would not have "other minds" as targets of their moral considerations. The profound difference between the two worlds of autistic and non-autistic people indicates anticipatorily how extremely heterogeneous "existence conditions" are among robots and humans. Barnbaum could not give an answer to the problem of what contents the ethics would have that could treat those two worlds morally equally. What she showed is that non-autistic people should not exclude that type of autistic from the moral community, however difficult it is to find ethics covering the two worlds. But, although her conclusion is intuitively right, her argument is not effective in regard to robots, because her argument tacitly depends on the "approximate sameness" of natural conditions of the members, which cannot be expected to hold among robots and humans.

Finally, the last point I have arrived at is that we should make artificially anew a moral system which has the following characteristics rather than look for ethics depending on some natural conditions as Hart pointed out. The new system would include robots, humans, autistic people, non-autistic people, and all other groups of peculiar beings, insofar as they have minimal folk psychological understandings of others. And these folk psychological understandings would be guaranteed by the attitudes that respect others as independent moral agents and by the recognition that others have their own independent minds and interests. Ironically enough, the core of the new moral system in this robot-century would be Mill's famous principle of "harm to others," which urges that we are permitted to do anything unless it does harm to other moral agents, whatever purposes, desires, intentions, feelings, or preferences we have. Of course we have to read this principle as demanding every moral agent to respect all other agents' freedom to act in every context as far as he/she can.

Notes

[1] According to the fourth edition of the American Psychiatric Association's *Diagnostic and Statistical Manual of Mental Disorders* (DSM-IV, 1994), a diagnosis of autism requires at least two signs from A, one sign each from B and C, and at least six signs overall as shown below.

A. Qualitative impairments in reciprocal social interaction as manifested by at least two of the following:
   1. impairment in multiple nonverbal behaviors such as eye-to-eye gaze and facial expression
   2. failure to develop peer relationships appropriate to developmental level
   3. lack of spontaneous seeking to share interests or enjoyments with others
   4. lack of social or emotional reciprocity.

B. Qualitative impairments in communication:
   1. delay, or lack of development of spoken language
   2. impairment in the ability to initiate or sustain conversation despite adequate speech
   3. stereotyped and repetitive, or idiosyncratic use of language
   4. lack of varied spontaneous pretend play or social imitative play appropriate to developmental level.

C. Restricted, repetitive, and stereotyped patterns of behavior, interests, or activities:
   1. preoccupation with one or more patterns of interest, with abnormal intensity or focus
   2. compulsive adherence to nonfunctional routines or rituals
   3. stereotyped or repetitive motor mechanism
   4. persistent preoccupation with parts of objects.

[2] We have several scenarios making up the false belief tests. As Barnbaum puts it, according to the "Sally and Anne Test," children are asked to consider the following story (Barnbaum, 2008, p.22). Sally and Anne, often represented by puppets, play with a marble, which they put in one place, for example a basket. Sally then leaves the room, and Anne moves the marble from the basket somewhere else, for instance into a box, before Sally comes back. After observing this, the test subject is asked, "Where will Sally look for her marble?" or, in some

cases, "Where will Sally think the marble is?" (Baron-Cohen, 1995, p.70f). Children with an intact theory of mind give the correct answer. By contrast, autistic children often say, "Sally will look for it in the box" because of their failure to understand that someone in Sally's position may have a false belief, while they have a true belief.

[3] Interestingly, Barnbaum also suggested a possibility of virtue ethics as a moral theory covering autistic and non-autistic people in a personal conversation with me at the International Conference on Social Brain: Autism and Neuroethics, in Kanazawa, Japan, on March 24, 2010. But the prospects of virtue ethics seem to be uncertain in the case of autism, too.

Acknowledgment

This work was supported by Grant-in-Aid for Scientific Research (B): 19320001 and 23320002, Japan and RISTEX, Japan Science and Technology Agency.

References

Asimov, I. (2000). *I, Robot*. New York: Oxford University Press.

Barnbaum, D. R. (2008) *The Ethics of Autism*. Bloomington, IN: Indiana University Press.

Baron-Cohen, S. (1995) *Mindblindness*. Cambridge, MA: MIT Press.

Benn, P. (1999). Freedom, resentment, and the psychopath. *Philosophy, Psychiatry, and Psychology*, **6**(1), 29–39.

Chalmers, D. J. (1996). *The Conscious Mind*. New York: Oxford University Press.

Dennett, D. C. (1987). *Intentional Stance*. Cambridge, MA: MIT Press.

DSM-IV (1994). *Diagnostic and Statistical Manual of Mental Disorders*, Vol IV. Arlington, VA: American Psychiatric Association.

Greene, J. and Cohen, J. (2004). For the law, neuroscience changes nothing and everything. In Zeki, S. and Goodenough, O. (eds.), *Law and the Brain*. Oxford, UK: Oxford University Press.

Hart, H. L. A. (1961). *The Concept of Law*. Oxford, UK: Oxford University Press.

Insel, T. R. (2010). The challenge of translation in social neuroscience: a review of oxytocin, vasopressin, and affiliative behavior. *Neuron*, **65**(6), 768–779.

Ioan, J. (2006). *Asperger's Syndrome and High Achievement*. London: Jessica Kingsley Publishers.

Kant, I. (1996a). Critique of practical reason. In Gregor, M. J. (ed.), *Practical Philosophy*, The Cambridge Edition of the Works of Immanuel Kant in Translation. Cambridge, UK: Cambridge University Press, pp. 153–271.

Kant, I. (1996b). Groundwork of the metaphysics of morals. In Gregor, M. J. (ed.), *Practical Philosophy*, The Cambridge Edition of the Works of Immanuel Kant in Translation. Cambridge, UK: Cambridge University Press, pp. 37–108.

Kass, L. R. (2003). *Beyond Therapy: Biotechnology and the Pursuit of Happiness*. New York: HarperCollins.

Kim, J. (1993). *Supervenience and Mind*. Cambridge, UK: Cambridge University Press.

Mill, J. S. (1969). Utilitarianism. In Robson, J. M. (ed.), *Collected Works of John Stuart Mill*, Vol. X. Toronto, Canada: University of Toronto Press, pp. 202–259.

Neumann, I. D. (2008). Brain oxytocin: a key regulator of emotional and social behaviours in both females and males. *Neuroendocrinology*, **20**(6), 858–865.

Index

action selection, 30, 37, 132, 134, 149, 152, 235, 244, 288
ADHD (attention deficit hyperactivity disorder), 202
affordance, 129–130, 132–138, 141, 152, 180, 231, 296
AI (*see* artificial intelligence)
AMD (*see* autonomous mental development)
amygdala, 134, 181, 279, 293–294, 306
artificial intelligence, 4, 59, 109, 218–220, 280, 287, 305, 323, 337, 350, 358
ASD (autistic spectrum disorder), 5, 190, 352–357, 359
Asimov, i, 6, 323, 325–329, 338–339, 345
asynchronous, 34, 43
attention, 28, 38, 47, 142, 145, 158–161, 165–167, 170–174, 180, 190, 196, 226, 228, 231, 235, 255–257, 260, 266–267, 279
attractor, 93, 219, 224, 282
attractor network, 91, 282
audition, 62, 157–158, 312, 329
auditory, 58, 68, 81, 91, 156, 236, 256, 261, 263
autism, 5, 178–183, 189–191, 197, 201–202, 205–207, 345, 352–354, 359–361
autistic, 6, 178–184, 186–192, 194–196, 201–202, 204–206, 208–210, 335, 354–357, 359–361
autonomous mental development, 5, 156–157, 163
autonomy, 59, 191, 206, 251, 255, 257, 277, 345
awareness, 275–280, 284, 295

back-propagation, 163
basal ganglia, 30, 37–38, 45, 134, 236–237, 254, 279, 283, 289, 293
BBD, (*see* brain-based devices)
BG, (*see* basal ganglia)
binocular rivalry, 310
brain-based devices, 3, 23, 289, 303–306, 310–311, 313–314
BrainBot, 5, 58–59, 62–68, 71, 77–82
Braitenberg, Valentino, 3, 23, 50

Capek, Karel, 3
categorization, 12, 309, 312
CDR (*see* cognitive developmental robotics)

central pattern generator, 34, 274, 289–290, 293
cerebellar, 292
cerebellum, 30, 44–45, 51, 237, 254, 289, 306
cognitive architecture, 5, 130, 134, 152
cognitive developmental robotics, 251–253, 255–259, 262, 264–268
cognitive map, 5, 132, 281–282
consciousness, 6, 261, 274, 278–279, 289, 295, 297, 303–304, 307–313, 316, 350–351
constructivist approach, 21, 251–252
CPG (*see* central pattern generator)
Cyber Rodent, 109–111, 117–118, 126

da Vinci, 331–333
Darwinism, 276
declarative, 130, 278–279
desynchronization, 27
desynchronize, 269
development, 6, 110, 133, 152, 156–158, 161, 163, 170, 173–175, 179–181, 190–191, 209, 217–218, 220–221, 224, 226, 228, 230, 232, 239–240, 251–259, 261–262, 264–265, 267–268, 281, 291, 339, 352, 358
developmental robot, 6, 157, 240
DNF (*see* dynamic neural field)
dopamine, 143, 175, 218, 233–237, 289, 306, 312
dynamic core, 297, 303–304, 309, 311–312, 315
dynamic neural field, 183–184, 186–187, 189, 194, 210
dynamical system, 6, 106, 219, 238, 288

EEG (electroencephalography), 251
efference copy, 260–261
embodied, i, 4–6, 30, 39, 81, 109–112, 118, 121–122, 125–126, 129–130, 133, 192, 197, 206, 219–221, 230, 240, 274, 278, 289, 304, 306, 312–313
embodiment, 4, 51, 217–218, 220, 226, 232, 239, 256–258, 278, 287, 316
emotion, 134, 178–181, 190–191, 194, 196–201, 206–210, 259, 261, 265, 267–268, 275–276, 278–280, 282, 293–294, 324, 335, 341, 346, 354–357, 360
empathy, 6, 178, 181, 255, 257, 259–261, 266–267, 356–357

Printed in the United States
By Bookmasters